INTIMATE STRANGERS

INTIMATE STRANGERS

Commercial Surrogacy in Russia and Ukraine and the Making of Truth

Veronika Siegl

CORNELL UNIVERSITY PRESS   ITHACA AND LONDON

Thanks to generous funding from the Swiss National Science Foundation, the ebook editions of this book are available as open access volumes through the Cornell Open initiative.

Copyright © 2023 by Cornell University

The text of this book is licensed under a Creative Commons Attribution-NonCommercial-NoDerivatives 4.0 International License: https://creativecommons.org/licenses/by-nc-nd/4.0/. To use this book, or parts of this book, in any way not covered by the license, please contact Cornell University Press, Sage House, 512 East State Street, Ithaca, New York 14850. Visit our website at cornellpress.cornell.edu.

First published 2023 by Cornell University Press

The epigraph to this book is an extract from "Anthem" by Leonard Cohen. Copyright © 1993 by Leonard Cohen and Leonard Cohen Stranger Music Inc., used by permission of the Wylie Agency (UK) Limited.

Library of Congress Cataloging-in-Publication Data

Names: Siegl, Veronika, 1985– author.
Title: Intimate strangers : commercial surrogacy in Russia and Ukraine and the making of truth / Veronika Siegl.
Description: Ithaca [New York] : Cornell University Press, 2023. | Includes bibliographical references and index.
Identifiers: LCCN 2023002729 (print) | LCCN 2023002730 (ebook) | ISBN 9781501769917 (hardcover) | ISBN 9781501771316 (paperback) | ISBN 9781501769931 (pdf) | ISBN 9781501769948 (epub)
Subjects: LCSH: Surrogate motherhood—Russia. | Surrogate motherhood—Ukraine. | Surrogate motherhood—Economic aspects—Russia. | Surrogate motherhood—Economic aspects—Ukraine. | Surrogate motherhood—Social aspects—Russia. | Surrogate motherhood—Social aspects—Ukraine.
Classification: LCC HQ759.5 .S544 2023 (print) | LCC HQ759.5 (ebook) | DDC 306.874/3—dc23/eng/20230126
LC record available at https://lccn.loc.gov/2023002729
LC ebook record available at https://lccn.loc.gov/2023002730

To Gundi and Walter,
in loving memory

**Forget your perfect offering
There's a crack in everything
That's how the light gets in.**

Leonard Cohen, "Anthem," 1993

Contents

Acknowledgments ix
Preliminary Notes xiii

Introduction 1

Part I

1. The Biopolitics of Motherhood 31
2. Secret Conceptions 56

Part II

3. Choreographing Surrogacy 83
4. Doing It Business-Style 112
5. Technologies of Alignment 136

Part III

6. Laboring with Happiness 165
7. Ambivalences of Freedom 193

Conclusion 217
Afterword: Surrogacy in Times of War 235

Appendix: Research Participants 241
Notes 249
References 257
Index 281

Acknowledgments

Many writers have drawn metaphorical parallels between the process of publishing a book and that of gestating and giving birth to a child—a parallel that seems all the more fitting when referring to a book on surrogacy. The process of "gestating" and "birthing" this book has certainly been exciting, joyful, and agonizing at once, and I count myself lucky for having the support of so many people who have accompanied me throughout the years from my first thoughts about this project in 2013 to the final publication of the book!

First and foremost, I want to thank my research participants, who have shared their lives, experiences, feelings, secrets, and thoughts and have provided me with invaluable insights. Thanks for your trust and openness—particularly to Lena and Katya as well as Teresa and Stefan.

I am also deeply indebted to the project team of "Intimate Uncertainties: Precarious Life and Moral Economy across European Borders," in the frame of which I carried out research for this book. The project was funded by the Swiss National Science Foundation (SNSF) and located at the Institute of Social Anthropology (University of Bern). I could not have wished for better colleagues than Sabine Strasser, Luisa Piart, Gerhild Perl, and Julia Rehsmann, who always made me feel part of a strong network of support and solidarity. A particularly big thank you to my supervisor and mentor Sabine Strasser. Sabine, I don't even have the words to express my gratitude for the way you sensitively encouraged, challenged, and guided me throughout the numerous ups and downs research—and life—always entails. Your feedback and perspective were always highly inspirational. I would also like to express my deepest gratitude to Gerhild Perl and Julia Rehsmann, whose unconditional help and friendship have been fundamental throughout the last years. Gerhild, special thanks to you for reading an earlier version of this book and helping me to identify and strengthen the book's main strands. Dear project team, you're the best, and I will miss our evenings with lively discussions, fondue, and wine!

I would also like to thank my research partner, Michele Rivkin-Fish (University of Chapel Hill, North Carolina), for reading parts of this book and allowing me to profit from her profound knowledge about motherhood and reproduction in post-Soviet Russia. A big thank you in this respect also to Christopher Swader (University of Lund), who helped me think through my material with critical comments and questions based on his own research on intimate economies in the post-Soviet space. I furthermore received great intellectual incentives from the members of the Graduate School of Gender Studies (University of Bern), coordinated by my colleague and good friend Tina Büchler, who has meticulously read and given critical feedback on some of my writings. Thanks, Tina, for all the great discussions but also for the many mountain tours, *Gipfeli*, and endless evenings at your kitchen table. Another big thank you to Eva Sänger (University of Cologne), whose perspective has opened new doors and who has a special talent for getting to the heart of a problem and offering a constructive solution—thanks, Eva! This also holds true for copy editor Julene Knox. Thank you, Julene, for your attentive reading and thoughtful refinement of my writing and my arguments. You helped me find the right words on so many levels, and this book wouldn't be the same without you.

Further thanks to Laura Affolter, Janina Kehr, Danaé Leithenberg, Sayani Mitra, Vera Mitter, Amrita Pande, Laura Perler, Sharmila Rudrappa, Kiri Santer, Carolin Schurr, Andreas Streinzer, Oleksandra Tarkhanova, Julia Teschlade, Diane Tober, Jelena Tošić, Anna-Lena Wolf, and Matthias Zaugg (in alphabetical order), who all provided either valuable feedback or important pieces of information and advice; to Ruben Flores, Lili di Puppo, Pavel Shelenkov, and again to Christopher Swader whose friendship and support were crucial during fieldwork in Moscow; to the Higher School of Economics in Moscow for providing me with an academic home during my fieldwork there, and particularly to Leila Ashurova for her continuous assistance in bureaucratic matters; to Christina Weis for sharing her insights about getting access to the field of surrogacy in Russia; to Olga Isupova for helping me in my search for research participants; to the Altra Vita IVF Clinic for opening its doors and allowing me to conduct participant observation; to the Swiss National Science Foundation, the Faculty of Humanities and the Institute of Social Anthropology (University of Bern) for financially supporting my research; to the Brocher Foundation (Hermance, CH) for allowing me to work on my manuscript on the shores of beautiful Lake Geneva as well as to Janina Kehr and the Department of Social and Cultural Anthropology at the University of Vienna for providing me with an intellectual setting and the infrastructure to complete the manuscript; and to Cornell University Press (particularly Jim Lance) for believing in this book as well as to the two anonymous reviewers for their truly profound engagement with the manuscript. Their critical and encouraging comments significantly shaped my book.

Parts of this book have been previously published. Parts of chapter 5 appeared in *Tsantsa: Journal of the Swiss Anthropological Association* 23 (2018): 63–72; parts of chapter 6 appeared in the *Anthropological Journal of European Cultures* 27 (2) (2018): 1–21; parts of the conclusion appeared in *Medicine Anthropology Theory* (2019); and a slightly different version of the afterword was published in German on the platform of *GeN-ethisches Netzwerk* (2022). I thank the editors and anonymous reviewers for their comments on these pieces and the publishing outlets for their permission to republish them.

A big thank you also to all of my friends who directly or indirectly supported me during the last years that were challenging in many respects, most of all Tina, Eva, Chrisi, Valerie, Birgit C., Birgit P., Laura, Gerhild, Julia, Sabine, as well as to the Ä-Weg Collective, my cousin Dorothea, and my partner Matthias. You all mean the world to me!

Last but not least, I want to thank my parents, Gundi and Walter Siegl, who were an inexhaustible source of support and care in my life until they passed away unexpectedly in the summer of 2019. This book is for you.

Preliminary Notes

All my research participants' names are anonymized, unless explicitly stated. I refer to them using their first name and father's name, which is the common form of respectful address in Russia and Ukraine; or first and last name, which is more common in Spain and Germany but is also how some of the Russian and Ukrainian professionals introduced themselves to me. However, concerning surrogates and intended parents, I move to using their first names only, as our relationships and the issues we talked about were relatively intimate.

I conducted my fieldwork in Russian, Spanish, English, and German—languages I have mastered to different levels but all well enough to engage in conversation and conduct interviews. In most cases I could therefore offer my interlocutors the opportunity to communicate with me in their first language. The translations I present in this book are my own (though I am very grateful for the occasional help of friends and colleagues!). I tried to stay close to the original formulations but took the liberty of adjusting terms and phrases so that they would make sense in English. For the sake of consistency, I also carefully modified quotes spoken in English by nonnatives, while always being careful not to change their meaning. Where I deemed it appropriate and significant, I included the original wording in parentheses and italics. My transliteration of Russian words is based on the Library of Congress system, with slight variation. I treat Russian and Ukrainian names more flexibly in this regard, drawing on common ways of spelling a name, for example "Lena" rather than "Lyena."

In presenting quotes, I furthermore use three dots to signify speech trailing off; three dots after a full stop to indicate a pause; and three dots in square brackets when I have left out words or sentences. I also use square brackets when I add words to quotes. Parentheses mean that I am providing additional information or clarifications on what is said or how it is said. Italics within a quote indicate words emphasized by the speaker, unless noted otherwise. This applies to quotes from my ethnographic material as well as from the literature.

In Russia and Ukraine, highly binarized understandings of sex and gender persist and remain tied to narrowly defined ideas about femininity and masculinity. This leads to a mostly unreflective predominance of cisgender perspectives, particularly in the field of reproductive medicine. Surrogates, for instance, are expected to be cisgender, and in the context of my research all of them were. I draw on the binary terminology of "men" and "women" in order to reflect this cisgender perspective and, moreover, in order to make the gendered aspect of reproductive labor visible—while, of course, acknowledging that further gender identities exist.

The time of my fieldwork in Moscow—September 2014 to July 2015—was marked by military conflict between Russia and Ukraine and economic sanctions by Western countries on the former. This led to a significant devaluation and a highly flexible exchange rate of the Russian ruble (₽) over the respective months. Thus, ₽1 million—which was the salary many of the surrogates in my research received—equaled US$27,000 (or €21,000) at the outset of my fieldwork in September. Thereafter the ruble's value fluctuated, and at its lowest point the same amount equaled only around US$15,000 (or €12,000). For the sake of convenience, I have not indicated this span in the book but rather calculated the median value of ₽1 million between the highest and lowest exchange rate at US$21,000 (or €16,500).

INTIMATE STRANGERS

Introduction

Larissa Osipovna interrupted our conversation and pointed to a man walking past with a small boy and girl. "These are his children," she said. "Twins, born through surrogacy. Amazing, right?" She smiled, gazing at the passersby until they disappeared in the slow but steady stream of visitors moving through the *inviTRA* International Fertility Fair. It was the third such fair in Spain, and this year, 2015, it was taking place in a hotel in the center of Barcelona. Organized by the online magazine and community *inviTRA*, the fair was aimed at intended parents.[1] Around forty stakeholders from the field of assisted reproduction had come to promote their services and products: surrogacy advocacy groups, authors of children's books on assisted conception, research groups, and—most of all—commercial actors in the field. The exhibition hall reflected the vast international network that has developed around infertility issues in the past twenty years: clinics and agencies from Spain, Ukraine, Russia, Mexico, and the United States, as well as agencies operating globally, presented their fertility programs, ranging from basic in vitro fertilization (IVF) treatment, through egg and sperm donation, up to all-inclusive surrogacy packages. While here and there a few photos of happy babies and pregnant bellies decorated the stands, most representatives foregrounded their special offers and price lists. No reproductive desire seemed out of reach—clients just needed to find the country with the right legislation and the right prices.

The surrogacy market is highly volatile but also flexible and innovative in adapting to new challenges or legal changes in one country by "realigning" its parts elsewhere in the world (Whittaker 2019). At the time of the fair, numerous

1

transnational agencies and clinics were promoting Ukraine, which was quickly developing into one of the most popular surrogacy destinations worldwide.[2] Larissa Osipovna's Kyiv-based agency profited from this development. As an agent, she orchestrated the entire process: she facilitated arrangements by selecting surrogates and monitoring their pregnancies, accompanying foreign intended parents through the surrogacy process and keeping them up to date, and organizing the medical procedures in collaboration with specific clinics in Kyiv.[3] Her client roster was growing, not least due to her cooperation with a lawyer from Barcelona, who took care of the legal paperwork for Spanish intended parents.[4] Today, the Ukrainian agency's website is available in fifteen languages, showing that it mainly caters to intended parents from Europe but also attracts clients from Israel, China, and Brazil.

Larissa Osipovna had just vented her anger about the vast amount of films and books that presented surrogacy as a "bad thing." Sad and scandalous stories sold much better than happy ones, she lamented, and most people simply did not understand what surrogacy was about—especially journalists, who usually published "bullshit," either because they did not invest enough time in researching the topic or because they had never experienced infertility problems themselves. "If you are the happy mother of a child, yes, you will know that the problem (i.e., infertility) exists ... but you will *never* feel the same as a mother who has lost her uterus due to a doctor's negligence. Who in the world can judge?" She looked at me sadly. "Who can blame a woman for wanting to be a mother? ... This is a truly amazing experience, and they are deprived of it." People who shared this understanding would inevitably be in favor of the practice itself: "Those who understand, they accept surrogacy; those who don't understand, don't accept it." She hoped I would write about the emotionally challenging path to parenthood and that my research would make governments with "stupid" laws that prohibited commercial surrogacy realize that there were many couples who needed this form of assisted conception and would undoubtedly create "amazing families." "It's good that you have so much time for your research," she continued. "You will talk to a lot of people and not make such *stupid* mistakes, I hope."

My interview with the agent Larissa Osipovna was one of the many fieldwork moments that made me feel somewhat uncomfortable. She too easily divided people into innocent, infertile women who just wanted to experience the happiness of motherhood and those who deprived them of this basic right. Many of my research participants expressed a similar position: either one was for or against the practice; either on their side or against them.[5] I was, consequently, often confronted with the assumption that I was doing research in order either to defend surrogacy or to criticize it. Both assumptions were burdensome and obstructive, as both brought their own distinct problems, including the expectation that

I would carry truth into the world as well as the direct denial of access, because I might make "*stupid* mistakes" and write something negative about surrogacy. Like Larissa Osipovna, many supporters of surrogacy framed the "side" people took not as a matter of political or moral conviction but as one of the "right understanding." I encountered this expression over and over in the course of my research. Some of my research participants explained that they themselves lacked the right understanding at the beginning and needed to achieve it in the course of time through thorough engagement with the topic—on an intellectual, emotional, and corporeal level. Reaching the "right understanding" required work on the self and on others. I will conceptualize this effort to reach and transmit the "right understanding" of commercial surrogacy as ethical labor, for it was clearly intended to turn ethical doubts into positive ethical certainties. It was this kind of labor that Larissa Osipovna was doing on me—and that I had experienced in so many other situations—as she was trying to "seduce" the ethnographer, as Antonius Robben (2012) might say, into adopting her understanding. Events such as the inviTRA fair offered spaces for circulating specific understandings in a transnational context that would then become part of a global repertoire of ethical labor.

The notion of the "right understanding" suggests that there is some kind of truth about the ethics of surrogacy, and supporters and opponents alike often presented themselves as monopolizing this truth—even though their truths differed a great deal. Intrigued by these appeals to moral truth, I started to wonder: What are these truths and why are they necessary? In what "understandings" are they grounded, and do these vary across different cultural contexts and social positionalities? How do those within and at the fringes of the surrogacy market—including surrogate workers, intended parents, doctors, psychologists, agents, advocates, and opponents—create, define, and circulate truths and with what aim? Whose truths are visible and matter, whose are obscured?

These are the questions that I seek to unravel. With this book, I am partly adhering to the demands some of my research participants placed on me to give space to their understanding and their truth about surrogacy. In doing so, however, I neither leave these truths unchallenged nor do I launch a fact-finding mission. Rather, I take my research participants' vulnerabilities, anxieties, and desires upon entering the field of surrogacy as a starting point to examine how specific words, metaphors, arguments, narratives, and logics are turned into truths. I challenge the shades of truths and nontruths, ranging from small secrets to blatant lies, in order to see not only what is foregrounded but also what is concealed in the moral economy of commercial surrogacy in Russia and Ukraine—two of the few countries in which this practice is currently legal and regulated, for citizens and foreigners alike.

Surrogacy as Moral Battleground

The topic of commercial surrogacy is rarely met with indifference. It often provokes a mixture of fascination, voyeuristic interest, and moral judgment, and the attention it receives by far exceeds its actual use (Harrison 2016, 9). Most people know little about the workings of this growing industry or about the experiences of its participants. And yet, many have an opinion on surrogacy, even a surprisingly strong and emotional one.

It was this affective force and my own ambivalent position within the cacophony of opinions that drew me to this topic. I embarked on my research from the perspective of a young woman in her late twenties who knew she wanted to have children eventually but not any time soon, and for whom infertility was not a direct issue of concern but nevertheless a distressing thought that loomed large. As such, I could empathize with the intended parents' wish for a child, but I hesitated to embrace the stories of unclouded happiness and harmony spread by surrogacy supporters. At the same time, I was deeply troubled by the economic imbalance many surrogacy arrangements seemed to rely upon, but also dissatisfied with the paternalistic images of surrogates that were cast by opponents. I wanted to know more, to understand how intended parents and surrogates grappled with the possibilities and restrictions in their lives and how "ethics" was negotiated at the "nodes of desire" (Nahman 2008), where the parties come together in their quest for a better life, be it a life with a child or a life with temporary financial security. I was curious what my perspective as an empathic, yet critical, feminist anthropologist could add to the ongoing debates about commercial surrogacy and other kinds of intimate labor.

Intimate labor describes a type of labor that is linked to touch, closeness, and care and that "denies the separation of home from work, work from labor, and productive from nonproductive labor that has characterized capitalist globalization" (Boris and Salazar Parreñas 2010, 2). Following this definition, surrogacy can be seen as intimate labor par excellence (see also Pande 2014; Rudrappa 2016a; Rudrappa and Collins 2015; Whittaker 2019): it is labor that attends to the needs of others, that is closely connected to one's feelings and body, that is reproductive and productive at the same time; and it is a kind of labor one cannot go home from at the end of the day. As the case of surrogacy shows, intimate labor is increasingly commodified and incorporated into a transnational market, linking providers and receivers over great geographical distances (Constable 2009). Such commercial uses of intimacy are marked by a complex dynamic of subjection and empowerment, often entailing stigmatization, bodily and emotional risk, and economic exploitation (Hofmann and Moreno 2016).

Speaking of surrogacy in terms of "labor" and "commercialization" fits particularly well with the Russian and Ukrainian contexts, where surrogates embrace their role as wage workers and are also strongly encouraged to do so by the other actors involved. As I will show throughout the book, this understanding is shaped, on the one hand, by the prevalence of high levels of economic inequality, coupled with a pragmatic and often disillusioned stance toward these inequalities, a neoliberal ideology of self-reliance and self-responsibility, and a highly gendered labor market—a setting that privileges a consumption-oriented and instrumental approach to surrogacy and other forms of intimate labor. On the other hand, the understanding of surrogacy as a work relationship results from a bio/political and religious discourse that morally promotes motherhood while condemning infertility and assisted reproduction. In this context, surrogacy needs to be practiced in secrecy, and emotional entanglements between the two parties are often not welcomed. Intended parents and surrogates thus have to remain strangers toward each other, despite the fact that—or one could even say, precisely *because*—they are so intimately connected. These aspects set Russia and Ukraine apart from such regional contexts as the United States, India, or Israel, where discourses and practices of commercial surrogacy are shaped by notions of love, altruism, and sacrifice, and where women experience their position as surrogates as highly meaningful (Berend 2016; Deomampo 2016; Jacobson 2016; Pande 2014; Rudrappa 2016a; Teman 2010)—aspects I will continuously return to in the course of this book.

Surrogacy remains one of the most morally disputed and polarizing practices within the field of intimate economies as well as assisted reproduction. Anthropologist Elly Teman (2010, 7) has argued that surrogacy constitutes a "cultural anomaly" that causes anxiety because it moves childbearing from the intimate sphere to that of clinics and markets. As such, the practice constitutes a battleground for different convictions, faiths, hopes, desires. Many have intervened in public discourses about surrogacy and assisted reproductive technologies (ARTs), triggering heated debates among medics, ethicists, religious institutions, gay rights activists, feminists, and many others.

The emergence of these debates was closely linked to the rapid development of ARTs from the 1980s onward. Concerning surrogacy, it was at exactly this time that technological advances made it possible to split the baby-making process into three parts: genetics, gestation, and social parenting. While previously only traditional surrogacy had been possible (where the carrier also contributes the egg cells, making her a genetic relative to the child), the new technologies gave rise to so-called gestational surrogacy, in which the surrogate did not contribute her own egg cells (Markens 2007).[6] The possibility of extracting egg cells meant that the fertilization process could now take place outside the body (in vitro) and, hence, the intended mother could use her own egg cells or those of an egg provider. Somewhat paradoxically, the fragmentation of what could be termed "motherhood" made it easier to define "ownership" and thus (legal) parenthood, for now the issue of intent was put center stage. At the same time, the fragmentation reduced the emotional risks around the surrogate becoming a carrier: for surrogates, because they were not giving away "their" children, as well as for the intended parents, who were now not taking in "somebody else's" child (Spar 2006). The new technological advances radically questioned the supposed biological "facts of life," opening up new forms of non/relatedness (Franklin 1998, 2012, 2013; Strathern 1992a, 1992b). This also meant that the surrogate's genetic contribution became irrelevant, providing the possibility of cross-racial and cross-ethnic surrogacy arrangements for the mostly white middle-class couples who could afford such infertility treatments (Harrison 2016; Twine 2011). These factors contributed significantly to the quick growth of the reproductive market and its global expansion.

These developments were accompanied by increasing criticism, not least from feminist scholars and activists. Their positions were—and still are—highly diverse. The FINRRAGE network (Feminist Interventional Network of Resistance to Reproductive and Genetic Engineering), founded in the mid-1980s, was an important and particularly radical participant in the early debates on ARTs. While FINRRAGE members such as Gena Corea (1985) or Maria Mies (1986) rejected the new developments as a patriarchal and colonial instrument of oppression, feminists such as Shulamith Firestone (1970, 195) highlighted the potential of ARTs to "liberate women from the tyranny of reproduction" and accordingly from patriarchal hegemony. Others lined up with free-market supporters, arguing that reproductive labor was a form of work and that nobody should interfere in women's employment choices (Shalev 1989). Debates generally evolved around what philosopher Michael Sandel (2013) has termed "the corruption critique" and "the coercion critique." The former states that subjugating children to a market logic is harmful to human dignity. The latter stipulates that women are coerced into this kind of labor by poverty. Questions of coercion—and hence exploitation—became particularly prominent with the internationalization of surrogacy and gamete sales, leading to debates about "trafficking in women" and "baby farming." Many scholars have problematized the "outsourcing" of dangerous or at least burdensome reproductive procedures, such as surrogacy or egg provision, to low-income countries (Cooper and Waldby 2014; Pfeffer 2011; Twine 2011). Applicable to all forms of ARTs, the debates seem to climax when talking about the "rent-a-womb" industry, as critics have called it.

At the beginning of my research these controversies were revived after several surrogacy cases triggered worldwide indignation. One of these involved Baby Gammy, a child born in 2013 with Trisomy 21 and left by the Australian parents with the Thai surrogate. Another was a controversial rescue operation during an earthquake in Nepal in 2015, in which newborns were collectively evacuated by their Israeli intended parents while the surrogates were left unassisted in Nepal. These stories and the media attention they attracted led to a number of legal changes in the surrogacy market, mostly in 2015 and 2016. Thailand as well as Nepal, and later Cambodia, closed their doors to international clients (Whittaker 2019). Also India, the "mother destination" for gay couples, changed its legislation to restrict surrogacy to Indian heterosexual couples as intended parents, who can find an altruistic surrogate among their relatives (Rudrappa 2010, 2016b). The events might also have affected the European Parliament, which in 2015 referred to surrogacy as "exploitation" and against "human dignity."[7] Moreover, in 2016 the European Council rejected a proposal that would have envisioned the international regulation of surrogacy and, as many feared, would have been understood as general approval of the practice (Starza-Allen 2016).

Resistance to and contention about ARTs have also spread within civil society across Europe. In 2015, women in Spain published the manifesto *No Somos Vasijas* ("We are not containers"), and around the same time the international campaign Stop Surrogacy Now was launched. While these initiatives call on national governments and the international community to ban surrogacy, surrogacy researchers warn that an abolitionist stance would drive the market underground, while a shift toward altruistic surrogacy within the family (as in India) could increase the surrogates' vulnerability due to familial duties and dependencies (Pande 2016; Rudrappa 2016b).

Legal scholar Joan Williams and economic sociologist Viviana Zelizer argue that "to commodify or not to commodify" might not always be the most appropriate question. They call for a shift "away from the Hamlet question toward an examination of the social conditions that frame market exchanges" (Williams and Zelizer 2005, 373), an examination that can only take place by looking at the specific contexts in which surrogacy occurs. When I started my research in early 2014, there was still little empirical research on surrogacy, but researchers—anthropologists and sociologists in particular—have quickly filled the academic vacuum, most likely prompted by increased public debates around surrogacy.

Researching Surrogacy within and beyond Anthropology

Today, there is a rich corpus of literature that explores commercial trans/national surrogacy, including ethnography-based monographs focusing on the United States (Berend 2016; Jacobson 2016; Ragoné 1994), India (Deomampo 2016;

Majumdar 2017; Pande 2014; Rudrappa 2016a), Southeast Asia and Thailand (Whittaker 2019), Israel (Teman 2010), and Russia (Weis 2021a). Scholars have revealed the manifold reproductive mobilities (Schurr 2019; Speier, Lozanski, and Frohlick 2020) involved in surrogacy and other forms of assisted reproduction that emerge from fundamental differences in legal regulation and treatment costs (Pennings 2004, 2009; Shenfield et al. 2010). Recent work has followed the movements of the different actors and bodily substances involved, shedding light on the global trajectories of homo- and heterosexual single people and couples seeking surrogacy in the United States, Mexico, India, or Thailand (Førde 2017; König 2018; Lustenberger 2016; Majumdar 2017; Pande 2014; Rudrappa 2016a; Schurr 2019; Teschlade 2019; Whittaker 2019) or egg provision in Spain and the Czech Republic (Bergmann 2014; Perler 2022; Speier 2016); of single and lesbian women seeking sperm provision in or from Denmark and Belgium (Adrian and Kroløkke 2018; Dionisius 2015; Pennings 2010); of globally traveling egg providers from North America or South Africa (Kroløkke 2015; Pande and Moll 2018; Tober and Kroløkke 2021), surrogate workers from the former Soviet republics traveling to Russia (Weis 2021a), or reproductive substances moving around the globe, such as egg cells traveling from Romania to Israel (Nahman 2011).

Taken together, this scholarship has illustrated the scale of regional, national, and global entanglements. It has also shown the crucial influence of information technologies and online communities on the growth of the reproductive market (Berend 2016; Speier 2011; Whittaker 2019) and emphasized how notions of gender, class, race, ethnicity, and ability inform and shape the dynamics of commercial surrogacy (Deomampo 2016; Harrison 2016; Pande 2014; Schurr 2017; Twine 2011; Weis 2021a; Ziff 2017) and gamete provision (Almeling 2007; Bergmann 2012; Perler and Schurr 2021; Speier 2016; Tober 2018; Vlasenko 2015), whether transnational in scope or not. Moreover, scholars have revealed how the new constellations produced through third-party reproduction require complex and challenging negotiations of relationships, kinship, and belonging between the different parties involved in surrogacy and gamete provision (Gunnarsson Payne, Korolczuk, and Mezinska 2020; Konrad 2005; Majumdar 2017; Mamo 2007; Pande 2009, 2015; Smietana 2017a, 2018; Teman and Berend 2018; Teschlade and Peukert 2019). ARTs thus have the potential to simultaneously disrupt and reproduce social norms around family, heterosexuality, and reproduction (Dumit and Davis-Floyd 1998).

Given the contentious nature of surrogacy, much research on this topic has implicitly or explicitly addressed how different market actors grapple with the moral questions at stake. Some of the empirical work that has zoomed in on this question draws on analytical concepts such as frames, framings, and frameworks. These concepts emphasize that moral engagements always take place in relation to social and cultural discourses and norms but can also actively contribute to them by creating new moral understandings (Smietana, Rudrappa, and Weis 2021). Susan Markens (2007, 2012), for instance, has analyzed media coverage of surrogacy in the United States, illustrating how the social problem of surrogacy and the proposed "solutions" are not self-evident but rather defined through "discursive frames" within which surrogacy is supposed to be understood. Focusing on the actors involved in surrogacy arrangements, Sharmila Rudrappa and Caitlyn Collins scrutinized how U.S.-American intended parents and Indian agents draw on and circulate "moral framings" of compassion and altruism that allow them to counter the common critique that they are exploiting poor Indian women. These framings, they argue, are "systematic to and constitutive of transnational surrogacy" (2015, 942).

The dissemination and streamlining of such moral framings have been facilitated through the numerous online fora and social media platforms for intended parents and surrogates, as also argued by Zsuzsa Berend in her study of U.S.-American surrogates' interactions on an online platform. She details the negotiations that surrogates engage in and shows how such platforms give rise to new collective meanings but also "teach women what to expect, want, and dream of" (2016, 11), thereby resulting in "new types of social control" (6). Other researchers have also emphasized the ways in which the surrogacy market tries to socialize surrogates into particular understandings of surrogacy—be it as a "labor of love" conducted by U.S.-American surrogates (Jacobson 2016) or as God's (financial) gift to poor and humble Indian surrogates (Pande 2010). These understandings also bring with them novel ways of conceptualizing the body and its parts, for instance by conceiving the surrogate's uterus as "oven" for the intended parents' "bun" (Teman 2010) or as "empty space" to be rented out (Vora 2013).

Comparing Israeli surrogates' experiences and narratives across time, Teman contributes another crucial insight: As opposed to the digitally less connected surrogates she had worked with previously (Teman 2010), the surrogates in her follow-up study could rely on a "dominant narrative of experience" that was "readily available to read, consume and retell" (Teman 2019, 285). The growing presence of online media had given rise to a "single story" that depicted what the "perfect journey" (a term that itself had traveled from the U.S.-American context to Israel) was supposed to look and feel like, thus simultaneously normalizing and restricting possible narratives and experiences. In this context, the term "reproductive technology" entails more than the medical technology involved: it also points to the reproduction of specific understandings of these technologies (292).

This body of research has illustrated how meanings, narratives, and practices are actively negotiated, produced, and circulated between spaces and actors, not least through information technologies that accelerate such processes and contribute to normalizing and standardizing particular understandings of surrogacy. Moreover, this scholarship indicates that the commercialization of intimate relationships necessitates new understandings of what intimacy constitutes and what not. My book builds on this work by exploring these dynamics through the analytical lens of moral economies, bringing different approaches into conversation with one another. First, I lean on Edward P. Thompson's classic definition of moral economy as "popular consensus as to what were legitimate and what were illegitimate practices" within the sphere of work and economic exchange in specific cultural settings (Thompson 1971, 79). Thompson developed his ideas when analyzing the emergence of food riots in eighteenth-century Britain—a phase marked by the transition to industrial capitalism, and thus by radical economic change. As also observed in the context of reproductive technologies and their commercialization, such times of change offer valuable settings for the exploration of how the economic and the moral intersect and how moral meanings are negotiated and attached to particular economic practices (Narotzky and Besnier 2014; Palomera and Vetta 2016; Simoni 2016). Building on Thompson's work, Andrea Whittaker has emphasized another important aspect of moral economy in her analysis of the surrogacy market in Southeast Asia: the way "moral values are transformed into economic value" (2019, 52). So moral economy refers to a consensus on questions related to the economy within a particular group as well as to the mechanisms through which moral values can facilitate economic exchange. To understand the moral economies of surrogacy in their dynamics, a third definition is useful: that of anthropologist Didier Fassin, who defines the term as the "production, distribution, circulation, and use of moral sentiments, emotions and values, and norms and obligations in social space" (2009, n.p.). To Fassin, moral economies are "unstable or at least fluid realities traversed by tensions and contradictions" and "produce new forms of understanding the world" (2009, n.p.). As the existing surrogacy research has also shown, Fassin's broad definition emphasizes that notions of ethics and morality are not simply "out there" but need to be created and disseminated.

My use of "moral economy" thus always implies the three aspects elaborated above. Through this perspective, I aim to illustrate how words, metaphors, arguments, narratives, and logics are turned into truths by what I call "ethical labor"—a notion I will explain further on in this introduction. In referring to the notion of "truths" I want to stress the absolute certainty with which some narratives were presented and the interpretative sovereignty some surrogacy supporters and opponents claimed. Many did not merely offer their understanding of surrogacy, seeing it as one of many legitimate understandings or acknowledging the many ambivalences that lay at the heart of their understandings. Rather, as the introductory vignette illustrated, it was clear that their understandings were truth claims and that these often related to supposed antitheses (be it "truths vs. lies," or the "right vs. wrong understanding"). A focus on truths thus allows me to make sense of the many dichotomies I encountered during my fieldwork. Moreover, it permits moving beyond the semiotic and cognitive to include how truths are implicit in social practices, and are therefore reflected in embodied and habitualized ideas of "right" and "wrong."

With this book I aim to contribute to the existing work on surrogacy by showing how truths facilitate and accelerate market expansion into intimate spheres of life that play out on women's bodies as mothers and workers in Russia and Ukraine.

Commercial Surrogacy in Russia and Ukraine

The post-Soviet context remains a rather neglected area within the existing surrogacy literature, and relevant publications have only lately begun to emerge (e.g. Brednikova, Nartova, and Tkach 2009; Dushina et al. 2016; Guseva 2020; Guseva and Lokshin 2019; Khvorostyanov and Yeshua-Katz 2020; Kirpichenko 2017; Nartova 2009; Siegl 2015, 2018a, 2018b; Tkach 2009; Vertommen and Barbagallo 2021; Vlasenko 2021; Weis 2015, 2021a). This may be because this region has only recently, in the wake of the above-mentioned legal changes in the global surrogacy market, become popular with Western clients and hence more prominent within international debates around surrogacy. However, surrogacy in Russia and Ukraine has for a long time reached beyond national borders, because their legislation applies to citizens and foreigners alike: Ukrainian women regularly become surrogates or egg providers in the reproductive hubs in Moscow or St. Petersburg because of higher payments; Russian intended parents arrange surrogacy programs in Ukraine because of lower costs; intended parents from countries with stricter laws travel to Russia and Ukraine in search of surrogate workers; and some agencies have branches in both countries or cooperate with agencies and clinics in other countries. The surrogacy markets in these two countries are thus tightly connected with each other. These connections were slightly unsettled when the military conflict between the two countries erupted in early 2014.[8] From the perspective of Western clients, however, the conflict had limited influence: some Ukrainian agencies lamented the fact that foreign clients were anxious about coming to Ukraine but nevertheless asserted that the total number of surrogacy clients had continued to rise since 2015.

Russia and Ukraine have fairly similar legislation, but prices for surrogacy packages differ, so many foreigners opt for Ukraine. Due to low income levels in Ukraine, surrogacy is not an option for most Ukrainian couples, and almost all intended parents are foreigners. This is a crucial difference from the Russian surrogacy market, where intended parents are mostly—though not exclusively—citizens. While at the time of my research standard prices for an all-inclusive surrogacy package usually ranged between US$45,000 and 65,000 in Russia, similar programs in Ukraine cost between US$35,000 and 45,000—as opposed to US$20,000 to 45,000 in India (Rudrappa 2016a) or the US$80,000 to 150,000 in the United States (Berend 2016; Harrison 2016; Jacobson 2016; Smietana 2017a). Occupying a middle ground in terms of costs between the two grand surrogacy players at the time, agencies in Russia and Ukraine also promoted their countries as *moral* middle ground between the "ethically superior" but unaffordable United States and low-cost yet "ethically dubious" programs in such countries as India (see chapter 6). Moreover, Russia and Ukraine—as well as other eastern European countries (Speier 2016)—can offer "Caucasian" egg donors, making these destinations popular with intended parents seeking "white" babies (Vlasenko 2015; Weis 2021a).

The post-Soviet space has a history of assisted conception going back to the 1980s. In 1986 the first IVF baby within the Soviet Union was born in Moscow. In 1991, the first baby through surrogacy within the territory of the former USSR was born in Kharkiv, Ukraine; four years later, surrogate twins were born in St. Petersburg, Russia. Despite these early developments, the practice of surrogacy remained relatively unknown for over a decade. One of the Russian intended mothers I spoke with said there was hardly any information on surrogacy when she started looking into the topic in the early 2000s. The surrogacies of Russian celebrities such as singer Alla Pugacheva and a few cases of posthumous surrogacy (Svitnev 2016) made the practice a more public issue in the following decade. Despite increased visibility and availability, the number of surrogate births remains low: According to the most recent statistics from the Russian Association of Human Reproduction (RAHR), in the year 2019 2,573 IVF cycles were conducted in the context of surrogacy programs and 806 surrogate children were born (RAHR 2021). The numbers have been steadily increasing—at the time of my research, the number of children born through surrogacy amounted to 388 in the year 2014 and 510 in 2015 (RAHR 2016; 2017). Official birth numbers, however, are unreliable, as clinics are not obliged to share statistical information with state bodies or medical associations, such as the RAHR. This also holds true for Ukraine, where a total of 396 surrogacy cycles were documented in 2013–14 (Gryshchenko and Pravdyuk 2016).[9] Media reports surrounding the COVID-19 pandemic and the subsequent border closures in Russia and Ukraine (see conclusion) suggest that the number of surrogate births might be much higher.[10]

In 1995, the year of the first surrogate birth in Russia, assisted conception was incorporated into the Family Code of the Russian Federation and was elaborated in greater detail in a number of Federal Laws and Orders. According to these legal documents, heterosexual couples (regardless of their marital status) and single women have the right to use ARTs, irrespective of their age (Federal Law No. 323, 2011). In the case of surrogacy, intended mothers have to prove that they have a "medical indication," which can include absence or malformation of the uterus, numerous failed IVF attempts, or repeated cases of pregnancy loss (Medical Order No. 107, 2012). Due to a recent legal amendment, from January 2021 onward, at least one intended parent needs to be genetically related to the child born through surrogacy (Loktionova 2020), while previously no genetic link between intended parents and child was required. According to the Family Code (1995), the intended parents' name can then be listed on the child's birth certificate, which means that there is no need for a court ruling or an adoption process. However, they can only do so once the surrogate has formally given up her parental rights in writing after delivery. This means that according to Russian legislation, the birth mother—namely, the surrogate—is always the legal mother of the child upon delivery. The surrogate has the right to abort the child during the pregnancy or to keep it after giving birth, while the intended parents are not obliged to take the child in after delivery.[11] The unenforceability of surrogacy contracts (Mouliarova 2019) thus causes high levels of uncertainty and anxiety for both sides in the surrogacy process (see chapter 2). However, a strict system of payments and sanctions ensures that surrogates adhere to the rules of the contract: During the pregnancy they only receive a monthly salary of ₽20,000–25,000 (approximately US$420–520), while the larger part of their salary (mostly ranging between ₽800,000 and 1 million, so roughly between US$16,500 and 21,000) is only paid out after delivering a "healthy" child and signing off maternal rights.[12] This usually means that surrogates receive little or no compensation if they miscarry, if the child dies during delivery, or if the child is born with disabilities or illnesses. Moreover, many contracts stipulate that if surrogates refuse to sign off their maternal rights, they will have to reimburse the intended parents for all their expenses (including the surrogates' payments) and additionally pay an exorbitant fine—something none of the surrogates in my research would have been able to do. In the absence of good legal regulation, the economic inequalities inherent in surrogacy arrangements ensure the surrogates' compliance (see chapter 4).

Concerning selection criteria for surrogates, the Russian law stipulates that they need to be "healthy" women, married or single,[13] between the ages of twenty and thirty-five, who have already given birth to at least one "healthy child" of their own (Federal Law No. 323, 2011). This last requirement—common in countries that allow and regulate surrogacy—serves several functions: It provides evidence of a "proven uterus" (Jacobson 2016, 35) and guarantees that the woman knows what it means to be pregnant and to give birth. Simultaneously, it is assumed that it will be easier for her to give away the surrogate child if she has her own child, and that any serious medical complications during the surrogacy program would not leave her childless.

Since single men are not explicitly mentioned in the law, their right to surrogacy remains fiercely contested (see chapter 1), and not all clinics work with single men. Nevertheless, they sometimes manage to circumvent such intraclinic rules by pretending to be in a relationship with the woman who is actually the surrogate. Such measures are often a mere matter of appearances, as the case of a gay couple in my research exemplifies: one of the men told me that "it's a don't ask, don't tell policy" (see chapter 6). Like this couple, many other gay couples and single men work with the famous Moscow-based lawyer Konstantin Svitnev, who has—by his own account (Svitnev 2012)—in the past decade successfully pushed through the right of many men to surrogacy and to be listed as the only parent to their children. However, this might soon change: As I detail in the conclusion, two draft bills were submitted to the Russian State Duma in summer 2021 that envision banning surrogacy for foreigners and single men.[14] Debates around restricting surrogacy erupted following a series of alleged child-trafficking cases Svitnev and his colleagues were charged with (Reiter and Rothrock 2020).

In Ukraine, surrogacy is mainly regulated by the Family Code and the 2013 Order of the Ministry of Health on Assisted Reproductive Technologies. While these laws are very similar to their Russian equivalents, there are three important differences: only married heterosexual couples are eligible for surrogacy; the surrogate has no right to the child she has gestated (the commissioning parents are automatically considered the legal parents of the child); and preimplantation genetic diagnostics and sex selection can be performed even with no medical indication (Druzenko 2013; Gryshchenko and Pravdyuk 2016; Guseva 2020).

Several scholars have argued that ART legislation in Russia—and this argument can be extended to the Ukrainian context—is "ambiguous and contains a number of hidden dangers" for surrogates and intended parents (Brednikova, Nartova, and Tkach 2009, 51) as well as "multiple inconsistencies and 'blind spots'" (Kirpichenko 2017, 234). It mainly regulates *who* can access these services or become a reproductive worker but says little about *how* assisted conception should be organized. Furthermore, legal infringements are not uncommon but seldomly result in state sanctions. While many of the professionals I spoke with welcomed the relative lack of state intervention in their field of work, anthropologist Michele Rivkin-Fish criticizes that women's interests, as intended parents or surrogates, are not adequately protected. The current legislation leaves the involved parties "to negotiate these relationships themselves, opening the way for conflict and manipulation rather than justice" (2013, 581) and gives private commercial actors a great "decision-making authority" (Kurlenkova 2018, 180).

Performing Ethical Labor

The weak regulation of surrogacy in Russia and Ukraine makes these countries a particularly productive context for studying the moral economy of surrogacy. Furthermore, gestational surrogacy constitutes a fairly new phenomenon, and public debates and legal policies lag behind the rapid medical developments. Participants in assisted conception can be seen as "moral pioneers," as Rayna Rapp (1999) has written, and Sharmila Rudrappa extended her argument by asserting that intended parents have "unleashed a whole new moral landscape" by pursuing surrogacy (2016a, 6). This landscape reflects dominant framings of surrogacy, but ARTs continue to constitute an "experiential system" (Knecht, Klotz, and Beck 2012) in which the rights and wrongs remain highly uncertain and contested. Consequently, the sphere of surrogacy provides considerable freedom in defining what moral conduct consists of and, consequently, in defining the truth of surrogacy.

According to Michel Foucault (1990, 1997), it is exactly this "freedom" that enables ethical practice. Going back to the Greek roots of the word "ethics" (meaning "character"), he states that ethics describes "the kind of relationship you ought to have with yourself, *rapport à soi*," which "determines how the individual is supposed to constitute [her/]himself as a moral subject of [her or] his own actions" (Foucault 1997, 263). Ethics thus relates to what Foucault calls "moral codes" but clearly goes beyond the unreflective following of rules.[15] He splits "ethics" into four explorable components, which can, according to James Laidlaw, be used as an analytical frame "of ethical reasoning and practice" (2014, 103): ethical substance, mode of subjection, ethical work, and telos. Of these, the third component, ethical work, is most relevant for conceptualizing how actors in the field of surrogacy create truth. It is the work "one performs on oneself, not only in order to bring one's conduct into compliance with a given rule, but to attempt to transform oneself into the ethical subject of one's behavior" (Foucault 1990, 27). Self-formation in order to become an ethical subject is a practice of the self and thus demands the subject to "act upon [her/]himself, to monitor, test, improve, and transform [her/]himself" (28).[16]

While I lean on Foucault's writing on ethics in this book, I speak of ethical *labor* rather than ethical *work*. Two reasons make this term more appropriate for my endeavor: Following Hannah Arendt (1958, cit. in Lambek 2010, 15), "labor" refers to the continuous and repetitive activities of daily life that are never entirely "done"; and following Susana Narotzky (2018, 31), "labor" is to be understood as work "in its relation to capital."[17] Hence, speaking of ethical *labor* stresses that it is a kind of labor that is economically productive and that has to be performed over and over again, never fully coming to an end. In the case of surrogates and intended parents, this ethical labor can go beyond childbirth and, hence, beyond the surrogacy arrangement per se.

The terms "ethical work" or "ethical labor" have also been employed analytically by anthropologists, who have explored how people ethically care not only for themselves but also for others or for the environment (e.g., Dow 2016; Feldman 2007). I take up the simultaneity of directing ethical labor toward the self and toward others but use the term to capture a practice that can be proactive as well as reactive and defensive, and sometimes—as in the case of the agent Larissa Osipovna—even strategic. Within a morally contested field such as surrogacy, ethical labor also entails forms of justification and protection. Likewise taking the moral contestedness of surrogacy as a starting point, Kristin Engh Førde has used the term "ethical work" in the context of surrogacy in India to describe the "projects and processes through which [intended parents and surrogates] aimed to resolve dilemmas and produce new understandings and positions to restore a sense of moral comfort" for themselves (2016, 31; see also 2017). My definition complements this work. I define "ethical labor" as encompassing the manifold kinds of labor—ranging from rhetorical justification and persuasion, through protective care toward others and oneself, and affective labor on others, up to bodily and emotional work on the self—employed to justify and uphold the morally contested practice of commercial surrogacy. As such, I contend that ethical labor goes beyond the individual but rather constitutes an integral part of the moral economy of commercial surrogacy.

Negotiating Access to Hidden Realities

Trying to capture the networks of trans/national surrogacy in Russia and Ukraine, I conducted multisited fieldwork between 2014 and 2017. The longest phase of continuous fieldwork took place between September 2014 and July 2015. In these eleven months, I was mainly based in Moscow. With its thirty-six registered fertility clinics, the city is the largest hub for assisted reproduction in Russia, followed by St. Petersburg with eighteen centers, according to the RAHR's statistics from the year 2019 (RAHR 2021).[18] Most surrogacy and egg-provision programs are conducted in private centers, since state clinics often have a shortage of potential surrogates and donors and, therefore, long waiting lists (Kurlenkova

2018). Despite the high number of infertility clinics in Moscow, accessing the field of surrogacy was difficult and draining, as it largely depends on the goodwill of institutional gatekeepers (Inhorn 2004). Moreover, issues around infertility and ARTs in Russia and Ukraine are shrouded in secrecy. While assisted conception was celebrated as a "triumph of the human mind over nature" in the Soviet Union, discourses from the 1990s onward have become infused with "moral panic" (Brednikova, Nartova, and Tkach 2009), and the public attitude toward assisted conception has become increasingly "hostile" (Isupova 2011). As I detail in chapter 1, these developments reflect the broader context of state intervention in matters of reproduction. Pronatalist rhetoric and incentives have been on the rise in the last decade and—concerning Russia—particularly since the "biopolitical turn" in 2012 (Makarychev and Medvedev 2015). The resurgent state concern with the nation's reproduction is connected to the increasing political importance of the Russian Orthodox Church, which has been actively campaigning against surrogacy since 2011 (Rivkin-Fish 2013). There have been numerous attempts to restrict or outlaw surrogacy in Russia—the latest in 2021—and some of my interview partners noted that public discourse on surrogacy had become increasingly contentious and aggressive since 2012 and 2013. These developments had a profound impact on my research.

One of my entry points were the numerous infertility clinics and surrogacy agencies in Moscow. With e-mails and phone calls being a fairly inefficient form of communication, I simply visited the clinics and agencies without advance notice. This was a time-consuming endeavor in itself. Although Moscow had been my childhood home for four years, I often got lost in the maze of winding backstreets and noisy six-lane roads, or in the huge courtyards with their multiple entrances and porches. Many times I returned home after several hours, without having found the place I was looking for. When I did manage to locate a clinic or agency, I was often quickly turned away. Reactions by members of staff ranged from hostility to amusement, aimed at shielding the sphere of surrogacy from dubious intruders. The issue of surrogacy was "hidden" and "protected," I was told, and they were therefore not interested in participating in my research. Members of staff often regarded my interest as inappropriate nosiness (*lyubopytstvo*). A recurring strategy was to reinterpret my inquiry by responding that they were not allowed to pass on private information about their patients—which was not what I had asked for. Many made clear that I had no right to engage with these issues and that speaking or writing about surrogacy was improper. As such, their responses per se could be read as a form of ethical labor, aimed at protecting the surrogacy market in general, and the vulnerable intended parents—often called *bio-roditeli* (bio-parents), even though they were not necessarily genetically related to the child—in particular. One fieldwork encounter was particularly telling in this regard. In an interview I conducted with Konstantin Pavlovich, the public relations representative for one of Russia's biggest agencies, he explained why he could not facilitate contact with the intended parents and surrogates that he worked with:

> This is medical information and in Russia there is a law that protects private medical information and any doctor has to keep this information a secret ... These are all highly personal issues; therefore, honestly, I wouldn't even ask them because *I don't have the right* to ask them for an interview. It's nothing personal: it's just that I don't have the right to share information about them.

In response I suggested that there might be patients who wanted to share their stories. "Maybe," he answered, "but I don't know that." He then repeated that he had no right to bother intended parents with such requests, as even bringing up the issue might cause pain and discomfort given the vulnerable position they were in:

> If *they* approached me and said "we want to talk to someone, find us someone," then yes. But like this, I just can't. These people are really in a very uncomfortable position; it's very difficult for them. For them to speak to someone and revisit all this (i.e., the painful history of infertility) unnecessarily (*lishnij raz*). Well, I just think that it would not be ethical to ask them that.

Konstantin Pavlovich saw it as his moral responsibility to protect intended parents from such intrusive requests as mine. He seemed to have fewer ethical concerns about the surrogates but nevertheless said he could not help me because "right now we don't have any surrogate mothers who would like to talk to anyone." Time and again, agents and clinic staff claimed to know what their patients and surrogates wanted. When, in another instance, I countered this claim by stating that several surrogates *had* already been willing to talk to me, the agency employee sent me away, saying that in that case I surely did not need their help. Elsewhere, a clinic employee told me to read about surrogacy online or go to conferences rather than waste her time, and another insisted that I would have to come to her clinic as a paying client if I wanted an interview. Yet another employee refused to talk to me but noted down the name of a doctor from a different clinic, who apparently liked giving interviews. "She needs the publicity," the woman said, handing me the scrap of paper, "but I don't." Some members of staff thus regarded giving interviews not only as ethically problematic but also as self-centered or self-celebratory. There also seemed to be a lack of trust in my assurance that I would maintain confidentiality. Regarding me as "inappropriately nosy," many members of staff were also suspicious about my true motives. Some clinics and agencies thought I might be working for another agency—a "spy," as one doctor said only half-jokingly—or that my research was funded by an institution or country with particular economic or political motives.

It is possible that the anti-EU sentiments that gained prominence in Russia in 2014 further contributed to this mistrustful attitude toward me. In the context of the recent revival of a rhetoric of exceptionalism and sovereign democracy (Bernstein 2013), foreigners—like me—who stuck their noses into Russia's "business" were not particularly welcome. Those clinic and agency employees who were willing to share their expertise and experience with me—and, thus, with a broader audience—were those who either hoped that their participation in my research would have a positive effect on their business (albeit indirectly) or who deeply cared about the intended parents and surrogates and hoped to contribute to destigmatizing surrogacy.

The clinics I visited in my first months of fieldwork included everything from more Soviet-style blocks and interiors up to those in baroque buildings, with soft leather sofas, white marble floors, and small chandeliers hanging from the ceiling. Such ostentatious clinics often had huge flat-screens on the walls of their waiting rooms, espresso machines in the corner, and quiet lounge music that created an atmosphere of refined relaxation. The Altra Vita IVF Clinic was somewhere in between. It was the first fertility clinic I visited and the only one that allowed me to conduct (participant) observation on site.[19] The clinic was founded in 2002 by Sergej Yakovenko, a doctor-turned-businessman.[20] In its early days, the clinic collaborated with agencies that recruited surrogates and took charge of the legalities. Later it took over these tasks, because—according to Sergej Yakovenko—"agencies do a bad job and charge a lot of money." Ever since, only the delivery of the child takes place elsewhere, in one of Moscow's birth clinics, and everything else is handled by Altra Vita.

Sergej Yakovenko had high ambitions and was planning to make his clinic the largest and "most humane" surrogacy clinic in the world, as he repeatedly told me. I soon realized that I was to be part of this plan. He wanted me to "include a small advertisement" in my publications, hoping that I could help his clinic gain prominence in the competitive global surrogacy market. The recent conflict with Ukraine had cast Russia in a negative light, at a time when he was intending to develop stronger bonds with his European and U.S. business partners and to attract more foreign clients. At the time of my research, the clinic had only a few clients from abroad, and almost all were in egg-provision programs, not surrogacy. It was clearly my position as foreign researcher that made a collaboration attractive to Sergej Yakovenko. This position proved to be advantageous in other situations as well, as some research participants felt reassured by the fact that

I would not publish in Russian and that information about surrogacy would thus remain to some extent inaccessible for most citizens.

It took half a year of long-drawn-out negotiations until Sergej Yakovenko and I finally agreed that I would not include "small advertisements" but that I would mention the clinic's name in my writings and presentations. In return, I was allowed to conduct six months of (participant) observation.

Beginnings

During my time at the Altra Vita IVF Clinic, I followed the daily routines of the so-called surrogate manager Natasha Sergeyevna. She was responsible for all surrogates up to the twelfth week of their pregnancies, when her colleague took over. Natasha Sergeyevna conducted the initial short telephone interviews with all "candidates," then organized appointments, made sure the surrogates received their hormone medication, accompanied them to medical examinations, gave telephone advice, communicated between surrogates and intended parents, and troubleshot in all kinds of situations.

In the months I spent at the clinic, I learned only a little about Natasha Sergeyevna. Personal questions often felt inappropriate, and her schedule did not allow for chitchat. She only once shared her passion for fridge magnets, when she asked me, with a twinkle in her eye, to bring her one from my hometown, Vienna—a wish I was happy to fulfill. On another occasion, while we were both waiting for a doctors' meeting to finish, Natasha Sergeyevna told me that she was a trained psychologist and for a long time had worked as a teacher. She was not originally from Moscow, but when her son started university, she and her husband had to move to the capital to find better-paid jobs. At the time of my fieldwork she had been working at Altra Vita for three years, living in the adjacent prefabricated buildings, where the flats for surrogates and egg providers were located. Being a psychologist was useful for her position at the clinic, as, according to her, she could quickly tell whether a surrogacy candidate was trustworthy and dutiful. It also seemed that her work as a teacher had left its mark: Natasha Sergeyevna's tone toward the surrogates was stern and educative when she explained the procedures and rules at the clinic, and she would often raise her right index finger, slowly flipping it back and forth in time with her words. Every now and then would she add a "Do you understand?" at the end of her sentences—a question usually reciprocated with a nod. A nod that was not always convincing, but then the atmosphere did not invite questions.

With Natasha Sergeyevna's help, I got to know many surrogates and surrogacy candidates who came to the clinic. If they agreed, I was allowed to interview and accompany them to their medical examinations, such as ultrasound. Establishing regular contact with the women was difficult as most did not live in Moscow but in the so-called regions or other neighboring countries (mostly Ukraine but also Belarus or Central Asian countries). They only came to Moscow for their regular check-ups and were usually in a great rush to get back home, as they had had to take leave from work and make sure someone was looking after their children while they were away. They only had to stay in one of the clinic's six flats in the first weeks after the embryo transfer as well as in the last weeks of their pregnancy. There was one flat for short-term visitors where approximately six women could stay, and turnover was very high. The other flats accommodated one or two people, usually surrogates whose intended parents paid the rent for them to live in Moscow during the entire pregnancy. This was the case for Katya Yefimovna and Lena Mironovna, whose pregnancies I followed until they gave birth in summer 2015.

The two women lived almost next door to each other but never became friends. Maybe they were just too different from each other. Lena Mironovna always had a big smile on her face, liked to joke around, and came across as a profoundly optimistic and carefree person. Her law degree did not translate into a good salary, so she and her husband temporarily moved to Moscow to find better-paid work, leaving their ten-year-old son with his grandparents. She was now looking for an additional income to her salary as a wedding photographer, had come across an advertisement for egg provision, and ended up becoming a surrogate instead. The couple did not desperately need the money but were happy to be able to save toward building a house of their own close to the city of Nizhnij Novgorod, a few hours from Moscow. In contrast to Lena Mironovna, Katya Yefimovna had opted to sell her egg cells first. She only decided to become a surrogate when she had to leave her hometown, Donetsk, unexpectedly in mid-2014 due to the armed conflict between Russia and Ukraine. Being Russian by ethnicity (*natsional'nost'*), moving to the other side of the border with her five-year-old daughter seemed like a good option. The surrogacy program provided her with the income she needed to later resettle in southern Russia, close to the Black Sea, until she could take up her job as a translator again. Katya Yefimovna often spoke of the surrogacy program as "rescuing" her but, nevertheless, deeply disliked Moscow and felt isolated living in a city she perceived as too big and populated by people who were "evil" and "unhappy." This feeling was shared by many other surrogates. City life outside one's home was marked by anonymity, hostility, and hurry, and in the many months Katya Yefimovna and Lena Mironovna lived in Moscow, they seldom ventured beyond the clinic's immediate surroundings.

The two women's stories are exemplary of the diversity among the surrogates and their experiences. All the women had already given birth to at least one child—due to the legal requirements—and around a fourth of them were single mothers. Many had become mothers at an early stage in life, and by the time they became surrogates, they were usually in their mid- or late twenties, had one or two young children, and almost all of them were working. While many had some form of college education or training, they worked in low-skilled and poorly paid jobs, for example as cooks, sale assistants, or cashiers. Their motivation to participate in a surrogacy program was primarily financial, as most were hoping to buy or build a flat or house with the money they received for carrying someone else's child to term. As already indicated, the surrogates framed their involvement mostly as a kind of work and the surrogacy arrangements per se were organized as a business relationship. I therefore follow Christina Weis (2015) in speaking of "surrogate workers" or simply "surrogates" rather than "surrogate mothers," even though the latter term (in Russian: *surrogatnaya mama* [singular] / *surrogatnye mamy* [plural]) was a self-description despite the fact that surrogates did not see themselves as mothers (see chapter 5). Some research participants also simply used the term *mamy* (mothers) or its diminutive *mamochki*, sometimes with the prefix *sur-/surr-*, with or without dash.

Unexpected Endings

Despite growing close and having "independent" communication with some of the surrogates working for Altra Vita, I remained at the mercy of the surrogate manager when it came to moving around within the clinic and making new contacts. Natasha Sergeyevna had some kind of sympathy for the endeavor, but her patience for facilitating these contacts was highly dependent on her mood and workload on the respective day, and I often felt like I was having to negotiate my access to the clinic every day anew, until I unexpectedly lost it for good.

One day, when I was about to leave the clinic and rush to an interview, the director's secretary asked me to follow her into the meeting room. It would just take five minutes, she assured me. It was a big, sparsely furnished room, with a long wooden table cutting across it. Eight people were sitting around it in silence, their gaze fixed on the tabletop. Some, like Natasha Sergeyevna, I had met and spoke with before; others I had merely crossed paths with in the corridor. The clinic's director, Sergej Yakovenko, sat at the head of the table. I took a seat. He looked me straight in the eye, the usual skeptical smile on his face. A few days before—halfway through the agreed time—my research at Altra Vita had come to a premature end. Two doctors had informed me that "our collaboration had ended" and that I had one week for final interviews and observations. They did not explain the change of heart, but now I was to learn more: Yakovenko was holding the list of interview questions I was obliged to share with him before speaking with the surrogate workers at Altra Vita. He shook his head. "All these questions can be answered in two days," he said, waving his hand across the paper. He did not understand why after three months of research I still did not have enough results. My methods were clearly inefficient. In fact, he still did not understand what the aim (*tsel'*) of my research was and how what I was doing could be called research at all. We had discussed this issue on numerous occasions before—in this very room, in his kitchen, in the clinic's corridors. The first time Sergej Yakovenko asked me whether I had collected enough results was only a week after I had started doing research at the clinic. He was a restless and impatient man and never seemed to really listen when I explained that anthropological research entailed long-term fieldwork, establishing relationships with people, becoming a "witness" (Goffman 1989) of their lives, in order to get a more profound and nuanced understanding. I always wanted to add that ethnographies were narrative, that they told stories, but held myself back, anticipating that this could undermine my position as an academic.

That day in the meeting room, I repeated my, by now, internalized definition of ethnography. Yakovenko began to chuckle. "Do you want to go with the surrogate mothers into their graves?" he asked in between laughing, looking for acknowledgment of his joke in his employees' faces. One of his secretaries gave a short giggle but quickly brought herself under control again, as if suddenly unsure whether her reaction was appropriate. Changing to a more empathic tone, Sergej Yakovenko suggested that I formulate a proper questionnaire of ten pages and just send it out to a few surrogates. The way I was doing research at the clinic was too time-consuming for staff, and he had realized that "we don't have enough time to control you." In the course of the three months, the surrogate manager's firm grip had loosened, and evolving relationships with surrogates enabled me to meet them outside the clinic. This was obviously not welcomed by the clinic.

When the meeting ended—not five minutes but an hour later—the secretary who had giggled approached me. Trying to comfort me, she said that the access I had enjoyed was exceptional and that I should not get too upset about it suddenly coming to an end. The secretary was probably right, as I was not able to move beyond conducting interviews in other clinics. I am grateful for these three months at the Altra Vita clinic. Taking part in hospital life provided me with important insights as well as with an implicit sense of how the process of surrogacy is organized, lived, and experienced over time.

New Beginnings

Having my contract terminated was unfortunate, but it happened at a time when I had reached some sort of empirical repletion from doing fieldwork at Altra Vita. I was no longer dependent on the clinic because the bonds with some of the surrogate workers were strong enough for them not to care about my lost status as clinic researcher. No longer being able to join them in the clinic or the surrogate flats—the newly installed surveillance cameras controlled not only the surrogates' but also my movements—we transferred our meetings from corridors and kitchen tables to nearby parks and playgrounds. Losing the clinic as a research site also allowed me to dedicate more time to the transnational networks of surrogacy. I had already conducted several interviews with intended parents and surrogacy agencies during and after the 2015 inviTRA fair in Barcelona but was now also able to arrange trips to Las Palmas and Kyiv, and later, in 2016 and 2017, to L'viv, Kharkiv, and southern Germany. The trajectories I could follow were shaped by the languages I was most fluent in—German, English, Spanish, and Russian—not just because I preferred working without translators but also because these were the languages that enabled me to read through online articles and comment sections, blogs, forums, and clinic/agency websites, in order to discern the "reproscapes" (Inhorn 2011) of surrogacy. Consequently, for my research, multisited fieldwork not only included connecting places but also connecting the real and the virtual.

As indicated above, the Internet plays a significant role in creating and shaping the moral economy as well as the networks of surrogacy. Given the secrecy and stigma characterizing surrogacy, it is also a place where individuals can anonymously seek information and encounter like-minded people. The virtual world was therefore a crucial site for recruiting research participants. I regularly scanned through the announcements of intended parents and surrogates on such transnational platforms as surrogatemother.com and surrogatefinder.com, or through the Russian platforms Probirka ("test tube"), Meddesk, and Ostrov Kenguru ("kangaroo island"). Given the high number of introductory messages I sent, the return was small; however, the effort was worthwhile, because the experiences of surrogates in so-called direct arrangements with intended parents significantly differed from those in mediated arrangements, that is, arrangements made through and controlled by an agency. The former enabled them to actively choose clients and negotiate conditions, while working with an agency usually meant standardized contracts and limited or no contact—a point I elaborate on in chapters 3 and 4. Around a quarter of the thirty-nine surrogate workers I spoke with in the course of my fieldwork were women who had experiences in direct arrangements (sometimes in addition to mediated ones); three-quarters, however, were women who had only experienced mediated arrangements, mainly through Altra Vita. Almost all of these latter women were first-time surrogates, not least because Altra Vita only accepted candidates who had given birth a maximum of twice.

As mentioned, agencies and clinics were unwilling to put me in contact with their clients, so online forums and platforms as well as personal recommendation played an important role in recruiting intended parents as research participants. The fact that I only managed to acquire six Russian intended parents—all of whom were women—reflects the stigma and moral panic around infertility and surrogacy. Keeping both these issues largely secret, intended parents were highly anxious that personal information could be leaked, endangering them and their future families (see chapter 2). In addition, some intended parents also felt at the mercy of the cruel and expensive market and were unwilling to share information for free, while "nobody does anything for us for free," as a woman looking for an egg donor replied to my interview request.

Overall, in addition to the thirty-nine surrogates and the six Russian intended mothers (five who were doing or had done surrogacy, and one who had done IVF with another woman's egg cells), I also interviewed twelve intended parents from Spain, Germany, and Austria, some of whom participated in my research as a couple. In total, I could capture the perspectives of nine couples (of which six had done or were planning to do surrogacy in Russia or Ukraine).[21] Most interactions with intended parents turned out to be limited to one-time narrative interviews, often via Skype. While following intended parents proved more difficult than following surrogate workers, I was lucky enough to get to know a couple from Germany who I could accompany virtually (via Skype) and physically (traveling with them to Ukraine) for over a year, from their decision to do surrogacy in Ukraine up to their final trips to Kharkiv and Kyiv after the birth of their twins.

Moreover, I conducted interviews with fourteen doctors (twelve in Russia, two in Ukraine); twenty-two agents—meaning agency directors/employees as well as private brokers—or lawyers (eight in Russia, eight in Ukraine, six in Spain); and two infertility psychologists (both in Russia). My material also includes two interviews with representatives of advocacy groups in Spain and two interviews with Russian opponents of surrogacy (one a clergy man, the other a former embryologist), all of whom were keen to change the public discourse or even the legal regulation concerning surrogacy in their countries. Last but not least, I interviewed eight representatives of six European consulates in Moscow and Kyiv, who were confronted with surrogacy cases once foreign intended parents needed the official papers to travel back home with their newborns. While these latter interviews are not central to the book, they did inform my research by providing valuable insights into the legal and bureaucratic aspects of transnational surrogacy.

In total, I conducted interviews and informal talks with 105 people who—in very different ways—played an active role in the field of assisted reproduction, mainly surrogacy, between 2014 and 2017.

The Structure of This Book

This book opened with a scene from the international fertility fair in Barcelona in 2015, which vividly captures the central question this book seeks to address: how the moral economy of surrogacy is shaped and sustained by the ethical labor of making and circulating truths. In the chapters that follow, I will explore this question by looking at surrogacy as a local phenomenon in Russia and Ukraine that is, nevertheless, entangled in translocal and transnational connections.

Part 1 lays the groundwork for understanding the moral economy of surrogacy in Russia and Ukraine by exploring experiences and discourses around motherhood and infertility in the post-Soviet context. It particularly zooms in on intended mothers, professionals, and religious opponents in these two countries (with a primary focus on Russia) and grounds their perspectives in broader debates and histories around pronatalism and the rhetoric of "demographic crisis." I show how the social pressures toward motherhood, the naturalization of the wish to become a mother, and the conceptualization of infertility as illness profoundly affect the sphere of surrogacy: Surrogacy needs to be legitimized and practiced in a way that does not disrupt social norms but promises to "save" the so-called traditional family (chapter 1). Moreover, violent Orthodox discourses that blame women for their own infertility and construct ARTs as a threat for the nation push surrogacy into a sphere of secrecy. This setting gives rise to carefully crafted practices of not telling the truth, omitting information, and appropriating/hiding the pregnancy that—in the current political climate—can be read as an ethics of care (chapter 2).

Part 2 focuses on the organization of surrogacy arrangements, foregrounding the perspectives of surrogates as well as the discourses about them. I detail how surrogacy in Russia and Ukraine is constructed as comprising anonymous business relationships, in which emotional entanglements between "clients" (intended parents) and "workers" (surrogates) are deemed dangerous. I develop this point by describing how and why surrogates enter the reproductive market and how the inherent uncertainties of surrogacy mean that they have to temporarily subject their bodies to a strict system of medical and social control (chapter 3). This system is legitimized and sustained by disseminating the image of surrogates as powerful, savvy, and dangerous entrepreneurs, while they are continuously depersonalized and their active labor is devalued (chapter 4). The surrogates themselves grapple with their position in these arrangements by engaging in specific "technologies of alignment" that allow them to de-emotionalize their pregnancies by strategically adopting apparent truths about the female pregnant body and, hence, becoming and remaining effective workers (chapter 5). Taken together, these chapters show how many market actors frame surrogacy as ethical only when based on a business project and economic exchange, because the context of stigmatization makes it necessary to erase the surrogacy experience from the biographies of those involved.

Part 3 of the book explores the shifts that take place once surrogacy involves intended parents who travel to Russia and Ukraine from western Europe and the agencies that facilitate their surrogacy arrangements. Focusing on these two groups of actors, I show how they culturally translate and affectively saturate truths to make them fit with a different set of moral concerns, one mostly focused on the surrogates' possible exploitation. In this context, the businesslike character of surrogacy becomes troublesome for some and needs to be countered by creating narratives and experiences of "happiness" (chapter 6) or by eagerly emphasizing the surrogates' free choice, while de-emphasizing the intended parents' choice in engaging in surrogacy (chapter 7).

I completed this manuscript in early October 2021, more than four months before Russia shocked the world by invading Ukraine in February 2022. The book's afterword picks up on this atrocious move and discusses the ongoing effects of the war on Ukrainian surrogates and the surrogacy market in general.

The chapters of this book illustrate manifold ways of making and circulating truths within the surrogacy market. These truths become part of a "repertoire" or "toolbox" that individuals can draw on to make sense of their experiences and to legitimize their actions. Moreover, the chapters reveal the particular "regime of truth" (Foucault 1987, 72–73) that sustains this moral economy—meaning, the regime that defines the discourses that are acknowledged as true or as false, the individuals that are ascribed the status of truth bearers, as well as the mechanisms and techniques regarded as appropriate in order to find or achieve truth. Taking into account the comparative perspective that this book offers reflects that the truths at stake can differ a great deal, as they are always negotiated in relation to specific social and cultural contexts.

However, as I will show, many of the truths I encountered seemed to rest on shaky ground. They were "fragile truths," so to speak, as they were fraught with tensions, inconsistencies, and contradictions, some remarkably evident, others hardly palpable. These truths, as I contend, are so valuable because they offer moral certainty in a setting of great moral contentiousness. And despite their fragility, they form the very foundation of the rapidly growing global market of commercial surrogacy in and beyond Russia and Ukraine.

Part I

1
THE BIOPOLITICS OF MOTHERHOOD

"A woman who can't give birth to a child is considered a cripple (*kaleka*) in our country," Olessia Valeryevna explained when she invited me to her spacious apartment for an interview. "You write this person off (*stavish' krest na etom cheloveke*); it means, this person is useless, good for nothing." Olessia was one of the six women I interviewed who had become or were hoping to become mothers through assisted conception. At the time of our interview, she had a nine-year-old daughter, who had been conceived with the help of an anonymous egg provider and a surrogate worker in Moscow. The image of infertile women as being "crippled," as "missing a leg" or being "invalids" appeared over and over during fieldwork. Using the words *stavish' krest na etom cheloveke*, which literally means "putting a cross on a person," Olessia even equated childlessness with a kind of social death. Such images were evoked not only by intended mothers but also by all sorts of actors, who commonly linked this understanding to the immense importance of motherhood for women's identity and role within society.

Starting from the notion of infertile women as "useless," this chapter sets out to explore the conditions that shape the moral economy of surrogacy in Russia and Ukraine. It scrutinizes the forms of "reproductive governance" and the ways the women in my research engaged with these—meaning, with the different mechanisms that "produce, monitor and control reproductive behaviours and practices," be they legislative, economic or moral (Morgan and Roberts 2012, 243). In the following, I therefore focus on contemporary and past notions of motherhood and trace how mothers have been deemed instrumental in reproducing the nation. The last hundred years of post/socialist history have witnessed numerous and far-reaching state interventions into women's reproductive lives. These interventions were and still are intimately tied to an omnipresent discourse of "demographic crisis." As a result, women in Russia—and many other postsocialist countries—are mainly addressed as mothers, and motherhood constitutes an important source of identity for women. While such state intervention has partly been enacted through coercive measures or incentives, the imperative of motherhood is ultimately imposed by what Foucault (1980) calls "biopolitics" or—in a somewhat blurry overlap—"biopower": a form of modern government that seeks to control the individual human body and the overall population. Biopower operates in the name of life and health, through specific "truth discourses" and the designation of authorities to speak the truth, through particular interventions in the population, as well as through the way in which individuals work on themselves and subject themselves to these truth discourses and interventions (Rabinow and Rose 2006, 197). Biopolitics thus governs through "practices of correction, exclusion, normalization, disciplining, therapeutics, and optimization" (Lemke 2011, 5) and constitutes a central element in Morgan and Roberts's (2012) concept of reproductive governance.

Here I explore biopolitics in Russia and Ukraine through the lens of reproduction and genetic kinship (Lettow 2015) and the vulnerability experienced by those who cannot comply with the dominant norms—particularly the norm of motherhood. This was a norm that some of the women I spoke with embraced and others severely criticized. Many women affected by infertility consequently undergo long, painful, and expensive medical treatments in order to conceive their "own" child. From a Foucauldian perspective, their experiences reflect the "dialectical force relation" between body and biomedical practice, as the latter can be at once enabling and repressive (Lock and Kauffert 1998, 7–8): while assisted reproductive technologies (ARTs) enable women to perform agency in the form of actively changing their lives to escape existential precariousness, such technologies also reproduce the social conditions that make them necessary in the first place. In the Russian and Ukrainian contexts—as well as in many other countries—assisted reproduction is not meant to disrupt social norms. Rather, as I show in this chapter, many doctors, agents, intended parents, surrogates, and others alike join hands in "naturalizing" (Thompson 2005) surrogacy by ethically framing their efforts as a medical solution to "save" the so-called traditional family and reproduce the "right" Russians. In this way, they buy into the biopolitical discourse that seeks to regulate who should and who should not reproduce. This discourse is not only shaped by the state itself but also by the Russian Orthodox Church, which has become a crucial biopolitical actor since the implosion of the Soviet Union and actively disseminates Orthodox "truths."

"A Life without Children Is a Lost Life"

Motherhood is regarded as an essential element of female identity in Russia. Scholars have argued that motherhood is "normative, and nearly obligatory" (Brednikova, Nartova, and Tkach 2009) or "compulsory" (Utrata 2015, 77–78). Along similar lines, Polina Vlasenko's research shows how Ukrainian women undergoing IVF treatments experience a "sense of handicap, self-hatred and unfulfilled femininity" (2014, 448). All the intended mothers I spoke with reported being subject to immense pressure to have children not only from their friends and families but also from official policies and discourse. The women dealt differently with this pressure. Some of them readily embraced motherhood as their own desire. For Rita Tikhonovna, whose surrogate was in the fourth month of pregnancy at the time of our interview, this desire was particularly connected to the wish to pass something on to the child and to live on in some way after death: "To remain childless—this is very *difficult*. There's no one to give your *love* to, you cannot . . . As my husband says: a life without children is a lost life. Nobody needs you. You die and you leave nothing behind." Galya Yanovna, whose five-year-old son had been born through surrogacy, spoke about having children as something she had never questioned: it was the normal thing to do—a common perspective on the wish for a child among (heterosexual) couples (Riggs and Bartholomaeus 2016, 2018). Nevertheless, she and her husband only started thinking about a family of their own when they realized that most of their friends and relatives of the same age had become parents: "Then we thought, OK, it's probably time to raise some kids." She was around twenty-five years old at the time, which, as confirmed by Olessia, would be considered a late age for first thoughts about children (see also Utrata 2015, 33–34): "I don't know, maybe this is some kind of Russian mentality or at least my generation's mentality," the latter said. "There is serious pressure (*davleniye*) on women. If you have a child after twenty-five, that's already considered late. And after thirty-five, women are simply not supposed to get pregnant." Galya's and Olessia's quotes reveal the social pressure involved in reproductive issues. Olessia was particularly critical of such expectations, but the interview with her made clear how she ultimately had to conform to them. This resonated with the experiences of one of the infertility psychologists I interviewed. Many of her female clients opted for ARTs not because they desperately wanted children themselves, but because they had simply given in to social pressure. This pressure could include constant questioning about offspring by strangers, who "like sticking their nose into other people's business," a female doctor asserted. According to her, one's offspring, or lack thereof, was such a public topic that people she barely knew asked her when she would be having children, because she was already in her late twenties.

Husbands also pressure women, and according to my research participants, divorce is not an uncommon response to the inability to get pregnant—not least because infertility is often assumed to be a woman's fault. Alisa Serafimovna, for instance, now mother of three children born through surrogacy, expressed gratitude about her husband not divorcing her: "In Russia, this happens a lot. When the woman can't have children, the men just leave." She recalled that her doctor—taking such an outcome into account—had asked her husband to leave the consultation room before confronting Alisa with the infertility diagnosis. He did not want to be the one who decided whether and when she would tell her husband. She did tell him, and he stayed with her, but he did not get overly involved in the surrogacy process. This lack of male involvement was an issue that most of the intended mothers mentioned. Only Olessia Valeryevna's situation was different, as it was primarily her husband who wanted the child, and his mother had imposed the most pressure: "She behaved like a moody little child. 'I want a grandchild!'" Olessia described her mother-in-law's attitude. "Not once did she ask me how I was feeling, why it didn't work out. She had just decided that obviously I didn't *want* a child." In fact, she was not too keen on having a child with her second husband, because she already had a daughter from her first marriage. But since children are an essential component of turning a couple into a family (see also Bärnreuther 2021), women and men who remarry are expected to have a child in their new marital unit, regardless of whether they already have children. Because these are second or third marriages, women are often too old to conceive naturally or carry a pregnancy to term. The importance of having children is also exemplified in the terminology my research participants drew on. One interview partner said—with some cynicism—that a marriage "demanded" (*tryebuyet*) a child, and in general many used such phrases as *mne/yei nuzhen rebyonok*, which translates as "I *need* a child" or "she *needs* a child." Rather than the expression "I *want* a child," the term *nuzhnyi* (necessary) illustrates that what is at stake is much more than a personal wish.

Dina Antonovna, another mother I interviewed, also had to struggle with the social pressure to have children. There were no examples of happy families around her while growing up, so having children was for a long time not on her agenda. She resisted the pressure, because she wanted to enjoy life, to do many "beautiful things" and work hard. When her partner eventually wanted children, Dina—who was around thirty-five at the time—thought, "well, why not?" Despite the fact that they had to turn to another woman's eggs in order to conceive, Dina was retrospectively glad that "it happened like that." Had she not gone through all the hardship of failed IVF attempts and hormonization, she might not have been able to appreciate her son as much.

Women like Dina are despised by many members of the Russian Orthodox Church (ROC), which has gained considerable power in post-Soviet Russia, particularly in the area of "moral governance" (Mishtal 2015). The ROC and its supporters have framed infertility as mainly self-inflicted. According to the ROC, unwanted childlessness, for instance, can be a "consequence of previous sins," such as, in Dina's case, postponing childbirth because of pursuing "worldly goals" (Tarabrin 2020, 181). According to Dimitri Anatolyevich, a priest in a small monastery in the south of Moscow, infertility could also be the consequence of promiscuity: "Most of these women have problems with infertility because they have had too many sexual partners before getting married or they have had too many abortions," he told me, reproducing a common assumption within the ROC (Onisenko 2020; Tarabrin 2020). Such assumptions also extend beyond religious circles. While abortion was the most common—and largely normalized—type of family control in the Soviet Union, in the 1990s activists from different camps started mobilizing against Russia's "abortion culture" by drawing on pronatalist and conservative discourses as well as on those around women's reproductive health and safety (Rivkin-Fish 2004, 2005, 2018). The view that abortion results in infertility has become widespread and coupled with a kind of moralism within Russian society: According to intended mother Rita Tikhonovna, every time she told someone about her infertility, she was asked how many abortions she had had—a question that might indicate this moralizing element. Such beliefs also left Father Dimitri wondering what would happen to society if deviant women reproduced with the help of assisted technologies.

The Russian Orthodox Church officially laid out its position vis-à-vis childlessness and assisted conception—as well as other socially relevant contemporary issues—in a document titled *The Basis of the Social Concept* (ROC 2000). Chapter 12, "Problems of Bioethics," reflects the ROC's somewhat paradoxical position concerning reproduction: While actively shaping the discourse of obligatory motherhood, the ROC encourages infertile couples to "humbly accept childlessness as a special calling in life" (12.4,1). Therapeutic and surgical methods of infertility treatment as well as homologous insemination (i.e., insemination with the husband's sperm) are acceptable from the ROC's point of view, but any form of extracorporeal fertilization is seen as unnatural and, therefore, "disagreeable with the design of the Creator of Life [*sic!*]" (12.4,1). From an Orthodox perspective, spiritual means should be the primary way for Orthodox believers to battle infertility—and "willing submission" to the "God-given Cross" of childlessness can even result in a "miracle," allowing the couple to eventually conceive naturally (Tarabrin 2020, 181). Echoing the ROC's document, the priest Dimitri Anatolyevich continuously stressed that rather than having children, the "physical and spiritual union of man and woman" is the purpose of a marriage. However, he also reiterated that there are good and bad reasons for remaining childless: "If you say, 'Why children? I want to live for myself, earn a lot of money, go on holiday and buy five cars,' then I would not approve of this."

Dimitri Anatolyevich's statement reflects the tendency often noted in religious talk that women had forgotten their "real position" in society. This was highlighted even more in my interview with Tatyana Vasilyevna. She was a trained embryologist but quit her job after working in an IVF clinic for around six years because she could not reconcile this profession with her religious worldview. Besides running a small art gallery in the center of Moscow, she had become an active opponent of surrogacy and other forms of ART, publishing articles and giving interviews on these issues. Tatyana Vasilyevna had a clear opinion on women's proper social function:

> Women should remember that they are women and men that they are men. Then there would probably be no need for assisted reproduction. A woman's function is to be a woman, a wife, a mother. Her responsibilities are the house and the family, and not to be a businesswoman. I can't sit at home all day either—I work. But first, you need children. And then what you do, you do it for them and not just to show the world how great you are.

This reminder that motherhood came before professional interests and developments also constituted part of the ROC's "Basis," where "the role of woman as wife and mother" and the "natural distinction" between men and women was emphasized (ROC 2000, 10.5,2). Tatyana Vasilyevna connected women's role as mothers to the bigger cause of the nation, stating that "if there are no children, there is no society, and there is no nation. And first and foremost, this falls on the shoulders of women." Her words are a poignant summary of pronatalist and nationalistic discourses about women, in and beyond Russia. Such discourses seize on women's capacity and duty as reproducers (Inhorn 2007; Kahn 2000), and on their ascribed role in raising children, to hold them responsible for the physical and spiritual continuity of the nation (Yuval-Davis 1997). While the state has long interfered in the reproductive lives of women in Russia, the focus on nationalism has gained new significance since the collapse of the Soviet Union, and in particular since the mid-2000s.

Reproducing the Nation

It is noteworthy that the mid-2000s marked a qualitative shift in reproductive politics in both Russia and Ukraine, with demographic concerns and motherhood taking center stage. In his annual speech to the nation in 2006, Russian president Vladimir Putin stated that the demographic predicament was "the most acute problem facing our country today." Linking this demographic situation to the unequal position of mothers within the family and the Russian labor market, he proclaimed that women who decided to have a second child deserved financial support from the state (Rivkin-Fish 2010; Rotkirch, Temkina, and Zdravomyslova 2007). The two-child family had also become a central image for Ukrainian politicians. In a speech dedicated to Mother's Day and the Day of the Family, then-president Viktor Yushchenko mentioned demography as one of contemporary Ukraine's most pressing issues. Just as in Putin's speech, his words reflected the way state support for women as mothers is constructed as central to demographic policy (Zhurzhenko 2012).

While the references in Putin's 2006 speech clearly signal a distancing from the socialist past, his arguments and recommendations reveal a continuity with socialist demographic policies (Rotkirch, Temkina, and Zdravomyslova 2007). Anxieties about the nation's demographic predicament have been articulated since the early days of the Soviet Union, given that the Union had suffered immense losses during the Civil War, the famine in 1921/22 and the two world wars (Rivkin-Fish 2003). Simultaneously building up a labor-intensive industrialization program, the state initially responded by encouraging—or rather obliging—women to enter the work force (Gal and Kligman 2000; Verdery 2013). This obligation was coupled with comprehensive socialist family policies and the establishment of childcare institutions. The socialist system was based on the concept of a "parent-state," thus on the concept of society as a family, with the Communist Party being the head of the family (Verdery 2013). One of the consequences was that men were removed from their position of patriarchal authority, while women's household responsibility remained unquestioned, despite state support. This led to a dynamic in which men were virtually excluded from the household and the sphere of childcare (Ashwin 2000, 2002; Issoupova 2000). As Sarah Ashwin stipulates, men "were to serve as leaders, managers, soldiers, workers" who "manage and build the communist system," while the state took over their role as fathers and providers. The women, on the other hand, were supposed to be "worker-mothers who had a duty to work, to produce future generations of workers, as well as to oversee the running of the household" (2000, 1). The Soviet gender order was constructed as a "triangular set of relations," in which men and women were structurally dependent on the state rather than on each other (2).

Such a gender order reveals that the often proclaimed Soviet "emancipation" of women did not challenge traditional gender norms. Rather, women were glorified as mothers who remained responsible for housework and childcare, and men were supposed to realize themselves in the public sphere, where they held the most important and powerful positions (Ashwin 2000, 2002; Holmgren 2013; Utrata 2015). This system institutionalized gender inequality in the labor market, which depended on women's involvement but profited from consistently underpaying them (Avdeyeva 2011).

While the party replaced the husbands and fathers as heads of the family and thus made women less dependent on men, this led to an "uneasy alliance" between women and the state (Gal and Kligman 2000) and provided the state with a new kind of access to women's reproductive labor. One measure to "honor" women's reproductive labor was the award of the "Maternity Medal" (for having five to six children), the "Order of Maternal Glory" (seven or more children), and the honorary title "Mother-Heroines" (ten or more children) (Zhurzhenko 2012). These measures were created by Joseph Stalin in 1944 but had no significant effect on the overall birth rate. By the 1960s, it became increasingly apparent that the Soviet Union's low birth rates were not merely an effect of the many lives lost to war and famine, as initially assumed. The expected baby boom after World War II had not materialized, and this realization called for different measures. State intervention in women's reproductive choices went hand in hand with a call for women to take up their national responsibility as mothers.[1] It was also in the 1970s and 1980s that concerns about the "feminization of men" and "masculinization of women" became louder, along with voices arguing for the return to more traditionalist gender roles (Ashwin 2000; Holmgren 2013; Kay 2002).[2] The realization that low birth rates were a result of women's double burden led to a shift in rhetoric from equality to difference between women and men (Gal and Kligman 2000). When in the mid-1980s Mikhail Gorbachev became the new leader of the Soviet Union and, in Rebecca Kay's words, "inherited a nation of exhausted women," his remedy for women's double burden was to advocate their return to the household, to their "purely womanly mission" (2002, 54).

Demographic anxiety continued and even grew considerably after the collapse of the Soviet Union, when fertility rates kept falling and resulted in an overall population decline in the early 1990s in Russia and Ukraine. This had numerous causes: the extreme economic and political turmoil of the late 1980s and early 1990s brought a significant decrease in production, high inflation, and a deterioration of public services, ultimately leading to increases in unemployment, alcohol and drug consumption, as well as social inequality in general (Gal and Kligman 2000; Rivkin-Fish 2003, 2011; Zhurzhenko 2012). These factors caused a sharp drop in the birth rate and a dramatic increase in the mortality rate, particularly male mortality.[3] Rather than tackling the root causes of the population decline, politicians and the Orthodox Church in Russia and Ukraine emphasized a return to "traditional values" to stop their nation from "dying out" (Rivkin-Fish 2005)—a rhetoric of panic that was also thriving in other post-Soviet nations, most of which were confronted with a fertility decline (for Poland, see Mishtal 2012, 2015; for Belarus, see Shchurko 2017).

This rhetoric was coupled with an increasingly ethnonationalist tone, constructing the nation as threatened by the invasion by ethnic others who reproduced much faster (Rivkin-Fish 2011; Zhurzhenko 2012). Such a dynamic clearly reflects how pronatalist ideologies do not address all women equally; rather, only some women are supposed to bear children, while others are actively discouraged or hindered (Pande 2014; Petropanagos 2017; Vertommen 2016; Wichterich 2018). In the post-Soviet context, both socialism and women were accused of destroying traditional national values. The political rhetoric and policy proposals of the 1990s, which coincided with the establishment of a competition-based market economy, were thus particularly directed toward driving women out of the labor force and back into the home (Verdery 2013). The state's agenda was presented as eradicating the "harmful Soviet 'experiment'" and "liberating women from an oppressive and unnatural 'over-emancipation'" (Kay 2002, 58).

From the 2000s onward—when Russia had stabilized economically somewhat—the state started to supplement pronatalist rhetoric with state welfare to increase the birth rate (Rivkin-Fish 2011; Zhurzhenko 2012). The most important measure was the program Maternity Capital (*Materinskii Kapital*). Implemented in 2007, the "flagship of the new Russian family policy" (Borozdina et al. 2014) targeted support toward women who decided to have a second or third child.[4] While birth rates went up following the implementation of Maternity Capital, it soon became evident that the material incentive had merely affected the timing of having children, not the number (Borozdina et al. 2016), since the measures did not challenge the root causes of low fertility.[5] The female body was thus instead instrumentalized for political purposes: as Michele Rivkin-Fish argues, cast as a "microcosm of the threatened nation," it could be made into "a useful biological-demographic tool for pursuing state needs" (2011, 415).

The "demographic crisis" has recently reemerged as top national priority. Demographers fear a significant population decline in the years to come—not least because many born during the baby boom after World War II are now reaching old age, while the low birth rate during the 1990s is reflected in a lower number of individuals of child-bearing age today (France 24 2020). In his address to the Federal Assembly in January 2020, Putin stated that Russia had entered "a very difficult demographic period." He expressed his great concern over the negative forecasts and asserted that it was "our historic duty to respond to this challenge" in order to "get out of this demographic trap" (Klomegah 2021). To reach this goal, the national project Demography (launched in 2019) was extended to run until 2030. One of its main aims is to increase the birth rate from 1.5 children per woman in 2019 to 1.7 by 2024.[6] As an incentive, Maternity Capital was extended to be given out even for first births, while fertility treatment will also be facilitated. IVF treatments have been covered by the state health insurance since

2013; in 2019, it became possible to get treatments at private clinics reimbursed, significantly reducing waiting times for prospective parents (Bowdler 2020).[7] Within the national project Demography, at least 450,000 couples are supposed to receive fertility treatment by 2024 (Beskaravajnaya 2020).

Moreover, several public and political figures have recently articulated somewhat absurd ideas regarding how to address the demographic problem. In late 2020, for instance, Russia's "Council of Mothers" proposed taxing women (approximately US$6.50/month) who "deliberately refused" to give birth to a child (Tickle 2020a). Another measure was proposed by a politician who suggested paying women to prevent them from having an abortion and, instead, encouraging them to give birth to the child and "give it to the state," which would then offer the child for adoption (Tickle 2020b). Both proposals were not widely endorsed, but the fact that these statements can be publicly made without causing much consternation indicates the degree to which such proposals in the name of the Russian nation have become normalized.

Overall, the situation in post-Soviet neoliberal Russia reflects that social and political problems are readily "demographized" (Schultz 2015, 339), that is, cast as demographic problems, while demography itself continues to be framed as determined mainly by individual behavior, which can be influenced through "monetized and individualized incentive[s]" (Leykin 2019, 153). Rather than adequately addressing structural problems, the state thus perpetuates the constant "crisis."

Genes and Masculinities

This historical and contemporary context is one crucial element in a complex entanglement of factors that led to the largely unquestioned value of mothering in Russia, and accounts for low rates of voluntary childlessness (Temkina 2010; Utrata 2015). Moreover, in her ethnography on single motherhood, Jennifer Utrata argues that having children is compensatory for women, as it offers them "a promise of security and fulfillment that is increasingly illusory in marriage" (2015, 77). While men come and go, motherhood lasts.

In my research, participants represented the drive for offspring as "base instinct" and as the ultimate purpose of life itself. A former surrogate asked rhetorically, "What should you strive for if not for this?" Life was thus about not merely having children but having genetically related children. Consequently, adoption was not an option for many couples wishing to become parents. As Maksim Antonov, one of the lawyers I interviewed, explained by means of comparison: "Adoption is not an alternative to [having your own child]. Coffee is not an alternative to fried eggs. And a cup of coffee is not an alternative to going to the Louvre. It's completely different." With this bizarre comparison, Maksim Antonov mocked the absurdity of expecting intended parents to opt for adoption rather than having a genetically related child.

The importance of this difference became particularly apparent during my interview with Galya Yanovna. While sitting and talking in her kitchen in Moscow, she showed me a picture of her son next to a childhood picture of herself. "Remember, I told you that I really wanted a biological child?" She gave me an expectant look, with a slight smile at the corners of her mouth. Reading her look as an invitation to comment on the similarity between her son and her, I nodded approvingly. "When I look at him," Galya continued, "I see myself when I was his age. He's an exact copy of me. I don't know why but this really makes me ecstatic. It just makes me really happy that he looks so similar to me." Even for Olessia Valeryevna, who explicitly stated that genetics did not matter to her (which was why she readily embraced her physician's suggestion for donor eggs), it seemed important to emphasize that already on the ultrasound screen she could see that her daughter's profile was "a copy of my husband's." According to Olessia, to say that she looked "very similar" to her father would be an understatement. "She is a real clone (laughs). She is a *real* copy of her father." This was not unusual, she continued: rather, in many cases of IVF, she had observed that the children very much resembled one of their parents. Galya's and Olessia's accounts could be read as efforts to claim belonging and relatedness. Even though they were not able to gestate their children, the emphasis on resemblance made clear who these children "belonged" to. Research on donor conception has shown that this emphasis legitimizes the child as part of the social family (Becker, Butler, and Nachtigall 2005), while creating distance from and erasing the third party involved (Nordqvist 2010). Techniques of "validating resemblance" are also common in surrogacy, as Teman (2010, 199) observes, interpreting them as "rites of integration" that turn a woman into a mother and a couple into parents. As the scene with Galya reflects, such techniques or rites also require public display and recognition of resemblance (Finch 2007)—in this case, I was the one who should confirm this resemblance by reciprocating her expectant look.

Alisa Serafimovna was also determined that she wanted to have "her" child, meaning a child that carried her genes. However, she only realized this when she visited an orphanage, having initially thought about adoption as an alternative: "I went, I looked, I played with the children.... But I understood that these are not my children, and they never could be. I just had this fixed idea that I would have to have my own child." One of the reasons why few intended parents consider adoption is the bad reputation of orphanages and their inhabitants. Orphans are commonly seen as victims of "antisocial" parents, who have struggled with alcoholism, drug addiction, and social marginalization. Such traits are imagined as having been passed on to the children, thus making them children with "bad genes" (Fujimura 2005, 17). Many of my research participants believed that taking a child from an orphanage was risky. They often pictured a child's genes as a kind of Pandora's box, as containing a person's "true" self (Harrison 2016) and their entire potential, which would inevitably "unfold" within the course of their life (van der Ploeg 2001, 65). "Genetics—this is a really scary thing," surrogate worker Katya Yefimovna said. "If you take a child from the orphanage, you don't know who they will be in fifteen years. . . . Just imagine that the mother is a prostitute and the father a drug addict: this is all passed down through the genes." One of the gynecologists I interviewed contextualized the bad reputation of orphanages in the 1990s. Before 1990, orphans were children whose parents had died, while afterwards the number of "social orphans"—children whose parents were alive but could not take care of them—had risen significantly. The political and economic turmoil in Russia in the 1990s had led to growing alcohol and substance abuse, which in turn increased the number of children given away for adoption. At the same time, the number of families who had the financial capacity to take in an additional child significantly decreased (Fujimura 2005). While the situation has slightly eased in the subsequent decades, Russia still has a high number of children, particularly of children with chronic diseases and disabilities, in institutional care. Poor state support and the lack of adequate training for caretakers means that these children often face neglect as well as physical and psychological violence (Disney 2015, 2017; Human Rights Watch 2014). It is likely that such factors contribute to intended parents' reluctance to seriously consider adoption if they have the financial means to opt for surrogacy and/or gamete provision.

Some of my interview partners stated that having genetically related children was more important to men than to women. One surrogacy agent, for instance, mentioned that she had never had a request for a sperm donor. According to her, women were flexible: they could quickly adapt to new situations and, therefore, more easily accept other children. Men, however, were more reluctant to accept somebody else's sperm: "They need to continue their line, their heritage. If you put a cuckoo's egg in the nest, they will feel uncomfortable." This was the case for Rita Tikhonovna and Olessia Valeryevna. Both considered adoption, but their husbands insisted on having a child they were genetically related to or no child at all. In Olessia's case, her husband played a crucial role in the surrogacy process. As already mentioned, she had a genetically related child from her first marriage. When things did not work out "naturally" with her new husband, she agreed to a few IVF treatments but then gave up. This was when her husband—who had no child of his own—got involved and suggested going for surrogacy. He took on all responsibility for finding a surrogate and an egg provider, and for organizing the process. Such male involvement, however, is rare. While women are generally more emotionally and organizationally involved when heterosexual couples engage in surrogacy (see, for instance, Berend 2016; Teman 2010), the Russian intended mothers seemed particularly isolated in this regard. Most of them had little more than the moral support of their husbands when going through their infertility treatments as well as the surrogacy process. When I asked Vera Romanovna about her husband's role in the ongoing search for a surrogate, she answered that "firstly, he has to earn the necessary money; secondly, he has to go to the clinic on a specific day to give his sperm." Vera was lucky to have a friend who had gone through surrogacy and with whom she could discuss every single step, because "my husband, of course, was no big help. He just didn't understand what was going on (laughs)."

Men were often seen as not understanding questions of reproduction, and it was generally accepted that this was not their realm of expertise and involvement. The exclusion of men from the family in Soviet times (Ashwin 2000; Holmgren 2013; Verdery 2013) offers a potential explanation for the alienation from the sphere of family life and childcare that men still experience today. This was also the reason why all the Russian intended parents I spoke with, and nearly all the authors of online announcements I encountered, were women. But it was not only reproduction that was generally seen as a woman's responsibility. In addition, the "failure" to reproduce was often projected onto the female body, as the earlier quotes from Dimitri Anatolyevich and Tatyana Vasilyevna (see also Isupova 2011) confirm. These factors made it difficult to treat or even speak about male infertility. According to the doctors I interviewed, men often reacted with aggression or denial to diagnoses of infertility, not least because such a diagnosis radically threatened notions of masculinity—a finding echoed in much anthropological and sociological work (Becker 2000; Inhorn 2003; Paxson 2003; Thompson 2005). Drawing on fieldwork in a U.S.-American IVF clinic, Charis Thompson (2005), for instance, has delineated how staff must constantly restore male pride and gendered "order" in this new context of family-making. Marcia Inhorn's (2003) research on IVF in Egypt has, furthermore, shown that men often experience infertility as "double emasculation," regarding their masculinity, on the one hand, and their patriarchal power, on the other—which can result in wife-blaming, for a couple's infertility is mostly grounded in the woman's inability to receive her husband's sperm, despite the high rates of male infertility in Egypt. This dynamic was also observed by one of the surrogates I interviewed, when she was reading through the online forums: "Men, they think they're superheroes and nothing bad can happen to their sperm. So if there's a problem, obviously the solution has to be found between the woman's legs."

Apart from being harmful to men's pride, resorting to other men's sperm brings with it the problem that the husband "completely falls out of the picture. He just pays, that's it," as doctor Mariya Alexeyevna said. While women can have either a genetic connection (in the case of surrogacy) or a biological one (through carrying the child but using eggs provided by another woman), or at least closely "follow" the surrogate's pregnancy, men do not have this opportunity or do not take it. All they can do is pay and provide sperm—a fact that significantly contributes to men's focus on genetic relatedness (Thompson 2005, 121). According to Mariya Alexeyevna, it was always a "catastrophe" when it became necessary to propose a second man's sperm to a couple. At her clinic, doctors only resorted to this when there was "really absolutely *no* way of using his sperm." Thus, while women are the ones who necessarily "embody" ARTs due to their reproductive biology (Inhorn and van Balen 2002, 14), in patriarchal societies they have to subject their bodies to even more medical interventions in order to "spare" their husbands.

Stories of Heroism and Pragmatism

The great importance of motherhood and genetic relatedness creates a situation in which women go to considerable emotional, physical, and financial lengths to conceive a child. Many intended mothers go through various IVF processes themselves, including extensive hormonal stimulation, before accepting surrogacy or somebody else's egg cells. The women in my research experienced their "quest for conception" (Inhorn 1994) in highly different ways: In the narratives of some, pain and suffering were put center stage; in those of others, assisted conception was welcomed as offering opportunities and possibilities.

Alisa Serafimovna's story certainly belonged to the former category. After my invitation to tell me about her life from the moment she first started thinking about children, Alisa spoke for half an hour without pause. She spoke with a certain pathos—slowly, quietly, punctuated with meaningful sighs. Her words felt heavy, as she recounted the seemingly endless failed attempts at getting pregnant but, then, pulling herself up to try again and again. The problems all started in her mid-twenties, when she suddenly experienced a thrombosis in her intestines that nearly cost her her life. She spent half a year in the hospital in an intensive care unit. No one believed she would survive. Alisa recalled that the most pressing issue for her was whether and when she could have children. She had only gotten married a month before the thrombosis. Doctors told her to forget the idea of having children once and for all, that she should be happy to have even survived this illness, but Alisa resisted their verdict: "I told them, 'No.' I said that

I had survived only *for this* (i.e., to have children) and this is why I won't listen to you." She visited almost all of Moscow's IVF clinics but most turned her away, saying that hormonal stimulation could have lethal consequences and they were not willing to take this risk. Being repeatedly turned down caused her great pain, but she eventually found new strength: "I cried a bit, then decided to take my future into my own hands once more and carry on." However, Alisa's bad luck continued until finally one of the doctors proposed surrogacy:

> I had to think about that for a long time. It was very difficult (sighs). I didn't know how I could trust . . . another woman (sighs), living far away from me (sighs), to carry my children. Let her live in my apartment? That would be even more difficult. To see how she carries [the child], and you're here, you can't do anything. For me, this was really difficult.

Despite her challenging situation, Alisa realized that she was getting older with each attempt and had to act soon. Money was not an issue for her and her husband, so she finally gave in to the idea of surrogacy.

As her story shows, it is not only the numerous IVF attempts that are painful, uncertain, and lengthy; the process of surrogacy itself can be just as challenging. Her surrogate lost a twin pregnancy in the twenty-sixth week. "I was ready to die," she stated. "I went home crying. . . . I couldn't talk to anyone, because nobody—apart from my husband and the *mama* (i.e., the surrogate)—knew about this. I somehow needed to carry on *living*, but it was very hard (exhales)." By now they had been through eight IVF attempts, and all of her extracted egg cells were used up. Again, doctors advised her "not to play with fire" and risk her life once more, but Alisa had lost all will to live anyway: "I told my husband that I will *not stop*: I will continue. He said: 'It's your decision, your life. Whatever you decide, I'll support you.'" She went through another round of hormonal stimulation, had egg cells extracted, and this time the surrogate pregnancy was successful and resulted in the birth of a son. Alisa wanted to forget everything that had happened up to her son's birth but then realized that she wanted a daughter. Her prior surrogate agreed to work with her again and became pregnant with twins upon the second attempt. At the time of our interview, her son was three years old, and the twins—a girl and a boy—were one year old.

In her story Alisa Serafimovna presented herself as a valiant heroine who fought for her dream to have children. The hormonal stimulation could have cost her life, but she "decided to take the risk" and "continue." After every failed attempt, she tried her utmost to escape the misery and find fresh hope. The image of the heroine was enforced by the way she spoke about her relationship with her surrogates, especially in moments of "failure." She said that she panicked when she received the surrogate's phone call about the miscarriage. But she did not show her panic, "because I knew I was *alone* at home. And nobody would help *me*. And that now I need to help *her*." Alisa acknowledged her surrogate's suffering, stating that "it was no easier for her than for me." They did not continue working with each other, but Alisa was again confronted with pregnancy loss with the second surrogate, this time only a few weeks after the embryo transfer. While the surrogate panicked, she tried to remain calm:

> She said that she can't continue, that this is an emotional trauma for her, that she wants to quit the program. I couldn't let this happen. By then I was so ready (*gotova*) for the birth of a child that I knew I couldn't go through the search for a surrogate mother again. I mustered all my energy to convince her to go for just one more attempt.... She listened to me and said: "OK. This is the last try."

Alisa not only had the energy and power to keep herself going but also to encourage her surrogates and lift them up, several times. Her narrative reflects her unwavering hope that—against all the odds—pregnancy might be achieved next time. Such hope perpetuates a vicious cycle of infertility treatments. The longer women have been trying, the harder it seems to give up. This dynamic could be attributed to a number of factors. One is the great uncertainty about why some attempts fail while others are successful, which in many cases makes it impossible to predict outcomes. Consequently, any new attempt is also a new chance. As doctor Mariya Alexeyevna told me: "If the patient asks me 'Is there a chance?,' I have to say 'yes.' Even if there is just a five or ten percent chance, there *is* a chance. And as long as there is a chance, they don't give up." Many "miracle stories," as she called them, can be found on the Internet, and clinics and agencies work hard to circulate stories about "miracle babies" (Franklin 2013), because they nurture their business. The lack of certainty makes the notion of hope all the more salient (Mayes, Williams, and Lipworth 2018, 50). Several clinic and agency websites reveal the fact that IVF—and all procedures involving IVF—has become a "hope technology" (Franklin 1997; Inhorn 2003). Hope can be made profitable (Becker 2000; Nahman 2010) through such websites, for instance by stating that "there is no absolute infertility! We treat even the most hopeless infertility cases." The clinic and agency websites offer surrogacy packages with such names as "Guarantee," "Success," or "Victory," and promise "a baby in your hands or your money back."[8] Such rhetoric casts infertility as a "tentative condition," meaning something temporary rather than definite (Franklin 1997, 1998). This leaves women with the sense of *having* to try everything possible (Sandelowski 1991), especially once they have already embarked on the process of assisted conception.

Some of the narratives I heard very much resembled "miracle stories." Alisa Serafimovna's experiences certainly did, and also Galya Yanovna's. With a slight tone of pride in her voice Galya told me that she had been one of her doctor's most difficult and stubborn cases. The image of the heroine was also invoked in her narration. When I asked what gave her the strength to keep on going for ten years, she drew a parallel to a phoenix rising from the ashes: "Well, like the phoenix, the bird: you die every time but then you clean your wings and continue to fly. Like that. Every time you find something [that nurtures hope]." Galya and her husband had been trying to conceive naturally since 1998—when she was around twenty-five years old—and then decided to opt for IVF. In the early 2000s, the first clinics had just opened up and there was no information about ARTs, meaning that patients had to "blindly trust" the doctor, Galya said. The hormone treatment necessary for overproducing and extracting egg cells had severe effects on her body. Within one month, she had gained ten to fifteen kilograms, her ovaries had suffered, and her endometriosis worsened. During the course of the treatments, doctors detected an early-stage cancer in her womb. Her husband—who had left her a few months earlier due to her infertility—returned upon hearing this diagnosis. After a treatment that damaged the inner lining of her womb, she lost faith in Russian medicine and decided to continue her IVF treatments in Italy, but finally returned, unsuccessful, to Moscow. Realizing that the effects of infertility and cancer treatment had reduced her chances of getting pregnant herself even further, she finally turned to surrogacy. Similar to Alisa, Galya described the process of accepting surrogacy as difficult. When her doctor brought up the idea, she immediately refused. She could not imagine another woman carrying her child and was worried about whether she could love a surrogate child as much as a child she had gestated herself. After a year, though, she gave it a try. At the time of our interview, she had a five-year-old son and could no longer relate to these worries. "Your maternal instinct sets in immediately," she stated. The path to surrogacy is long and burdensome, but afterwards you regret not having done it earlier, she added.

Alisa Serafimovna's and Galya Yanovna's efforts to stress their struggles in overcoming infertility can be understood as quests for legitimization—for seeking approval as women who had proven how much they wanted and "deserved" a child (see also Gunnarsson Payne and Korolczuk 2016). Their stories are thus a counternarrative to the image of the rich career woman who buys a child simply because she does not want to spoil her figure—a stereotype that pervades much public discourse about surrogacy in Russia. Alisa and Galya, however, emphasized their "motherly" nature in sacrificing their health in order to conceive themselves and only turning to surrogacy once there were no other options available to them. Their stories were similar to the narratives of women found in Polish IVF forums—narratives through which women sought to normalize assisted conception by foregrounding their diagnoses of infertility and their heroic fights for living a "normal" life having children (Gunnarsson Payne and Korolczuk 2016; Korolczuk 2014). They also resonate with the statements of Greek women using IVF, who emphasized their maternal heroism and sacrifice, making clear that this effort also makes for a strong and proud sense of identity (Paxson 2003)—even though, in contrast, the Russian mothers through surrogacy and egg provision felt it was not safe to share this with a broader public.

Dina Antonovna's and Olessia Valeryevna's stories were different. Theirs were not narratives of suffering but rather of opportunity and pragmatism (see also Lock and Kauffert 1998). Heavily criticizing the imperative of motherhood in Russian society, they were not ostensibly concerned with rehabilitating their subjectivities as women and mothers. They gave in to the pressure to produce offspring but were happy to find pragmatic solutions that involved egg provision (in Dina's case) and surrogacy with egg provision (in Olessia's case). The first thing that Dina said when we met was that the whole process was not emotionally difficult for her. She tried a few IVF cycles with her own egg cells but then convinced her physician—who originally wanted to keep trying with her egg cells—to immediately opt for another woman's eggs. "Life has taught me to find fast and effective solutions," Dina stated, and this was what she needed because, being in her late thirties at the time, she had the feeling that time was running out. Dina did not know how long the whole process would take, but she knew that she would only get older and therefore had to hurry up. "I devised a strategy in order to force (*forsirovat'*) this through as fast as possible," to invest the "maximum" from the beginning. Becoming pregnant with another woman's eggs was not a big deal for her, because this did not "disrupt the natural process in any way." Furthermore, it made things easier for her, because her own body was less exposed—"I just paid the money." Similarly to Dina, Olessia welcomed the options assisted conception offered. She only tried a few IVF attempts herself, first with her own and later with another woman's eggs. But she soon accepted that approaching the age of forty, she was probably too old to carry a child. When doctors offered surrogacy, the idea immediately resonated with her: "I felt enthusiastic," Olessia told me. "This is an opportunity! This is *great!*" In contrast to Alisa Serafimovna and Galya Yanovna, she did not suffer in this situation and she did not feel "ill." "Hope" was not a word that fitted her situation, she declared when I brought up the term. In her view, the word implied having little or no control over what happens, and this was not the way she felt. Rather, Olessia was a woman who had a "problem that needed to be solved."

Reproducing Norms and Elites

The doctors and intermediaries I spoke with also commonly discussed infertility as a "problem" that needed a solution. They were particularly vocal about emphasizing that it was a *medical* problem, as opposed to a moral or religious one. Kyiv-based agency director Sergej Petrovich, for instance, criticized how many people were opposed to surrogacy because they considered it to be "against God's will." However, for him, these two issues were completely unrelated:

> This is a medical problem, not a religious one. If we followed God's will with everything, then technological and scientific development would have stopped a long time ago. The question of morality is in no way connected to this: it is a question of medical art, of medical science, medical professionalism.

Sergej Petrovich claimed that religion and morality had no place in medicine; that these forces impeded science, progress, and development, which were, according to him, inherently positive ideas. Casting infertility and assisted conception as medical issues is a recurrent frame of legitimization in the post-Soviet context. Alya Guseva and Vyacheslav Lokshin (2019), for instance, have argued that professionals working in the fields of surrogacy in Kazakhstan employ a similar discourse of reasoning, distancing themselves from reproaches concerning morality and commercialization by emphasizing their medical—and therefore "neutral"—perspective. Such a perspective foregrounds the technical aspect of medicine. This, however, does not mean that such procedures should be available for everyone. Rather, the framing of surrogacy as a medical issue allows doctors and intermediaries to make surrogacy only available to those who were infertile for medical rather than social reasons, as would be the case for gay men. The fact that Vladislav Korsak, president of the Russian Association of Human Reproduction, also supported this claim (Kolesnikova 2021a) reflects that it was backed up by the official representative body in reproductive matters. The different evaluation of medical and social infertility, according to Sergej Petrovich, was that these men were "naturally" not meant to have children anyway:

> I think if some relationships are against nature, if nature didn't make it possible for homosexual couples to have children, then they shouldn't. [...] It's a different matter to help a married [heterosexual] couple that has infertility problems. This is a medical issue. We have to help such couples.

Thus, while professionals like Sergej Petrovich portrayed medicine as a value-neutral area, their practices—as well as legal regulation itself—were infused with and guided by moral values. While Ukrainian legislation clearly limits surrogacy to married heterosexual couples (Gryshchenko and Pravdyuk 2016), Russian legislation is more ambivalent in this regard. Stating that surrogacy is permitted for heterosexual couples (independent of marital status) and single women, the issue of single men is not mentioned in the law (Federal Law No. 323, 2011). This opens up considerable freedom of interpretation for practitioners. A significant number of doctors and intermediaries claimed that assisting single or gay men is "illegal," that the law "strictly and clearly" prohibits these men from using the services of a surrogate worker. Obviously, this is not true, and their claims can rather be seen as a way of referring to the authority of the law in order to circumvent sharing their own opinion on this question. Other research participants, however, were quite direct in affirming that they did not regard single and gay men as adequate parents. Often their comments entailed some skepticism as to why a single man might want a child in the first place: "We don't like single fathers, because we are not sure what they want and why they are looking for a surrogate," one of the doctors said, implying that single men had questionable motives. Similarly, another agent confirmed she was afraid to work with and did not trust single men who "suddenly" decide to have a child. As in this agent's statement, a single or gay man's desire to become a father was often seen as whimsical rather than well thought through. Furthermore, men were not regarded as capable of taking care of a child. "A single father—what's that? That's not a family," one doctor said, contrasting the idea of single fatherhood to the notion of the "complete" or "intact" family (*polnotsennaya sem'ya*, which literarily means a "family with full value"). Some even labeled assisting single fathers as "amoral" and dangerous. This was most salient in my interview with Russian doctor Pavel Viktorovich, who condensed different strands of critique when telling me how the famous Russian singer Philipp Kirkorov became a single father through surrogacy in the "pseudo-democratic" United States:

> One should not confuse democracy with permissiveness (*vsyedozvolyennost'*). What they do on the other side of the ocean, that's permissiveness. And what we do here, that's democracy. You understand? Think about it yourself. A man with an infant in his arms and without a woman: it's obvious that he'll take a nanny and a housekeeper...A child always needs a mother. Don't you agree? One father can't properly raise a child on his own. Have you studied any psychology? (I shake my head) What happens to a child that does not experience motherly affection in its early years? ... Do you love your mother? [me: "Yes."] And now imagine that you hadn't had her affection: you would be a completely different person. Hard-hearted and tough. You understand? (Laughs)

That's why raising children shouldn't be undertaken on a whim (*kapriz*) or for selfish reasons. That's the way it is.

Pavel Viktorovich's words imply that the interests of the child are violated through single male or gay parenthood, as men are not only incapable of childcare but also of offering the kind of love a child needed—motherly love. He also added that children need to grow up with clear images of masculinity and femininity. Distancing himself from countries with "laissez-faire regulation," Pavel Viktorovich promoted Russia as a true and responsible democracy, as opposed to the image of Russia as aggressor, which at the time—only a few months after the annexation of Crimea—permeated international debates.

Framing surrogacy as a medical issue and thereby excluding people who, according to Pavel Viktorovich, do not and *should* not have a womb (due to their sex) also allows assisted reproduction to be incorporated into the discourse of demographic crisis, with surrogacy presented as a solution. This was what agency representative Konstantin Pavlovich hinted at when he told me that maybe in four hundred years the Vatican would come to accept IVF, "if humankind has not died out without IVF by then." Konstantin Svitnev, a well-known family lawyer and director of Rosjurconsulting, an influential law firm facilitating surrogacy arrangements, takes these claims a step further. In an article entitled "The Right to Life," Svitnev states that if demography does not become the first priority of the Russian state, then soon "there will be no one to live in new houses, no one to be cured by new doctors, teachers will have no pupils, and no one will work in the country" (2006, n.p.). He then moves on to write that the "ethnic composition" of Russian society has become a big problem because ethnic non-Russians reproduce faster, while people from the "intelligentsia" have few children, which might lead to "socio-demographic 'skewness.'" While such nationalist rhetoric is also known to come from those with more conservative and traditionalist opinions, Svitnev (2006) uses it to argue *for* surrogacy, by claiming that this technology enables the "reproduction of the elite," because "only well-to-do and successful people can resort to the services of surrogate mothers." So while the Russian Orthodox Church paints a picture of moral decay and of the dissolution of the nation, Svitnev suggests that assisted reproduction not only contributes to population growth but also to making society wealthier, more "Russian," and more intelligent. His arguments reflect how the development and use of medical technologies are often embedded in a "narrative of progress, and of the betterment of humanity in general" (Lock and Kauffert 1998, 21). Svitnev's nationalistic and classist stance regarding access to assisted reproduction was not mirrored in my own empirical data, but considering his prominent role in the field of assisted conception, it can be assumed that his comments have a broad audience.

In regard to the financial background of the six Russian intended mothers I interviewed, only Dina Antonovna and Olessia Valeryevna seemed to smoothly fit into the category of economic "elite" mentioned by Svitnev. Dina stated that she was "lucky with money" at the time of the IVF program, which was why she opted for maximum comfort. She chose Moscow's most expensive clinic and spent ₽3 million (roughly US$120,000 at the time) over the course of the three years until she finally got pregnant. "Comfort" was also the term that came to my mind when I met Dina in the little café on the ground floor of the building where she lived. Making my way from the metro station to her home, I was not expecting this newly built gated community surrounded by a high fence. The neighborhood did not make a luxurious impression, but then again it was not unusual to find such well-guarded bubbles of privilege in the less exclusive areas of Moscow. I had to pass two security guards before entering her building, which included six hundred flats. The ground floor resembled a hotel. There were long corridors with sofas and plants, and numerous shops, ranging from a pharmacy to a small supermarket. Dina did not like Moscow and appreciated that her current living situation allowed her to leave home as little as possible. She did not even have proper winter clothes, as she could take the elevator directly into the garage, where her car was parked. Similarly, Olessia lived in a fancy and fairly new brick building surrounded by mostly old and somewhat neglected houses. Together with her husband and their child, she lived on one of the top floors. Entering the flat almost felt like walking into a prospectus: A huge glass frontage offered a view over the neighborhood; everything looked immaculate and modern, with only a few personal items lying around.

Rita Tikhonovna, Vera Romanovna, and Galya Yanovna, on the other hand, hoping to soon become mothers, rather emphasized their financial struggles. Rita did not belong to the social class for whom money was of no concern, she said with a laugh, adding: "I have to work a lot to be able to live." Galya too had to forego many things during the infertility programs and set clear priorities in order to save the more than ₽2 million (roughly US$70,000 at the time) she spent over time on the different kinds of infertility programs. Considering the overall costs of such programs, it was clear that—even though many women and couples surely had to save money in order to access them—those who could eventually afford them belonged to the wealthier section of the population.

Naturalizing the Traditional Family

State efforts to engineer women's reproductive lives have a long history in post-Soviet countries, and motherhood in both Russia and Ukraine can be regarded as the only "intelligible mode of subjectivation" (Vlasenko 2014, 446) presented by the two dominant biopolitical actors: the state and—since the collapse of the Soviet Union—the Orthodox Church. Within the broader biopolitical context described in this chapter it is no surprise that women who cannot reproduce are made to feel "crippled," like "invalids" or someone "missing a leg." The stories presented here make clear that the women were "complicit" in this mode of subjectivation: that is, they had either fully embraced the idea of becoming a mother and did not give up on this until they succeeded (which, as in Alisa Serafimovna's case, could have had life-threatening consequences); or they had reluctantly accepted the "need" to have a child and pragmatically followed all the necessary steps to solve their problem, as Olessia Valeryevna put it.

When infertility is presented as illness, disease, or even disability, providing a "cure" becomes a matter of course or even of entitlement (see also Paxson 2003; Sandelowski and De Lacey 2002)—as became evident, for instance, in agent Sergej Petrovich's almost sympathetic claim that "we have to help" infertile (heterosexual) couples. Such a framing, Margaret Lock and Patricia Kauffert argue, medicalizes a specific bodily state and thereby legitimizes "manipulation of the 'abnormal' body" (1998, 20). Assisted reproduction can, consequently, be cast as a "manifestation of our mastery of the vagaries of nature" (20)—as opposed to God's punishment for a sinful life that does not conform to "traditional" values, as the Orthodox Church would have it. In light of such reproaches, the medicalization of infertility can be regarded as an effort to naturalize assisted reproduction—thus to normalize procedures such as surrogacy by "making them seem like appropriate ways of building a family rather than monstrous innovations" (Thompson 2005, 141). Thompson shows how naturalization works in a fertility clinic through presenting specific practices as "unproblematic" and "self-evident" (80) and results in a "peculiar mixture of conservative and innovative, in which conventional understandings of gender difference and roles are deployed to domesticate and legitimate the new" (141). As this chapter has shown, such efforts at naturalization were very much present in my field site and constituted an essential component of my research participants' ethical labor of legitimizing surrogacy in light of harsh moral and religious critique.

Following Foucault (1980), biopower not only shapes the need for measures such as surrogacy but also determines the legitimate forms this practice can take. And it was precisely this "peculiar mixture" that manifested itself in the way my research participants framed surrogacy as a medical solution restricted to women and heterosexual couples. Professionals conducting assisted reproduction were innovative in their methods but drew on conservative values concerning gender and sexuality. Domesticating the "new," they had to reaffirm the old and bring "order to these novel sociotechnical settings" (Thompson 2005, 141). They did so by naturalizing women's desire to have a child but denaturalizing men's desire for the same; or by naturalizing women's biological capacity to bear and nurture children, while denying men the ability to take care of a child—a rhetorical move that the intended mothers themselves participated in. By delegitimizing single men and "nontraditional families," my research participants legitimized surrogacy for heterosexual couples. They claimed that they were not using such procedures *against* nature but were working *with* nature (Paxson 2003); they were merely "giving nature a helping hand" (Franklin 1997, 103) but not disrupting the natural order of things. In this way, (assisted) reproduction becomes a crucial site for negotiating the future as well as the past and the traditional (Franklin and Ragoné 1998, 11). Such a medical framing can, at least partly, be accommodated into an Orthodox perspective (Tarabrin 2020). Using assisted reproductive technologies in line with nature allows the foregrounding of the potential of such technologies to reproduce specific heterosexual norms of parenthood (see also Tkach 2009) and, thereby, to save the "traditional family" or, as some suggest, even the Russian nation per se, which was said to be going through yet another demographic crisis.[9] The omnipresent talk of crisis—be it in relation to demography or traditional values—was one of the dominant truth discourses perpetuated by the state and the ROC.

Picking up the notion of demographic crisis, lawyer Svitnev (2006) claims that surrogacy enables the reproduction of a specific class of Russians: the elite. His argument that surrogacy could prevent "socio-demographic skewing" is yet another example of naturalization, for assisted conception is presented as facilitating the natural—read "unskewed"—and desired growth of society. The economic imbalance between those who could afford such services as surrogacy and those who could not was striking. It was noted by many of my research participants, but it was taken for granted and not greatly problematized. Rather, the consumers paying for these services could be seen as "members of the deserving class" (Rivkin-Fish 2009). Exploring this dynamic in the context of women's health more broadly, Rivkin-Fish argues that the material privileges that became available to the educated middle class after the collapse of the Soviet Union were often legitimized as "moral restitution" for their dispossession under socialism: "Capitalism (and, by extension, the inequality and stratification of consumption that accompany it), the claim goes, will enable Russian society to return to a 'natural' (because not Soviet) form of social hierarchy" (85). Commercial surrogacy is, thus, not only naturalized through a medical framing but also through a framing that constitutes economic inequality as a given and as the logical result of people's different abilities to make a living (Iarskaia-Smirnova and Romanov 2012; Trubina 2012; Walker 2012). This approach to surrogacy is not only a question of rhetoric but also constitutes and shapes the moral economy of surrogacy:

It facilitates surrogacy arrangements in which the intended mothers' "illness," their wish for a nuclear family, and their purchasing power are put center stage, while the surrogates are attributed a marginal, almost technical, role as a paid worker. Simultaneously, the threatening and moralizing reproaches from the ROC and other conservatives make surrogacy participants worry about their and the children's future lives—a fear that often results in turning surrogacy into a secret and hidden endeavor.

2
SECRET CONCEPTIONS

I got to know Alisa Serafimovna through an announcement posted on the Russian online platform Meddesk in 2015:

> I am selling a set of strap-on bellies made of silicone, for the period 5–7 months and 7–9 months, including support underwear, made by the firm Belly Make. Clothing sizes 42–46. These are lucky bellies—I have three little children!!!

Maybe *know* is not the right word, for we never met but only spoke once, via Skype, with the video function turned off. She did not want me to see her face, and it is likely that she did not tell me her real name. Wearing the strap-on bellies she was now ready to sell, she had simulated two pregnancies and was not planning to tell anyone—including her three children—about the surrogacy programs. Her caution in this regard was not exceptional but common for women who had become mothers through assisted reproduction.

Intrigued by what I perceived as a drastic measure, in this chapter I explore how the biopolitics of motherhood intersects with the stigmatization of infertility and assisted reproduction in Russia. Some of my research participants emphasized that public attitudes toward these issues had taken a threatening turn. Intended mother Olessia Valeryevna remarked that a "catastrophic shift" had taken place, referring to the growing influence of the Russian Orthodox Church (ROC) and the subsequent retraditionalization and clericalization of Russian society and politics. Political and social scientists Andrey Makarychev and Sergei Medvedev (2015) argue that the year 2012 (when Putin started his third term as president) introduced a "biopolitical turn" in Russia. This turn marked an increasing concern with citizens' bodies and private lives, based on the need to protect "traditional values" from the moral threat coming from deviant "Others," such as people who reproduce through assisted conception.

The growing influence of religious actors and conservative views is not unique to Russia but can also be witnessed in other post-Soviet countries, most notably in Poland, where the Catholic Church has been a central biopolitical actor from the early 1990s onward, with a significant influence on reproductive politics. Building on the concept of "reproductive governance" (Morgan and Roberts 2012), anthropologist Joanna Mishtal argues that the Catholic Church operates through what she calls "moral governance"—a term that captures "how particular 'moral' discussions and mechanisms have been used to enact individual surveillance and political intimidation to maintain legislative control over reproduction" (2015, 20). Despite the many differences between the two countries, Mishtal's concept is useful to understand how morality can be powerfully instrumentalized, to affect the lives even of those who are critical of Catholic or Orthodox morality. One crucial way of doing so, according to Mishtal (2015), is through the dissemination of truth discourses. As previously indicated and further elaborated in the following, religious conservatives in Russia are very explicit about their views on surrogacy. Their truth discourses include accusing surrogates of selling "their" babies or arguing that infertility is caused by (women's) sinful behavior and that allowing such women to reproduce through assisted reproductive technologies (ARTs) would result in the birth of artificial "monsters." Ultimately, they predict, these developments would lead to moral decay and the nation's extinction. While doomsday scenarios of society's moral decay per se are not new in Russia (Rivkin-Fish 2005), they have gained a new quality in the past ten years.

In this chapter, I am interested in how this contentious environment affects the kinds of practices deemed legitimate in the moral economy of surrogacy (Thompson 1971). I show how this environment significantly contributes to turning surrogacy into a secret and hidden endeavor for the Russian intended mothers and surrogates (although here I will again mostly focus on the former), and how practices of not telling the truth, omitting information, hiding/simulating a pregnancy, and constructing alternative narratives of gestation and childbirth become not only morally acceptable but even necessary practices in order to avoid stigmatization and potential danger. I propose to read such practices as a particular form of ethical labor, which is informed by an ethics of care. As opposed to classical moral theories that are grounded in notions of rationality, autonomy, and independence (such as Kantian ethics or utilitarianism), an ethics of care emphasizes relationality and dependency (Gilligan 2003; Held 2006). Moral reasoning and judgment, therefore, take into account relations of care and responsibility toward others, particularly those in more vulnerable positions, but also toward oneself (Tronto 1994; Tronto and Fischer 1990). While "care ethics" is often used as a normative concept, I employ it here as an analytical lens through which to make sense of practices of secrecy as ethical labor.

Russia's Designated Others

While still not widely discussed in Russia, since the mid-2000s surrogacy and other forms of assisted conception have become increasingly visible. More information has become publicly available, and the topic regularly features on talk shows, in soap operas, and in media articles. The openness of some Russian celebrities about their surrogate pregnancies has certainly contributed to this trend: pop star Philipp Kirkorov, for instance, became a single father to two children born in 2011 and 2012, respectively, by a surrogate in the United States. Curiously, his former wife, the famous singer Alla Pugacheva, and her new husband, showman Maksim Galkin, became parents of twins born by a Russian surrogate just shortly after, in 2013, when Pugacheva was sixty-four years old (RIA Novosti 2013). Around the same time, there were also three incidents involving posthumous surrogacy that were widely discussed in the media. In all cases, young men affected by cancer had their sperm frozen before starting chemotherapy. None of them survived, and their mothers ensured they had offspring by hiring a surrogate and buying egg cells (Svitnev 2016). While these cases increased the public awareness of surrogacy, such awareness can have ambivalent effects, as it can easily provoke resistance and contestation, as the case of surrogacy shows.[1]

My research participants described contemporary public opinion on surrogacy in varied, even contradictory, terms. Several referred to a survey conducted in 2013 by the state-run Russian Public Opinion Research Center (VCIOM). Results showed that 76 percent of Russians thought surrogacy to be acceptable—60 percent if there was a medical diagnosis, 16 percent even without a medical diagnosis. Only 19 percent were completely opposed to it; 25 percent of respondents stated that they would turn to surrogacy if they could not have a child of their own, while 45 percent answered that they would turn to adoption. Only a month later, a similar study was published by the independent Levada Center, showing that 50 percent of all respondents deemed surrogacy acceptable and 34 percent unacceptable (*Sputnik* 2013). Some of my interviews with doctors and surrogacy agents reflected this widespread approval of surrogacy and assisted conception. However, such statements as "nobody is ashamed of doing surrogacy anymore" or that "surrogacy is not a taboo" were rare and must be treated with caution, as they were made by those actors who had a vested interest in communicating that foreign intended parents would encounter no problems when conducting surrogacy in Russia.

For the majority of my interview partners, especially the intended mothers I spoke with, the issue of infertility and surrogacy was clearly linked to considerable stigma and fear. While I cannot account for the significant difference between the VCIOM and Levada Center data, the gap between the survey data and my own could be explained by considering the "biopolitical turn" (Makarychev and Medvedev 2015) mentioned above. This turn can be related to President Putin's decreasing legitimacy: While his earlier success relied on the country's sustained economic growth, recession after the global financial crisis in 2008/9 contributed to increasing dissatisfaction within society. This dissatisfaction resulted in massive protests concerning the parliamentary elections (December 2011) and the presidential elections (March 2012), when the ruling party, United Russia, was accused of tampering with the results (Gabowitsch 2013). The protests—the largest Russia has seen since the collapse of the Soviet Union—were met with the counterstrategy of demarcating the loyal, silent "Putin majority" versus the negligible anti-Russian opposition, the latter allegedly financed by foreign enemies (Smyth and Soboleva 2014). This discourse idolized Putin as a strong leader who would ensure stability on all levels—a promise backed and spread by the ROC, whose primate, Patriarch Kirill, even spoke of Putin as a "miracle of God." After the protests, the relationship between the church and the state intensified, resulting in a "perfect harmony" (Anderson 2016) that was consolidated a few months later, when the feminist collective Pussy Riot performed their Punk Prayer in Moscow's famous Cathedral of Christ the Savior. Regina Smyth and Irina Soboleva (2014) argue that the staged character of the following trials as well as the greatly exaggerated court sentence reflected a symbolic politics meant to restore the regime's authority. They see the case as a significant turning point in the Kremlin's measures to reframe relations between the state and its (disobedient) citizens. At the same time, such interventions divert attention from the country's pressing socioeconomic issues by creating a sense of moral panic and threat coming from "designated Others" (Makarychev and Medvedev 2015, 51). Russia's "Others" are confronted with a strikingly similar state discourse around gender/sexuality, demography, and morality that attempts to cast an apocalyptic future that will destroy the Russian nation. While such discourses—and the respective interventions—usually target feminists or the LGBTQI+ community, I will show in the following that the medically infertile body and the "artificial" ART body (i.e., the body of the child born through IVF) are also significantly othered.[2]

The Moral Governance of Otherness

Considering these developments, it is no coincidence that surrogacy reemerged on the politicians' agenda roughly around the time of my fieldwork in Moscow. In 2013, State Duma deputy Yelena Mizulina—at that time head of the Duma's Family, Women, and Children Committee—spoke of surrogacy as the "most frightening phenomenon that threatens not only Russia but all of mankind with extinction" and repeatedly called for banning or severely restricting the practice (Krainova 2013).[3] In the following years, two further attempts to ban or restrict surrogacy were undertaken by Vitaly Milonov, Duma deputy and at the time member of the Legislative Assembly of St. Petersburg, in 2014; by Senator Anton Belyakov in 2017; and by a group of Duma deputies led by deputy chairman Pyotr Tolstoy in 2021 (Kuznetsova and Gubernatorov 2021).

Representatives of the ROC have also threatened to push for a ban on surrogacy, describing the practice as "mutiny against God" and "happy fascism" (Tétrault-Farber 2014). In its official document *The Basis of the Social Concept*, the ROC states that surrogacy entails "the violation of the profound emotional and spiritual intimacy that is established between mother and child" (2000, 12.4,2) and "traumatizes both the bearing woman, whose mother's feelings are trampled upon, and the child who may subsequently experience an identity crisis" (12.4,3). Moreover: "The use of reproductive methods outside the context of the God-blessed family has become a form of theomachism carried out under the pretext of the protection of the individual's autonomy and wrongly understood individual freedom" (12.4,4).

But surrogacy opponents not only draw on religious norms to counter the practice. As Emil Persson has analyzed in the context of homophobia, the "alternative modernity" envisioned by Russian traditionalists "embraces reason and science" (2015, 268). My interview with former embryologist and vocal Orthodox believer Tatyana Vasilyevna was particularly illustrative of how professional experience and supposedly scientific studies can be drawn on when claiming moral authority and truth. Tatyana Vasilyevna did so in order to support her claim that children born through IVF were inherently abnormal:

> Based on my own experience, I can say that these children (i.e., children born through IVF) are really different. They are just a bit strange when compared to normal children (i.e., children not born through IVF). Any person would see this straight away if you put these two kinds of children next to each other.

She went on to tell me that kindergartens and schools in numerous European countries commonly single out children born through IVF and put them in separate classes in order to study their behavior.⁴ From Tatyana Vasilyevna's perspective, this is an important safety measure:

> To me it seems that we are creating little Frankenstein [monsters]. They are less emotional; they are more susceptible to others' influence. They don't have an opinion of their own. If you tell them "Stroke the cat!," they will stroke the cat. If you tell them "Hit the cat!," they will hit the cat. We don't know how this could be made use of. We don't know what they will be like once they grow up, so we should not ignore this aspect.

Tatyana Vasilyevna is not alone in making (up) and circulating such "truths." An online article from the Russian newspaper *Pravda* (Sudakov 2011b) cites family and infertility psychologist Galina Maslennikova, who stipulates that children born from "medical experiments" such as ARTs have "immense difficulties in approaching their peers and get along very badly with their mothers." The mother, in return, "has no maternal instinct" and thus "the majority of mothers" who conceive through assisted reproduction end up putting their children in an orphanage. The author also suggests that children born through surrogacy receive no love during gestation and thus end up as "spiritual invalids." Consequently, these children will be unable to form a "normal family" in the future. Many religious opponents of ARTs furthermore claim that children born through IVF have no soul. While Tatyana Vasilyevna implied that she could not know whether this was true, she emphasized that doctors could create people in a physical sense but could not give these people a soul. It would only be a matter of time before this question could be answered, she said. However, according to her, the reasons for "spiritual invalidity" go beyond whether or not a person has a soul; the rupture of the maternal bond is also problematic: "In the womb the child has an intimate and deep connection to the mother. When a child is torn from the mother, it experiences a psychological trauma. This is obvious; we don't even have to talk about it. That's just the way it is," she claimed. Drawing on her medical expertise as an embryologist, Tatyana Vasilyevna furthermore argued that IVF will inevitably result in the "degeneration of humankind." One of the reasons for this degeneration is the fact that while natural conception needs "strong" sperm cells, IVF programs also use "weak" ones that would not otherwise "make it."⁵ Tatyana Vasilyevna's words echoed hostile positions on ARTs in the health sector. In 2009, well-known pediatrician Alexander Baranov—who is also a full member of the Russian Academy of Medical Sciences and honorary president of the Union of Pediatricians of Russia—publicly stated that 75 percent of the children born through IVF had birth deficiencies and concluded that the state should not invest in ARTs (Interfax 2009). More recently, Lyudmila Ogorodova, a pediatrician and former vice-minister of education, told the media that "we know for sure" that children born through IVF fell behind in terms of physical and neuropsychological development and that they suffered from "very serious defects" that significantly altered quality of life (Beskaravajnaya 2020).

While I cannot evaluate how widespread such claims really are, the fact that they are disseminated by influential individuals and news outlets might mean that they fall on fertile ground. This was certainly the case for Olessia Valeryevna's pediatrician, who asked her for double the fee, claiming that IVF children are generally sicker and therefore need more medical treatment than "normal" children.

Such arguments can be read as central to strategies of "moral governance" (Mishtal 2015). It is thus not surprising that Orthodox truth discourses in Russia are strikingly similar to those perpetuated by the Catholic Church in Poland. Even though IVF is accepted by the Polish majority, the Catholic Church works hard to construct a "distinct category of 'IVF children'" whose "genetic otherness" is said to threaten the Polish nation (Korolczuk 2016, 127). Church representatives as well as Catholic doctors and scientists in Poland have repeatedly compared children born through IVF with monsters, who are prone to physical impairments and mental problems, even experiencing "survivor syndrome" regarding their "unborn siblings" (i.e., embryos that were not chosen for implantation) (Maciejewska-Mroczek and Radkowska-Walkowicz 2017). In 2013, a Polish priest and professor of law even stated that children born through IVF displayed a "tactile crease" on their foreheads, reflecting their genetic defect (Maciejewska-Mroczek 2019). Just like their Russian counterparts, these actors often draw on biomedical terminology and refer to scientific studies or authoritative medical figures to underline their arguments, without, however, providing evidence (Maciejewska-Mroczek 2019; Radkowska-Walkowicz 2012).

While many of the above-mentioned statements can be easily dismissed as "fragile truths" that have no scientific foundation, there is indeed much uncertainty concerning the health of children born through IVF. Epidemiological research (Berntsen et al. 2019; Halliday et al. 2019; Magnus et al. 2021; Mitter 2020) has shown that children born through ARTs tend to be smaller in terms of size and weight at birth than those conceived "naturally" and that they have an increased risk of certain developmental issues and cardiovascular problems such as high blood pressure. However, causal links seem difficult to establish, since the prevalence of these risks could also result from parental health and low fertility, from the hormonal treatment for the stimulation of oocyte growth in the woman or the manipulation of gametes and embryos in the laboratory (e.g., in the process of freezing or pregenetic testing), as well as from the number of embryos transferred (Berntsen et al. 2019; Mitter 2020). Moreover, in many cases risk is only higher at a specific age and disappears once the children reach adolescence

(Halliday et al. 2019; Magnus et al. 2021). In short, while much remains unknown and studies partly contradict each other, there are currently no indications that IVF procedures severely affect the health of children.

"Nature is not stupid," Tatyana Vasilyevna continued our conversation on ICSI. "If the sperm were not supposed to make it, then there is a reason and we shouldn't take this decision into our own hands. If we do, we will have to bear full responsibility for whatever happens." She argued that "if people's attitudes toward marriage, family, children, love—not 'free' love but normal love—do not change, then, I am afraid, this will not end well." Father Dimitri, the Moscow priest I interviewed, shared this opinion: If people "live in a society that allows itself everything, where they live outside the family (i.e., adultery), drink, take drugs, use assisted reproduction, then this society will gradually crumble," he said. Such doomsday scenarios are common in the religious discourse on surrogacy and are frequently combined with a lament for the loss of traditional values and fear of the moral decay of society as a whole. Mentioning assisted conception alongside adultery, alcoholism, and drug abuse clearly adds moral weight to this issue. Dimitri Anatolyevich perceived the development of assisted conception as a great threat, "because today, with assisted reproduction, any woman can have a child, no matter how sinful her life has been. She can do whatever she wants, because she doesn't have to fear the consequences of her amoral behavior." From this perspective, assisted reproduction leads to an erosion of overall morality, as people will lose the moral framework for their behavior. According to Father Dimitri, the solution to infertility is thus not to invent new technologies but to "select the proper path in life." Tatyana Vasilyevna also emphasized that Russians need to return to "values"—"values that start with the family, the people, the nation, the country" rather than with "omnipresent cosmopolitanism." For religious traditionalists in Russia, the term "cosmopolitanism" has a distinctly negative connotation: it stands for such evils as feminism, homosexuality, or IVF, which are said to come from "the West" and to be inherently anti-Russian. Dimitri Anatolyevich regarded this as a result of the "propaganda for a life of freedom" that he observed in his country.

In my interviews, the term "propaganda" popped up a number of times in interesting ways. According to the *Oxford English Dictionary*, it describes "information, especially of a biased or misleading nature, used to promote a political cause or point of view."[6] However, what my interlocutors described often did not seem particularly biased or misleading. Rather, they were mere instances of, for example, homosexuality or IVF being mentioned in conversation, made publicly visible, or disclosed in some other way. This conflation becomes all too obvious in the case of Russia's so-called Gay Propaganda Law (Federal Law No. 135, 2013), which was instituted in the wake of the "biopolitical turn" (Makarychev and Medvedev 2015). The law aims at "protecting children from information that advocates values opposed to those of the traditional family" and is formulated in such a broad manner as to turn any signs of queer existence into a criminal offense. The formulation can lead to absurd situations such as the inquiry of a concerned citizen in the region of Chelyabinsk, who wanted to know whether the rainbow-colored lamppost in his town violated the new law (Nechepurenko 2013). It also became clear in the way surrogacy opponent Tatyana Vasilyevna used the term. In her eyes, the increased "propaganda" for assisted reproduction in the Russian media, especially in TV series and feature films, was proof of the "strangeness" of IVF children: "It is common knowledge that a good product does not need advertisement," she stated. "So if they start making propaganda for a product, you know that there's something wrong with it." While I do not know which specific series and films Tatyana Vasilyevna had in mind, the above-mentioned example with the lamppost raises the question of whether these really "advertised" IVF or whether they merely included characters who had used assisted conception.

"Virtually No One Trusts Strangers"

Given the harsh moral critique and the strong apocalyptic commentaries by conservatives in Russia, many intended parents—as well as surrogates—keep their involvement in assisted conception secret. The church's recent intervention has destroyed the efforts of many supporters and users of ARTs to normalize these practices. When intended mother Galya Yanovna entered the field of assisted reproduction in the early 2000s, these procedures were still rather new, and the ARTs community that had formed through the various online platforms—mainly Probirka—actively fought against the prevailing prejudice. "We tried to change things," Galya said. Doctors and patients gave interviews in newspapers and magazines and on television, with the aim of "proving" that children born through IVF were normal.

In the meantime, things had changed but not for the better, as Galya had hoped. While only a few years previously she had not been afraid to disclose her use of IVF (although not of surrogacy!), at the time of our interview she was no longer as open about these procedures. Demography scholar Olga Isupova, whom I interviewed in 2014, confirmed this shift. She stated that due to the political situation and the economic crisis in Russia, "people are generally more aggressive and less happy now," searching for any outlet for their emotions. This reduced interpersonal trust even further, which, according to Isupova, had already experienced a significant drop from the 1990s in Russia. "Virtually no one trusts strangers," she commented on the contemporary situation. According to the European Social Survey (2017), Russia is the third least "stranger trusting" country within Europe. In this sense, Russian society has very low levels of "thin" interpersonal trust (Khodyakov 2007) and can generally be classified as a "low-trust society" (Radaev 2004).

When I asked my interview partners how they explained their low trust in others, some emphasized that people in Russia "really liked to judge others," as Dina Antonovna phrased it. She framed this trait as a continuation of the Soviet past:

> In the Soviet Union they built lots of these five-storey houses—they were everywhere. Outside *every* entrance there were two benches . . . and every one of them was occupied by *babushkii* (i.e., grandmothers). Five or six *babushkii*, and every time somebody passed by they were like "Look who comes here" and they discussed absolutely everything. So this is where this interest in other people's lives comes from: this aggressive and impudent habit of sticking your nose into other people's business.

Similar statements were made by other research participants. Doctor Mariya Alexeyevna was among those annoyed about what she termed the "pathological interest in interfering in the lives of others." Referring to the Soviet legacy, she—half-jokingly—drew a parallel with Russia's past as a "country of councils" (*strana sovyetov*). With this analogy to the meaning of "USSR" (Union of Soviet Socialist Republics), Mariya Alexeyevna was playing on the Russian word *sovyet*, which means "council" or "assembly" as well as "advice," "recommendation," or "suggestion." "We are still such a country of *sovyets*. Everybody gives *sovyet* to everybody, especially concerning medical things. How to get pregnant, how to give birth, and so forth. In this sense, people are not well versed in how to behave toward each other." Dina shared this opinion, stating that Russians simply show no respect for other people's feelings or secrets. Among her friends, however, it was different. In contrast to the "masses" (*massa*), her friends were more reflexive (*dumayushchiye*), educated, and tolerant and did not stick their noses so much into other people's business (*nye tak sil'no lezut v chuzhuyu zhizn'*). In a way, Dina could be seen as evoking the Soviet notion of "culturedness" (*kul'turnost'*), which delineated such characteristics as good education, proper moral behavior, self-responsibility, or health consciousness. Being "cultured" meant being "civilized"; it was a form of capital that served as a marker of distinction from the lower classes and still does so today (Patico 2005; Rivkin-Fish 2009).[7] *Kul'turnost'* was something that Dina attributed to herself and her friends but not to the "masses," who did not know how to behave properly toward others.[8]

Considering this lack of mutual respect, doctors and surrogacy agents actively discouraged intended parents from sharing their thoughts and experiences with others, because "you can't avoid someone somewhere spreading something," as Mariya Alexeyevna said. Galya Yanovna, for instance, told her new partner only that her child was born through IVF, not through surrogacy:

> I'll tell you why. Today everything might be great, you have a wonderful relationship, big love . . . but what will happen after that? Nobody knows. People work like this: when there's a conflict, they try to hurt you. . . . And I wouldn't place that trump card in their hands . . . Maybe I think the worst of people, but I just don't want to take any risks.

Surrogates were also discouraged from sharing such information. Contracts often included a paragraph stating that they were not allowed to talk to anyone about their job. Some agencies tried to keep surrogates apart from one another, warning that information could be leaked. Surrogates were also advised not to reveal that they were gestational carriers when they went to a public clinic for their regular check-ups, as they ran the risk of being insulted or treated badly by medical staff. These forms of discrimination were not necessarily outright. Ukrainian surrogate Alyona Timofeyevna, for instance, mentioned that the staff in the maternity clinic where she gave birth for a German couple, subtly—through single words, gestures, or looks—but continuously, let her know that they disapproved of what she was doing. "People come into your life and go again," Raya Antonovna, another surrogate, mentioned. "Today we might be friends but tomorrow we might not; so you never know what will happen to the information you give to others." Other than that, surrogates often stipulated that their lives were nobody else's business, and they did not want to risk being judged. Some, like Raya, also believed that telling others would bring them bad luck:

> I don't know what they (i.e., friends) might think about surrogacy, but I like them and I don't want to have a reason not to like them anymore. So I simply don't tell anyone. And anyway, I think that the fewer people that know, the higher the chance of success (i.e., getting pregnant).

At least this had been her experience in the last fifteen years: "If I talk too much about something, then it will definitely *not* happen," she said with a laugh. Similarly, intended mother Rita Tikhonovna was worried about "scaring her luck away" by sharing too much information, and also Vera Romanovna mentioned being afraid of the "evil eye" (see also Teman 2010, 116): "You never know how people will react. Maybe they won't say anything to my face but then they'll go around discussing my life with others. So in order to avoid this negative energy, it's better not to tell anyone."

"I'm Not Deceiving Anyone, Right?"

None of the Russian intended mothers I spoke with were entirely transparent about how their children had come into being. However, the degree of non/transparency varied—between the women themselves as well as within a temporal frame, at different stages of their lives. As mentioned, Galya Yanovna was initially open about her IVF procedure (though not about the surrogacy), while later being more careful about sharing information in public. The same held true for Olessia Valeryevna. Eleven years previously, when in the process of surrogacy, she had told most of her neighbors, colleagues, and friends; reactions were mostly positive or indifferent. But then the family moved to another area of Moscow and decided not to share this part of their biography. After the bad experiences with the pediatrician who wanted to charge an extra fee for examining her child, Olessia had also decided not to tell any other doctors: "When I am asked about the pregnancy, I calmly answer all questions. I don't give a detailed description of what happened; I just mention the facts. So I'm not hiding anything, I just don't mention that it wasn't me who was pregnant." Olessia stuck to the same strategy when talking to friends and family. It seemed important to her to distinguish between "hiding" and "not telling," and to stress that she was *not* hiding. She later partly relativized this statement, when saying: "I guess you could call this 'hiding' but, honestly, I didn't go to great lengths to do this. Nobody would ever think that maybe this was surrogacy or egg donation. It just doesn't occur to them. So it's a question of not telling anyone rather than 'hiding.'" Galya similarly emphasized the notion of "not telling," when she said with a mischievous smile: "I'm not deceiving anyone, right? I'm just not telling the whole story." Later on in our interview Olessia stated that sometimes things she said were not entirely true but that she would not call this lying, because at the moment of speaking she herself believed what she was saying:

> Well, you understand, I never lied. [. . .] Yes, there were moments [. . .] when I only realized afterwards what I had said. When I say: "After I had given birth to her . . ." (sighs), only later did I realize that it wasn't like that [. . .]. So I didn't lie in that moment, you understand? I had just forgotten (laughs).

For Olessia, "hiding" and "lying" clearly had negative connotations that she wanted to distance herself from. She implied that "hiding" and "lying" were much more active than "not telling." Furthermore, she saw "lying" as a deliberate act. By drawing these distinctions, Olessia could be seen as engaging in what Susan Gal (2002) calls an "indexical recalibration" of un/truthfulness. Indexicals are linguistic expressions that depending on context, can refer to different things or meanings, and that form part of an oppositional pair. This opposition can be "recalibrated," which means that the same opposition can be found again within the individual categories themselves, however, referring to a new set of contents. Regarding truth as an indexical means that rather than an absolute, it becomes a relative notion that can change its meaning and moral implications. In this sense, truthfulness might be seen as opposed to untruthfulness, but once you zoom in on and recalibrate the notion of untruthfulness, a new distinction could be made between truthfulness ("not telling") and untruthfulness ("lying" or "deceiving").

Dina was also "not telling" many people about her IVF with donor eggs. However, she emphasized that it was not common to discuss problems with others, particularly those related to "making children":

> There are many things we don't discuss with others. That doesn't make them secrets. They are just *not interesting* for others or they are too intimate. [. . .] It's not especially about whether or not you've had IVF. It's generally just *not common* to talk about *exactly how* we do this (i.e., how we get pregnant). [. . .] This is considered to belong to the personal sphere. [. . .] I also wouldn't want anyone to *dump* (*obrushit'*) these private problems on me.

Everybody had their difficulties, she concluded, which they should resolve for themselves. For Dina, bringing up infertility problems was not "sharing" but rather "imposing" intimate details on someone. These details were thus not necessarily secrets; rather, there was no point in talking about them because, according to Dina, they were of no interest to others. This assumption corresponded with intended mother Vera Romanovna's response, when I asked her whether she spoke with friends about her search for a surrogate. "Why should I? My friends can't give me any advice (*sovyet*). Exactly what should I talk to them about? This information has no value for them." The only people who knew about the surrogacy were her husband and one friend.

Involuntary childlessness was a lonely affair for most of the women I spoke with. Considering the important role of motherhood and the associated "tragedy" of infertility, many did not feel like they could or wanted to share their experiences with many people. Isupova's analysis of online conversations on the platform Probirka confirms that women feel uncomfortable sharing information about their infertility with friends and family, because often they had not received the kind of emotional support they would have expected and needed. Consequently, the majority kept their infertility a secret (Isupova 2011). However, most of the women I interviewed did not regard this secrecy as a burden. Vera, for instance, said she had no "urge" to tell anyone, and Olessia implied a comparable attitude when she said: "To be honest, I also don't talk about having a cold with everyone;

there are a lot of things I don't talk about with everyone." Similar to the Russian gay men and lesbian women interviewed by David Tuller (1996) and Laurie Essig (1999) in the early 1990s, the idea of "coming out" was not something Olessia, Dina, and others aspired to or even wanted—for both groups of "Others" disclosure of this kind was not regarded as necessary for a meaningful relationship with friends and the broader family (Rivkin-Fish and Hartblay 2014). It was a kind of disclosure inevitably linked to sexuality and, as such, belonged to the "personal" or "private" sphere (*lichnaya sfera*), as Dina pointed out. From the perspective of my research participants, the notion of the personal or private sphere emerged as something that needed and deserved protection. Their accounts are reminiscent of the meaning the private sphere had in Soviet times. Within a setting of tight state control and intervention, it was a space of retreat, safety, and freedom that was fiercely defended by the people (Funk 2004; Gal 2002; Ritter 2001; Rivkin-Fish 2005).[9] Similar to the LGBTQI+ persons interviewed by Irina Soboleva and Yaroslav Bakhmetjev (2015), the intended mothers wanted to become "invisible" to the state and their fellow citizens.

Within the limits of nondisclosure, online forums bridge the gap between the personal/private and the public. These offer anonymous spaces of exchange and solidarity (Brednikova, Nartova, and Tkach 2009) and play a crucial role in creating communities that would not otherwise exist (Isupova 2011; Speier 2016; Whittaker 2019).[10] Probirka is the most important discussion space among these online forums. It was founded in the early 2000s by a number of intended mothers who longed for the opportunity to share their experiences. One of the mothers I interviewed became a forum user in the year 2005 and gradually became an "activist," as she put it. Once a month she met up with other women. Later, she became a moderator on the site, then administrator and editor. Among other things, she initiated small competitions, in which women could win free IVF attempts. She continued working for Probirka until 2012, a few years after the forum was bought by one of Moscow's big surrogacy agencies. There were numerous conflicts with the new owner: while she saw her job as serving the needs of the users, the new director was a "businessman" mainly interested in profit. He would, for instance, ask her to remove the bad ratings of clinics that had paid for advertisements on the forum, while his own clinic always "received" very positive ratings. She did not regret having left Probirka, since the pregnancy was long enough ago that she felt the topic was now "closed" for her. She nevertheless remained in contact with many of the women she had got to know there, and they still meet once a year. Dina Antonovna also used to be a frequent forum user. Many of her current friendships were with people she had met on these platforms. In the early days, around fifteen to twenty years ago, only "the most well-off and most educated" people used IVF, Dina said—it was something for the "elite." People talked about life, about books, different interests, about everything. Now, these forums had become "for the masses," for the common people (*lyudi iz naroda*), partly due to the government's subsidization of IVF programs. Dina was clearly part of the "elite," and while I could not discern what she thought of the "massification" of IVF procedures, her words illustrated the community-building character of forums—possibly more in former times, when the community was smaller and less diverse than it is now.

Rita Tikhonovna was the only intended mother in my research who clearly suffered from not being able to discuss her infertility and treatments with friends and family. She had recently started sharing some information with her closest friends, telling them she was looking into the option of surrogacy but not that her surrogate was in the fourth month of pregnancy. "I'll only tell them when the child is born, when I'm holding it in my arms. Because you never know whether it will go well until the end," she said, alluding to the uncertainties inherent in assisted reproduction. Only her husband and parents knew about the pregnancy. The latter had struggled to accept that their daughter was having a child with the help of a surrogate: "They are from the postwar generation; they have a completely different mentality. In their day, there was hardly any technology, even just fixing teeth was difficult." In the end, however, they understood that "this was the only option." Olessia Valeryevna, on the other hand, had decided to circumvent this process with her husband's mother by simply avoiding seeing her for about a year. Luckily, the child looked a lot like its father, which made the mother-in-law happy enough not to bother her with unnecessary (*lishniye*) questions.

The Un/wanted Visibility of Pregnancy

The full force of the intended mothers' anxiety about other people's reactions becomes apparent when considering the lengths to which some go, such as simulating entire pregnancies. Intended mothers Galya Yanovna and Alisa Serafimovna had both worn strap-on bellies (*nakladniki*) during "their" pregnancies. The latter had done the "full simulation," as she said. "If you do that, you have to go the whole way." That is why she accompanied her surrogate to the doctor's appointments, to know exactly what was said and recommended. The time with the surrogate furthermore enabled Alisa to observe her movements: "I imitated her, I copied her, I looked at her and repeated all that she did." It helped that Alisa often had pregnant friends around her—there were many examples she could learn from. Her husband was also an attentive observer and gave her advice every now and then. "The simulation was necessary, for my own peace of mind, for my emotional well-being, and also for the people around me. Because they weren't ready to accept this." Alisa would not let others touch her strap-on belly, but even had they done so, nobody would have questioned its "realness": she had a high-end silicone product that even took on her body temperature. She was also lucky with the season—the peak of the pregnancy was in winter, so she could wear thick clothes on top of the belly.

Galya Yanovna had also simulated "her" surrogate pregnancy, from the third month onward. She had bought the strap-on belly at a theatre accessories shop in Moscow but told me that they could also be found in online shops. The belly she used consisted of two parts—a small belly and a larger belly—that could be worn alone or together, in order to create an even larger belly for the final months of pregnancy. "There is no way someone could tell the difference; it even has a belly button," she laughed. The *nakladniki* were not totally comfortable, so Galya decided to continue her work from home and leave the flat as little as possible. She had gained a considerable amount of weight anyway, due to the hormone treatment, and when she met with her friends in the early months of her surrogate's pregnancy, they were already commenting on her "round belly," even though she was not even wearing the strap-on. Like Alisa, Galya mentioned that wearing the belly comforted her psychologically—it helped her to "feel" the pregnancy. She even kept the surrogacy secret from her mother, who stayed at her house for two weeks during the time of the program—a detail she told me with a satisfied tone. She seemed proud of all the elements in this hiding game. Galya had kept her strap-on bellies just in case she wanted a second child. But when I asked to see them, she shied away: "They are hidden somewhere in the depths of the wardrobe," she said, suggesting that it would take too long to look for them.

Surrogates were also confronted with the challenge of concealment; however, they had the reverse problem of needing to hide their pregnant bellies. While most of the moralizing critique concerning surrogacy was directed toward the intended parents, the surrogate workers also came under fire in public debates. They were portrayed as greedy and needy women selling their babies and bodies. This is also an image perpetuated by the Russian Orthodox Church, which equates surrogacy with prostitution (Rivkin-Fish 2013). According to the priest Dimitri Anatolyevich and the former embryologist Tatyana Vasilyevna, surrogates are "abnormal" women, for any normal woman would develop a maternal bond with the child and could therefore not give it away. In light of these reproaches, most surrogates I spoke with did not want too many people to know about their pregnancies. Many of the women from smaller towns whose programs were located in the capital, like Oksana Yevgenyevna, thus welcomed the obligation to move to Moscow between the thirtieth and thirty-second weeks of pregnancy. When I met her in the clinic flats, she had just moved to Moscow for the final weeks of her pregnancy, as stipulated in her contract. She lived with other surrogates in one of the apartments the clinic provided. She did not like Moscow as a place to live but enjoyed the anonymity. Originally from the area around Mariupol, in Ukraine, Oksana had told her friends and family that she was in Moscow to earn money, where she had found a job as a babysitter, watching over a two-year-old child. Many Ukrainian women work abroad, even many of Oksana's friends, so her absence did not raise suspicion. Women often work as nannies or cleaners for two or three months and then travel back home. The day before our interview, Oksana had Skyped with her mother, careful not to reveal her belly in the Skype window of her telephone. Surrogate worker Lena Mironovna had also told her family and friends that she was in Moscow working as a nanny. She spent the entire pregnancy in the capital, having decided to leave her ten-year-old son with her parents in the Russian city of Nizhnij Novgorod; this was the easiest way to keep the surrogacy secret. She and her husband regularly sent him carefully staged pictures. On her camera, Lena showed me the photographs her husband had taken a week before, when it was her twenty-ninth birthday. One of the pictures showed her behind a big tree, with just her head peeking out. In another picture Lena held a giant bunch of flowers in front of her, covering her belly. Most surrogates, however, did not hide the surrogacy from their children, as they were usually quite young and would, so the women hoped, soon forget about the pregnancy.

Surrogates who spent the first five months of pregnancy in their hometowns had to think of more elaborate concealment measures. Olga Georgyevna told me that her husband was the only one who knew about the surrogacy. Her parents and brothers lived far away from her hometown, Belgorod in Russia, so it was not unusual that they hardly saw each other, and she managed to postpone meeting up until after the pregnancy. She hid from other people, rarely leaving the house: "When we are invited somewhere, my husband always just says, 'Olga got ill,'" she told me and laughed. And when they had guests, she retreated into one of the rooms and her husband said that she was not at home. Like intended mother Galya Yanovna, she seemed almost proud. Her own two children had not noticed the pregnancy, which surprised even herself, considering the size of her belly at the time. Other surrogate workers decided not to hide the pregnancy and postponed thinking about a good story to tell until after the birth of the children. Ukrainian surrogate Katya Yefimovna, for instance, decided to "play *Santa Barbara*" for her family. Alluding to the famous U.S.-American soap opera featuring scandals and intrigues, she said she did not hide the pregnancy but also did not say that the child was not hers. Eventually she disclosed the surrogacy to some relatives. When I asked how they had reacted, Katya simply said that they did not approve of her decision but that their opinion did not matter to her.

What struck me was a seeming contradiction between many of the surrogates' efforts to conceal the fact that they were surrogates and their strikingly indifferent attitude toward public opinion, when asked about it. They often reported that they neither knew nor cared what others thought, or simply commented that "everybody has their own opinion. Some are in favor; others are against it. We can't forbid anyone to have an opinion." I frequently heard such statements in the course of my fieldwork—for instance by surrogate worker Ksenia Demyanovna, a twenty-one-year-old single mother from Ulyanovsk. She had traveled the thirteen hours from her hometown to Moscow for a medical examination the day before and had asked me to accompany her to the Pokrovski Monastery, for fear of getting lost in the city's maze of streets. The monastery is visited by people—especially women—who want to start a family. Ksenia wanted to queue up in front of the famous icon of the Matrona of Moscow in order to place a written note there with her wish for a new boyfriend or husband—not for a successful surrogate pregnancy, as I had initially thought. Assuming that she must be a believer, I asked Ksenia what she made of the Orthodox Church's condemnation of surrogacy. She seemed to not know about their critical stance. "The church opposes surrogacy?" she asked, but then quickly added with a shrug that she actually did not care. She was not the only one to give me such an answer, and the reason for this can probably be found in the words of another surrogate: public opinion did not matter to her, she said, as "nobody else will give me this money." Implying that she needed the money so urgently that other people's opinions would not stop her from doing surrogacy, her words hinted at another possible cause for indifference: she could not afford to care much about public opinion. Consequently, this ostensible indifference seemed like a protective shield and therefore not so much a contradiction but rather a measure that complemented hiding the surrogate pregnancy.

"Suddenly, They'll Be Throwing Stones at Our Children"

In view of the largely negative public discourse on assisted reproduction, the intended mothers I spoke with all voiced concerns not only about what society might think of *them* but also how this might affect their children's future. Olessia Valeryevna, for instance, asked herself what might happen to her child if she openly spoke about the surrogacy—"I don't want to test it. That's why this information is private." She later mentioned: "What will it be like in ten years? I don't know. [...] Suddenly, they'll be throwing stones at our children or they won't be giving jobs to children born through surrogacy, you understand? This troubles me." Olessia's words—similar to those of surrogate worker Raya Antonovna cited above—reflect that her thoughts on transparency were closely linked to issues of trust in others and that she negotiated these in relation to an imagined future (Khodyakov 2007). She needed to simultaneously configure numerous "life plots," living with an "acute 'what if' sensibility," as Cheryl Mattingly (2019, 20) would say, or with the sense that "anything can happen"—a notion Anna Kruglova (2016) develops in her analysis of everyday morality in Russia. Faced with radical uncertainty concerning the future, Kruglova's research participants "tuned themselves" (*nastroit' sebya*) into a mode of vigilance, constantly on the lookout for sudden dangers coming their way.

From the perspective of the mothers I spoke with, there seemed to be too many dangers coming their way. To Olessia Valeryevna it didn't make sense to tell her daughter the truth and then ask her to remain silent about it: "What for? This would mean that I pass the problem onto the child. 'You know about this but, please, keep quiet.' It's better that I keep quiet about it myself . . . I just don't know how to talk about this in our society," she said, alluding to the fact that there were no acceptable social scripts for such "reproductive storytelling" (Nordqvist 2021). The way Olessia "talk[ed] about this" was—as mentioned above—through leaving out pieces of information or "constructing phrases." She did so not only with family, friends, and strangers, but also her daughter:

> I don't know what effects these constructed phrases might have later but I know that the risks of telling her now [about the surrogacy] are higher. When she asks, "Mama, was I in *your* belly?," I say, "Yes, you were in *the* belly" (my emphasis). I'm not deceiving her; I'm not lying. Of course I wouldn't make up a whole story, but I'm just stating the facts.

Olessia shrugged her shoulders and gave me a conspiratorial smile—"I'm a psychologist, Veronika, this is my daily bread. Constructing phrases is not difficult for me." Not all intended mothers were as clear about this issue as Olessia. Their children were still young—the eldest being nine years old at the time of our interview—so they would still have time to think about what to do. Galya Yanovna had originally planned to tell her son about the surrogacy but had become increasingly unsure about this. She would have to see how the political situation developed in Russia and whether the government's idea of banning surrogacy would be put into practice or not.

But anxiety about the political changes in society was not the only reason why intended parents were reluctant to reveal to their children how they had come into being. While they mostly mentioned no reservations regarding ARTs in the interviews, when it came to telling their children, a certain worry about the emotional damage this might cause came to the fore. Alisa Serafimovna, for instance, stated that "if I tell my children, I don't know what that would do to their psyches. If I put myself in their position, I certainly wouldn't want to know something like that."

Doctors confirmed that many intended parents feared their children would experience some kind of psychological trauma, and some, such as Anton Feodorovich, seemed to share this opinion:

> In America now people are obliged to tell their children when they turn 18 that they were born with the help of a donor. So you have to say "John, actually, your dad is not your dad. Your dad is donor IX-51-Q-15," and the child has the right to search for the donor. Honestly, I think that this is too much. I don't think this is the right approach. A child's psyche is very vulnerable; there is a high potential for suicide; it is really a very difficult issue. I, personally, I really don't see any need to say there was IVF or there was no IVF. It's not important. Maybe if they ask. But in the end, they are born the same way, just a little bit differently.

This quote illustrates that while doctors and parents were clearly in favor of assisted conception, some of them thought that such procedures were emotionally harmful to children, at least under conditions of transparency. However, a federal law on disclosure in the United States does not exist. While such laws have been implemented in many European countries—for example Austria, Germany, Sweden, and the UK—in the United States only a few states have followed this path, while in the majority of the country providing donor information remains subject to the goodwill of individual clinics and sperm banks (Hellman and Cohen 2017; Vaughn 2020). What Anton Feodorovich seems to be referring to is rather a specific Western ideal: while nondisclosure was for long deemed to be in the best interests of donor-conceived children, secrecy came to be seen as increasingly problematic and detrimental to the child from the 1980s onward (Nordqvist 2021, 680). Today, there appears to be a certain consensus in Europe, North America, and Australia that a child has the right to know its genetic origins (see also United Nations OHCHR 1989) and that disclosure is generally beneficial to the child (Tober 2018, 153–55). Petra Nordqvist (2014, 2021) has critically commented on the pressure and stress that the new moral imperative causes for parents, arguing that disclosure is not an individual matter but is tackled in a relational context, under careful consideration of how this might impact existing networks and connections. Research from the United States and the UK has shown that parents remain highly uncertain about how and when to disclose (Becker 2002; Nordqvist 2014, 2021), and a significant number of (heterosexual) parents decide against full disclosure in the case of gamete donation (Golombok et al. 2002; Murray and Golombok 2003; Readings et al. 2011). This is often different in surrogacy, because it is less easy to hide the lack of a gestational than a genetic link; most parents from the above-mentioned regions of the world therefore do disclose the surrogacies, be they altruistic or commercial (Deomampo 2016; Jacobson 2016; Jadva et al. 2012; Majumdar 2017; Rudrappa 2016a). The Russian context, however, is different, and the contemporary climate makes disclosure risky. Consequently, while many Western parents might feel a "moral obligation to talk" (Nordqvist and Smart 2014, cit. in Nordqvist 2021), the Russian mothers in my study felt an obligation *not* to talk, believing that their children had the right *not* to know.[11]

Gay Becker (2002) has argued that questions of disclosure are tightly entangled with the parents' wish to establish normalcy within their families. As Anton Feodorovich, quoted above, implied, not being "normal" could, consequently, be seen as a potentially disruptive and traumatizing element in children's lives. Also particularly telling in this regard was an interview with infertility psychologist Aleksandra Denisovna. When I asked her whether she recommended to parents that they tell their children about the IVF procedures, her friendly attitude suddenly changed to anger:

> Why should you tell a child that "we don't know where you're from"? "You came out of a test tube"? You would uproot this child; you would destroy his foundation. Why would you want to do that? The child will carry this pain with him all his life.

She gave me an accusatory look, as if the question per se was problematic. Then she continued:

> The most important thing is the health of the child. This is more important than positive advertising and propaganda. Why would you say to everyone: "My child was born through IVF; look how great he is!" Why? . . . Most parents spare their children this painful information.

Just as many intended parents did not consider it "necessary" to tell others about surrogacy, it was also often mentioned that it was "not necessary" to tell the children, because "they don't need this information." The question of whom to tell about surrogacy thus often revolved around the issue of what specific purpose this information could have. Concerning the children, parents saw no point in telling them, given they would then need to keep this information secret, as highlighted by Olessia Valeryevna. Aleksandra Denisovna did not deem it healthy, because it would "uproot" the child's identity. And Anton Feodorovich referred to the harmful effects of assisted conception but then quickly downplayed the procedure itself by stating that it was actually "not important" how a child came into being and, thus, "not necessary" to tell her or him. The issue of "propaganda," brought up by Aleksandra Denisovna, was also interesting. As mentioned above, it generally refers to particularly invasive and manipulative behavior. However, it also implies a politically charged move in the *public* sphere, while Aleksandra Denisovna obviously thought that surrogacy should remain in the *private*, supposedly apolitical, sphere. In this context, the term furthermore implies an element of egoism and boasting, of being politically rather than morally motivated (Rivkin-Fish 2004).

Either way, doctor Anton Feodorovich suggested that with time all questions and worries connected to infertility and its treatment tended to lose importance for those involved. This was also reflected in my interviews with the mothers, who stated that after the birth of their children the issue of surrogacy had quickly slipped to the back of their minds. The fact that so few people knew about their surrogacies facilitated the process of forgetting. Galya Yanovna recounted that just days after the delivery of her son, she had nearly forgotten that she had not been the one who gestated him—"You just forget (*zabyvayetsya*)," she said. The Russian expression *zabyvayetsya* implies that something just happens, beyond your control. She had also never again thought about her ten years of suffering during the various infertility treatments and stated that it felt like all that had happened in another lifetime. She assumed this to be some kind of automatic "psychological protection."

Forgetting about surrogacy can be seen as another—perhaps subconscious—strategy for dealing with its contested nature. This "forgetting" is enabled by processes that settle in much earlier, already during pregnancy. For some intended mothers, knowing the surrogate and being involved in the process allowed them to appropriate the pregnancy by feeling pregnant or experiencing the symptoms of pregnancy themselves. The interview with Galya Yanovna revealed that wearing a strap-on belly helped her to simulate a pregnancy not only for the benefit of the outside world but also for herself: "I was pregnant in my head. Yes. My child was not in my belly. But I was pregnant. And, hmmm . . . this is a really astonishing thing." In our second interview, she described this feeling in more detail:

> This is an amazing thing, but everyone experiences it: There is some kind of autosuggestion (*samovnusheniye*), yes, I can't describe it in any other way. You experience a slight nausea, in the mornings you feel sick. Then there are moments in which you start feeling somewhat uncomfortable, [. . .] you feel something in your womb.

The feeling of being "pregnant in the head" was so strong that she *felt* her own belly being pregnant beneath the strap-on, that she did not just walk like a pregnant woman but *felt* pregnant when walking. Simulating pregnancy also entailed going shopping for maternity clothes and always being conscientious about not lifting heavy bags when other people were around. Galya enjoyed this feeling—it made the whole surrogacy psychologically easier for her: "I can't say that I felt [emotionally] uncomfortable with these strap-ons, absolutely not. [. . .] Quite the opposite: psychologically, I looked at myself in the mirror and I saw myself pregnant," she said and laughed. "And psychologically, this made me feel better." Galya had also experienced "some kind of distant connection" with her child. She sensed when her surrogate was not feeling well. Once, nervousness suddenly overcame her, and when she called the surrogate, the latter said that she had just been to the doctor's because she was experiencing contractions in the uterus. According to doctors and agents, some intended mothers become so close to their surrogates during pregnancy that they come to share the same physical and emotional states. Even Olessia Valeryevna, who was not particularly close to her surrogate, told me how surprised she was when she experienced hyperemesis (nausea) when her surrogate did and that she knew before the delivery that her child would be born that very day.

Such experiences and practices of "feeling" the pregnancy are not uncommon in surrogacy arrangements, particularly when surrogates and intended mothers have a close relationship, which is often the case in North America or Israel (Ragoné 1996; Teman 2009, 2010; Toledano and Zeiler 2017). Elly Teman (2009, 2010) even shows how the Israeli women she interviewed engaged in what she calls a dyadic body-project, in which the pregnancy was detached from the surrogate body and shifted toward the intended mother. She sees such practices and sensations as couvade and, as such, as an "ongoing process of embodied claiming" (Teman 2010, 151). Couvade-like practices such as the "shifting body" are thus "a way for the intended mother to mark her territory, to claim the child, and to claim the route of production of the child as her own" (177). As the Russian case emphasizes, such claiming practices are not merely directed toward the outside but also toward the inside, in order to facilitate internalization and forgetting.

Processes of "forgetting" also seemed to be at work when the intended mothers were telling me their stories, in which the surrogates they worked with were hardly mentioned. When the intended mothers did speak of them, it was as "my surrogate," often without saying their name, without giving this woman a personality in the sense of describing who she was and what she was like. It was often only upon my questioning that they told me more about the women who had carried their children and the relationship between them. In a social setting that does not allow the surrogate to become part of the birth narrative of the children, it also became necessary to cut ties between intended mothers and surrogates. All of the Russian intended mothers were no longer in contact with the surrogates. "I am grateful, but I wanted to close this door on what has happened," Galya Yanovna said. Olessia Valeryevna also stated: "This is a closed topic. And this is also why it was better to end the relationship with the surrogate mother. Because ... how would I explain her to my child?" Thinking of surrogacy relations as temporary was also something encouraged by the commercial and medical actors, and largely embraced by the surrogates.

Secrecy as an Ethics of Care

In a biopolitical context in which women are primarily addressed as mothers, the inability to perform this role has painful consequences. This is especially so when women are blamed for their own infertility, for having had too many abortions or having led a sinful life.[12] The growing role of the Russian Orthodox Church in state affairs means that the church has great power in exerting "moral governance" (Mishtal 2015) by circulating such supposed truths and thus shaping public discourse, legislation, and, ultimately, the lives of intended mothers, surrogates, and the children born through such arrangements.

The intended mothers and surrogates I spoke with clearly distanced themselves from the ROC's position on issues of (assisted) reproduction, at times mocking the church's panacea of praying when confronted with unwanted childlessness. However, even though many of them were not strict Orthodox believers, they did believe in some kind of higher power and, as a result, the church's harsh critique might leave traces of uncertainty in their lives, as to whether they had acted immorally in choosing surrogacy. Intended mother Alisa Serafimovna, for instance, hinted at such uncertainty when she said that if surrogacy were a sin, then she would face the consequences "up there," pointing toward heaven; and surrogate Lena Mironovna also asked herself retrospectively whether she had committed a sin. But even those who were not spiritually or emotionally affected by the ROC's discourses had to carry the consequences of a form of "moral governance" (Mishtal 2015) that spread aggression and anxiety.

The contentious setting makes an open discussion about infertility and surrogacy almost impossible. Assisted conception is thus shrouded in secrecy and needs to be concealed by alternative truths. As I have shown in this chapter, the hostile attitudes call for "recalibrations" (Gal 2002) of un/truthfulness in relation to issues of disclosure. Taking seriously the fears and concerns of my research participants, I suggest viewing practices of imitating and appropriating the pregnancy, of "not telling the whole truth" and "omitting information" through the analytic lens of care ethics. According to Joan Tronto and Berenice Fischer, caring activities include "everything we do to maintain, contain, and repair our 'world' so that we can live in it as well as possible." This world encompasses "our bodies, our selves, and our environment, all of which we seek to interweave in a complex, life-sustaining web" (1990, 40). From this perspective one could say that truth is not necessarily a value and end in itself that must be articulated in all circumstances; rather, my research participants evaluated ethical questions of non/disclosure in relation to the potential effects this might have on their particular "worlds"—more specifically, on their and their children's mental and physical health and safety.[13] They took decisions about non/disclosure not as mere individuals but as persons embedded in a web of social relations and dependencies that they did not want to endanger (see also Nordqvist 2014, 2021).

Following an ethics of care, the women were "acting for self-and-other together," as Virginia Held writes, for "the well-being of a caring relation involves the cooperative well-being of those in the relation and the well-being of the relation itself" (2006, 23). The women's secrecy practices can thus be viewed as an ethical labor of care toward themselves and the children. The intended mothers perceived it as a moral responsibility toward their own children to spare them from burdensome information or from endangering them through sharing information with others. They needed to cultivate a state of "vigilance" (Kruglova 2016). This moral stance was supported by doctors and psychologists, who on the one hand downplayed the "necessity" of telling a child that it came into being through an IVF procedure, while simultaneously expressing great concern about the emotional damage this might do to the child, potentially "uprooting" the child and "destroying" its existential foundation.

But where did the intended mothers' "world" start and where did it end? Who was within and who outside their limits of caring? Taking the broader political perspective that Tronto (1994) calls for shows that an ethics of care is entangled in relations of power and inequality in many contradictory ways. On the one hand, the ethical labor of secrecy helped intended mothers to "repair" their "world" (Tronto and Fischer 1990, 40) shaken by infertility and to remain "invisible" (Soboleva and Bakhmetjev 2015) to potentially harmful others. On the other hand, these practices can be seen as a powerful mechanism to render invisible the subjectivity and the labor of the surrogate workers—the social and political climate produced the necessity to conduct the surrogacy program in a way that left no traces. The surrogates were a disruptive element that needed to be erased from the family biography (see also Rudrappa 2016a). The intended mothers "appropriated" the pregnancies and thereby performed the ideal of the traditional nuclear family. As time went by and memories faded, some mothers came to believe their own "narratives" and said they had forgotten that they ever participated in such a thing as surrogacy. The surrogates, therefore, formed only a temporary part of the intended mothers' "life-sustaining web" (Tronto and Fischer 1990, 40), and in many cases they did so merely as a means to an end.

Part II

3
CHOREOGRAPHING SURROGACY

Natasha Sergeyevna was a busy woman and on her feet the entire day. She was a bit stout, in her late forties, and her movements were slow but always somewhat hectic. Her whole body spoke of exhaustion from endless trips up and down the stairs, and back and forth along the clinic corridors. But during short breaks she never took a seat in the corridor—"I wouldn't have the energy to get up again," she once told me. Natasha Sergeyevna was one of the surrogate managers—or "curators" (*kuratori*) as they were sometimes called—of the Altra Vita IVF Clinic in Moscow. As such, she was responsible for coordinating the surrogacy arrangements at the clinic. Her constantly furrowed brows expressed that she was expecting trouble at any moment. She often complained about surrogacy candidates who made appointments but then never showed up, or those who did not answer their phones even though they were obliged to be available around the clock. "But this is just what they're like," she would say, shaking her head.

Through Natasha Sergeyevna, I was able to experience everyday life at the infertility clinic and follow not only her working days but also those of the many surrogates she introduced me to. In this chapter, I explore how the various actors carefully "choreographed" (Thompson 2005) their lives and the lives of others—primarily those of the surrogates—so a healthy child would be born at the end of a surrogate pregnancy. This choreography is all the more fragile because infertility treatments, in general, and surrogacy arrangements, in particular, are marked by manifold uncertainties. In light of this, Natasha Sergeyevna's comment on the surrogates' unreliability reveals only part of the picture, as it can also be read as a direct expression and result of these uncertainties. Understanding uncertainty as a condition in which future developments and outcomes cannot be calculated or anticipated (Knight 1921; North 2010; Strasser and Piart 2018), I am here particularly concerned with the impossibility of predicting the near future in the context of surrogacy. Many months and failed attempts can pass between the different steps involved—deciding to become a surrogate, entering into a specific agreement, becoming pregnant, keeping the pregnancy, and giving birth to a healthy child—which has a profound effect on the organization of surrogacy and the lives of those involved.

Largely based on ethnographic fieldwork at the Altra Vita IVF Clinic, this chapter focuses on how surrogates enter the reproductive market as "pragmatic realists" (Utrata 2015) and how they negotiate its many uncertainties for themselves as well as with clinic/agency staff and intended parents. Following the surrogates and their attempts to get pregnant, I show how—in a context where pregnancy outcomes are referred to by some as more a matter of "miracles" than "medicine"—surrogates are instructed to take care of their bodies as if they were frail "crystal vases," as Natasha Sergeyevna once said, which demanded maximum care and control. The intrinsic uncertainties morally justify a system of control through payment schemes and accommodation rules that ensure the surrogates' compliance. Overall, the chapter illustrates everyday life in the reproductive market, where women come together with the hope of escaping either the financial pressures of their lives or the pressures of (as yet unachieved) motherhood. Both groups of women need to constantly manage their expectations, flexibly adapting to changing circumstances, and often play numerous games at the same time.

Following Surrogate Pregnancies

Of the thirty-nine surrogates I spoke with in the course of my research, about two-thirds worked for the Altra Vita IVF Clinic in Moscow. Many had chosen this clinic because of its good online reviews and because of the high salary it offered to surrogates. Some had also had positive experiences with selling their eggs at Altra Vita and thereafter decided to enter a surrogacy program. The clinic was situated in the southwest of Moscow, just outside the inner *koltso* (belt), one of the big streets surrounding the center. It was hidden behind a black metal gate that opened onto a small courtyard dotted with patches of green, a few trees and benches, and a snack machine that visitors passed before taking a pair of blue hygiene shoe covers and entering the building. The ground floor of the clinic comprised examination rooms as well as the so-called "men's rooms" (where men left their sperm samples) and the "clean area" (*chistaya zona*). The latter included operating theaters (where procedures such as hysteroscopy and embryo transfers were conducted), rooms where patients could recover from medical procedures, and the clinic's laboratory and cryobank (where frozen sperm and egg cells as well as embryos were stored). There was also a separate room for VIP patients, containing two beds with gold-colored linen, an illuminated slab of agate stone, and a wardrobe, adorned with agate and crystal handles.

The door from the reception area opened onto a clean, quiet corridor. Altra Vita had no separate waiting rooms, so patients waited on the blue plastic benches that lined the hallway. Most stared into space or occupied themselves with their phones, only occasionally looking up when someone walked by. The patients were mainly women, some visibly pregnant, others—so I assumed—hoping to get pregnant on these very premises. The many paintings that decorated the clinic's walls were probably meant to nurture these hopes. While many other clinics had pictures of laughing infants and happy parents, Altra Vita dedicated its walls to the slightly irritating artworks of a Russian painter: a naked woman swimming amid thousands of tiny sperm; a flying stork with a bundle in its beak, again against the background of sperm; a small baby lying on top of a cabbage—alluding to the Russian popular belief that babies can be found in cabbages. The feeling these pictures and the entire atmosphere conveyed to me was not one of hopefulness. The silence, the stares, the whispering, the anonymity seemed to tell a different story. And yet, every now and again, I would see a woman with a bunch of flowers, a small present, and an almost imperceptible smile on her face, as if not to offend all those still waiting and hoping—two central experiences that accompany infertility treatments (Bärnreuther 2019). These women, however, stayed beyond my reach, as I was not allowed to speak with them. Just like in other clinics and agencies, Altra Vita's director protected his paying clients from "nosy" researchers like me.

The first floor of the clinic mainly housed a big room for staff meetings and other events, of which the most memorable during my research was the celebration of International Women's Day on March 8—a widely celebrated national holiday. The long conference table was loaded with rich platters of cheese, cold sausage, and pickles as well as bottles of wine and cognac, while YouTube videos of songs by Queen and ABBA were projected onto the empty walls. There was also a huge bunch of red and pink tulips, and every woman, including me, received a small bouquet of flowers. This joyous event was a bizarre contrast to the silence and seriousness that characterized everyday life at the clinic on all other days.

Next to the meeting room were the administrative offices, such as that of the surrogate manager Natasha Sergeyevna. She was the first point of contact for women interested in becoming surrogates. In a short telephone conversation, she would set out the basic requirements and conditions, and if both sides were interested, the specific woman then came to the clinic as a *pyervichka*. This term derives from the Russian adjective *pyervichnyj*, meaning "initial," "basic," or "primary," and was used by the surrogate manager for candidates at their first visit. All candidates then underwent a second interview and their first vaginal ultrasound. The questions covered many biographical aspects and were oriented toward obtaining information on their own and family illnesses, operations, and accidents; number of children (including date of birth and weight at birth); number of abortions and miscarriages; commencement and regularity of menstruation; as well as questions concerning education, job, marital status, and much more. Women's height and body mass index were also taken into account, because they should not be "too small and not too big," as one doctor said. Surrogacy candidates should also not have had any abortions or C-sections or "harmful habits" (*vrednye privychki*) such as drinking, smoking, or taking drugs, and preferably no tattoos or piercings. If women passed these initial examinations, they went through a more detailed ultrasound and gave a blood sample, to check for diseases such as HIV, hepatitis B and C, among others. Moreover, they had to undergo a psychological screening, in which it was determined whether the surrogacy candidates were reliable and compliant, and whether they had the "right understanding" of surrogacy. Ideally, the candidate should pass all these examinations and then sign the contract with the clinic. In mediated arrangements, which most at Altra Vita were, contracts were usually made between the clinic and the surrogate on the one hand and between the clinic and the intended parents on the other. Contracts were standardized, and surrogates had limited say concerning the conditions of their work. They could, however, determine whether they wanted one or two embryos to be transferred, whether they would want to live in Moscow during the pregnancy, and whether they would be willing to quit work during this time. At Altra Vita, the monthly pay surrogates received was intended to be mainly spent on food products, which was why intended parents who did not want their surrogates to engage in wage labor were required to provide additional compensation for this loss of income.

Immediately after the signing of the contract, the surrogate received a hormonal injection that marked the beginning of the hormonal stimulation known as the "preparation." If the embryo transfer was to be conducted with fresh eggs, the menstrual cycles of the intended mother (or egg provider) and surrogate had to be "synchronized." The intended mother (or egg provider) was hormonally stimulated, so her ovaries would release several eggs at once rather than just one. The extracted eggs were fertilized in vitro with the husband's sperm, and the resulting embryos left to develop for around five days.[1] By then, some would have died; the most visually "even" were chosen from the remainder, and the rest frozen. From the former, one or several embryos were transferred into the womb of the surrogate, whose uterine mucous membrane had usually been hormonally stimulated for two to four weeks in advance. At Altra Vita, in almost all cases only one embryo was transferred. In other clinics, usually two and sometimes even three were transferred, of which, if all three lodged and survived, one would usually be "reduced" within the first twelve weeks of pregnancy—in many cases a contractually defined precondition for becoming a surrogate.

Natasha Sergeyevna would introduce me to the surrogates who came to the clinic, and if they agreed, I was able to interview the women and accompany them to their medical examinations. Almost all surrogates gave their consent, but I felt like the surrogate manager's way of asking left little room for declining her request. Furthermore, initially she sat in on the interviews, as the director had instructed her to prevent unsupervised conversations between the surrogates and me. In this sense, the surrogates were also protected by the clinic but in fundamentally different ways from the intended parents. It seemed like the clinic protected intended parents because of their vulnerability, while they protected surrogates because they might leak compromising information. Being under supervision meant that my early interviews were brief and technical, as neither I nor the surrogate workers felt at ease. Some seemed to express their resistance by providing me with only one-word answers. It did not help that these interviews took place in consultation rooms, where Natasha Sergeyevna sat me in the position usually occupied by the doctor, which seemed to suggest that my questioning was part of the official selection process. After these interviews, she would usher us out and seat the surrogate and me at opposite ends of the waiting corridor, so that we would not chat in her absence.

Luckily, her firm grip soon loosened, and I had more time and space to tell surrogates about my research project and seek their consent in more sensitive ways. Almost all were willing to tell me about their lives and experiences. We often had several hours to talk before and between their appointments, even if we sometimes had to do so in low voices, so that other patients could not overhear our conversations. The long and uncertain waiting hours illustrated the "politics of waiting" (Hage 2009a; Rehsmann 2018; Ticktin 2013) in such spaces as clinics, where doctors' time is usually more valuable than that of patients, and particularly—so it seemed to me—that of surrogates. In light of the long waits, most surrogates enjoyed having someone to entertain them, and they often asked me as many questions as I asked them. Some were personal, but most concerned the surrogacy process itself, as they were reluctant to articulate their concerns about the medical and emotional uncertainties the program entailed to the surrogate managers or other staff members. They were keen to find out how things worked at the clinic, had questions about other surrogates' experiences, how long it would take to get pregnant, who the intended parents might be, and what I knew about options and payments in other clinics and agencies.

My mornings usually started on the sofa on the first floor, where I waited for Natasha Sergeyevna and tried to anticipate what might happen during the day ahead. The sofa was right next to her office, which guaranteed that she would come by sooner or later. This place was my retreat: it was where I returned to numerous times during the day, having lost her or when waiting between appointments. There were several hours of waiting every day, and at times I felt like I had sunk into the cushions so deeply that I also would not be able to get up again. On good days, Natasha Sergeyevna approached me on the sofa, informing me of the day's appointments. Then she seemed to enjoy her involvement in my research and often commented on the different surrogates we spoke with in the course of the day. "Today, we're not lucky with the surrogates: they're not very talkative," she once whispered to me with a smile after a stilted interview with one of the *pyervichki*. At other times, though, Natasha Sergeyevna merely bestowed a terse "good morning" on me as she walked past, seemingly oblivious to the fact that I was waiting for her. On these days she would deny me access to the same appointments she had allowed me to attend the day before.

The months at the clinic remained highly challenging but provided me with invaluable insights into the uncertainties surrogates experienced before and in the course of their pregnancies as well as into why and how they entered the reproductive market.

Making a Living by Making Life

Zhenya Pavlovna was wearing white underpants and a thin strappy top. She was sitting at the kitchen table with one leg crossed over the other, looking me deep in the eyes. "You probably want to know why we do surrogacy?" she asked, and without waiting for an answer she continued: "Nowhere else in Russia can you earn one million rubles [at once]. . . . For us, the material aspect is essential. There is no such thing as everybody being kind in this world and me going for this for noble reasons. Nobody does this for noble reasons." Sonya Vitalyevna, who had come to join us in the kitchen of one of the surrogates' flats at the Altra Vita IVF Clinic, shared this opinion: "If I need money, I'm willing to give my kidney. Or part of my lungs. You just start thinking about these things." She put a bowl of dates on the table and invited me to take some. The dark rings under her eyes made Sonya look tired; her day visit to the clinic in Moscow involved an early start and a twelve-hour round trip by train from her hometown of Lipetsk. She was now "in preparation" (*v podgotovke*) for the embryo transfer. Zhenya had already had her embryo transfer a few days earlier and was staying in the capital until she could take the pregnancy test in about two weeks' time. These were the clinic's conditions, because having the surrogates on site made it easier to control the process. But Zhenya did not mind—she enjoyed the time away from home and from her everyday household obligations in Smolensk, a city roughly four hours west from Moscow. She was also happy that the clinic handled all communication with the intended parents—"What do I need this personal contact for? I do my job and get money for it; that's all I need to know," she told me, shrugging her shoulders.

The conversation with the two women was one of my first with surrogates in Moscow. At this early stage of my fieldwork I was taken aback by their directness. Considering the delicacy of the topic and having read up on how surrogates frame their involvement, motives, and expectations in other parts of the world, I had not anticipated such a plainspoken statement as Zhenya's. Surrogates in the United States, for instance, refuse to see surrogacy as work, emphasize altruistic motivations and their enjoyment of pregnancy, and feel uneasy talking about financial issues (Berend 2016; Jacobson 2016; Ragoné 1994; Ziff 2017); Indian women clearly articulate economic motives when becoming surrogates but understand themselves not as workers but as caring and sacrificing mothers, who experience surrogacy as a meaningful endeavor (Pande 2014; Rudrappa 2016a; Vora 2009); and Thai surrogates stressed that the surrogate pregnancies brought them not just a welcome income but also Buddhist merit (Hibino and Shimazono 2013; Whittaker 2019). In all these cases, the economic aspects of surrogacy were presented either as not being central or as something that was decisive but did not turn the women into self-interested workers—echoing the widespread expectation that women who provide reproductive services or substances are at least partially motivated by altruistic reasons (Almeling 2007).

The surrogates I met in Russia, however, were very explicit about their financial motives, and self-interest was not deemed a morally problematic notion. Almost all regarded surrogacy as work and spoke of "working" (*rabotat'*) or "collaborating" (*sotrudnichat'*) with a certain clinic, agency, or intended parents. Zhenya Pavlovna was thus not alone in taking such an approach toward the surrogacy. Also Lena Mironovna confirmed: "All surrogates do it for money. Even if somebody tells you they do it for charitable reasons, that's just blah-blah. This is Russia! 99.9 percent do it for the money." This was the "mentality" here, she said, quickly adding that things might be different if Russia's economic situation were more stable or if the government provided more financial assistance and housing, especially for single mothers. Maybe then women would not go to such lengths as to "sacrifice" their health for money:

> I would never sacrifice my health if there was no financial necessity. But we need a flat and I know there is no other way of earning this amount of money. I'm just being realistic. I'm not one of these people with their heads in the clouds; I look at life objectively and I know I have to choose between the options given to me.

Lena and her husband, Aleksej, wanted to buy a flat in order to achieve some financial stability. Considering the tremendous economic and political turmoil Russia had witnessed in the previous thirty years, renting a flat was a risky endeavor because prices could suddenly rocket and the currency could be devalued. The couple had moved to Moscow to find work for one year, because salaries there were higher than in their hometown, Nizhnij Novgorod, a city located on the banks of the Volga River, about four and a half hours from Moscow. Their ten-year-old son was staying with Lena's parents in the meantime, thus making visible the care chains (Deomampo 2016; Hochschild 2000) that often result from such migratory care work. Looking out for job opportunities, she had read about the possibility of becoming an egg provider and earning ₽50,000 (roughly US$1,000) in Moscow.[2] At the clinic, she was turned down for medical reasons, but she accepted the alternative offer to become a surrogate. Several of the women I met had been egg providers before becoming surrogates, opting for the "fast" money of selling eggs first and only entering the surrogacy program once their financial situation had somewhat improved. Like Lena, many others wanted to invest their prospective salary in buying a flat or building a house. However, while taking part in one surrogacy program used to be enough to achieve such an aim, this was no longer the case—especially not during and after the economic crisis that hit Russia in 2014, while I was doing fieldwork. Several women were frustrated about the steep fall of the ruble during their pregnancies—the revenue from the process would be worth much less than at the point of signing the contract.[3] For many, having a flat or house of one's own was considered very "basic" and essential, from not only the financial but also the emotional point of view. Katya Yefimovna, for instance, a Ukrainian surrogate, stressed that "having your own little corner" was one of the most important aims in life. For Zhenya Pavlovna, on the other hand, surrogacy was more about having extra money on the side (*lishnij den'gi*). She already had a home and earned enough to cover daily costs. But while she had envisaged achieving a certain level of material well-being before turning thirty, this had not yet materialized; so Zhenya, now twenty-nine years old, decided on surrogacy. Material possessions were important to her. When choosing a job she had always prioritized higher earnings over whether she liked the work. "I don't know, I can step beyond myself. Even emotionally. The important thing is to prepare yourself emotionally." Hinting at the notion of "being prepared," Zhenya stated that she would do anything to improve her financial situation.

For other surrogates, surrogacy was more a matter of financial survival. Lyuba Dmitriyevna, for instance, could barely make ends meet. A twenty-five-year-old single mother to a child with a severe disability, most of her money went to medication and checkups for her son. They lived in a small town close to Minsk, Belarus, in "primitive conditions," as she put it, but she wished to make her home cozy with the salary she would receive for the surrogacy. She wanted to install water and gas in her house and buy a few nice pieces of furniture. Sonya Vitalyevna also struggled financially in everyday life. Working in a canteen (*stolovaya*), she earned only ₽8,000 (roughly US$170) a month, and her husband's salary as an electrician was not much higher. They had to take care of two children and her elderly mother-in-law. The five of them shared a one-room apartment that cost them over half of their monthly income. No, there was no "plan B," she replied with a laugh upon my asking about this—surrogacy was the only possible way to earn such a large amount.

For Sonya, the amount of money she received for the surrogacy (₽1 million as salary and ₽20,000 as monthly allowance) was around thirteen times her yearly salary. Most of the surrogates, however, were in a more financially stable situation: Carine Lvovna, for instance, from the Russian city of Kostroma, close to Moscow, stated that she made ₽20,000 per month working in a factory, meaning that the surrogacy payment was only five times her annual income; and Mariya Yegorovna, who worked in a flower shop in Moscow, could earn two and a half times her yearly income through the surrogate pregnancy. The meaning this money had in quantitative terms thus varied greatly, not least depending on the living costs in the different parts of Russia and Ukraine.

The importance of the financial incentive that drew women to surrogacy was one of the reasons why almost all perceived their involvement as "work." Katya Yefimovna was one of the few who objected to this term. Being a surrogate required no qualifications and, anyway, women were "predestined to give birth," she said. Another surrogate stated that pregnancy was enjoyable and that she associated "work" with unpleasant activity. Both of these women also described surrogacy as "salvation," because they were at a point of crisis when they entered the program. Katya, for instance, had decided to become a surrogate a while before but wanted an arrangement that would allow her to remain at home. However, being Russian by ethnicity (*natsional'nost'*), when the armed conflict between Russia and Ukraine started to affect her hometown, Donetsk, in summer 2014, she decided to leave the city. She took the northbound train with her five-year-old daughter—a painful departure, for she had to leave behind a newly purchased apartment, a well-paying job, some of her family, many of her belongings, and the feeling of having a place she could call home. The way she spoke about her old home and her new life in Moscow revealed that she felt relegated to the position of a refugee without means. "This is all very difficult," she said, but she nevertheless considered surrogacy to be a good option in her situation, for the clinic provided her with a place to live and with an income.

A woman's decision to become a surrogate in countries such as Russia, Ukraine, or Belarus has to be seen in the context of the postsocialist "backlash" concerning gender equality (Turbine and Riach 2012). The capitalist "shock-therapy" of the 1990s resulted in lasting disillusionment for many—during this time, income inequality doubled and 40 percent of the population became impoverished (Remington 2011). These effects hit women harder than men. They were pushed to the margins of the labor market and back into the private sphere, receiving little financial state support (Funk 2004). Single mothers—which around a quarter of the surrogates in my research were—in particular needed to work hard to get by and find adequate childcare. Even though the fathers of their children were legally required to pay alimony, they rarely did so or, if they did, the sum was hardly a significant contribution—the laws were seldom enforced and to avoid taxes many men did not officially register all their income anyway (Utrata 2015, 63). Moreover, while the Russian and Ukrainian governments employed various methods of rehabilitating "the mother," there were no serious efforts to counter discrimination against women in the labor market (Turbine and Riach 2012; Utrata 2015; Zhurzhenko 2012).

Despite these conditions, research on Russian women's lives reflects their pragmatic, self-reliant, and tenacious take on economic hardship. Women tend to downplay gendered discrimination and stress individual responsibility for shaping their lives (Ashwin 2002; Kay 2002; Turbine and Riach 2012; Utrata 2015). Jennifer Utrata's ethnography on single motherhood in Russia is particularly insightful for understanding the social position of women who become surrogates and their attitudes toward life. Observing and wondering about why single mothers seldom complained about their material difficulties, Utrata argues that many were so accustomed to these difficulties that they had become "part of the routinized crisis that characterizes Russia" (2015, 85). What is more, alongside the remnants of the Soviet ideal of the "superwoman," who easily mastered waged labor and household duties, a new "form of gendered neoliberal ideology" has emerged in the post-Soviet era, in which individuals are held responsible for their own fate and, thus, also their own failures in making ends meet (96). These aspects have given rise to an outlook on life marked by what Utrata calls "practical realism" (chap. 3): many of the single mothers in her study recognized the limited options they had in life, were bleak about receiving support from men or the state, and stressed "taking what they can get." An important asset of practical realism is flexibility and adaptability, making it possible for women to quickly respond to changing life situations, for instance by pursuing several strategies at the same time (114–18). Being a practical realist also entails avoiding complaints and taking pride in successfully handling material hardship. These findings overlap with those of Vikki Turbine and Kathleen Riach (2012, 180), who found that the women they interviewed framed their struggles in work and life as individual rather than structural. They did not, however, want to appear as "helpless victims," reflecting the broader Russian cultural norm of women as "innately patient and with an ability to cope with prolonged difficulties" (180). Thus, while employment remains central to women's identity in Russia, women define themselves rather through the ability to survive and care for their families than through a particular job (Ashwin 2002; Utrata 2015). They are, therefore, more likely than men to take on jobs with low status and low salaries (see also Patico 2009) and express a "gloomy 'realism' in relation to opportunities, against the background of a fatalistic acceptance of the status quo" (Ashwin 2002, 29). The notion of "practical realism" can thus be seen as central to many women's lives, not just when they are single mothers. Moreover, Utrata (2015) points to the difficulties of establishing clear boundaries to what being a single mother really means, because men are often absent from family life. This was particularly evident in Katya Yefimovna's case: She was married to the father of her daughter, but they were in an on-off relationship that seemed to me mainly dependent on his mood and his need for money. On the rare occasions when she mentioned him, she emphasized that he was good for nothing, and the way she spoke about her life made clear that her everyday struggles were those of a single mother. Also some other married surrogates indicated that it was mostly them who had to support the family financially.

In general the above-mentioned research mapped well onto my own conversations and interviews with surrogates, who were well aware of their limited options. They had accepted that their lives had not "turned out" the way they had imagined when they were children, as Sonya Vitalyevna stated, and they had decided to "look at life objectively," as Lena Mironovna said. However, while such terms as "gloomy 'realism'" and "fatalistic acceptance of the status quo" (Ashwin 2002) seemed fitting in many of the situations I encountered, the negativity of these expressions might also conceal the fact that these were women who were actively trying to change their lives and to escape the feeling of "stuckedness" (Hage 2009b). As "practical realists" (Utrata 2015), they weighed their options and made pragmatic decisions, flexibly adapting to the ever-changing circumstances of their lives. Similar to the women who became surrogates in South and Southeast Asia, surrogacy was not the kind of job they would do without financial necessity, but it represented a feasible alternative to other strenuous or demanding employment options (Rudrappa 2016a; Vora 2013; Whittaker 2019).

By entering the surrogacy market, women create value from their reproductive capacity and property (Cooper and Waldby 2014, 83–87) and engage in a kind of self-commodification that has become somewhat accepted in parts of the post-Soviet space. This development is closely linked to the shift from a socialist to a market economy. The latter was accompanied by a tremendous increase in inequality and the sudden abundance of expensive goods, which led to the rise and legitimation of materialist values and self-interest (Swader 2013), and, in turn, a "more individualized, rationalized, consumption-oriented culture," also in relation to intimacy and the body (Swader and Obelene 2015, 252). Christopher Swader and Irina Vorobeva (2015, 324), for instance, have shown how practices of compensated dating in Russia, Ukraine, and Belarus—as opposed to other regions in which the topic has been researched, such as Latin America—are marked by de-romantization and plain economic language, while both parties display agency and creativity in the way they negotiate and practice their relationships. Women, for example, frame themselves as "investment projects" and men as "start-ups," while men speak of "collecting" girls like they were collecting cars (Swader et al. 2013). In the field of partner and marriage choices, Anna Temkina and Elena Zdravomyslova (2015) make similar observations, arguing that a new "instrumental script" has emerged in post-Soviet Russia, in which sexual life is framed as an economic and calculated exchange. While such an attitude did exist in Soviet times, it was not accepted, while now it has become "widespread and legitimate" (309). The moral economy of surrogacy is thus informed by a broader moral economy, in which the intersections of the economic and the intimate are not necessarily problematized and in which an instrumental approach to social relations is not uncommon.

Entering the Reproductive Market

Most of the women had been aware that such a thing as surrogacy existed before considering working in this sphere themselves. The topic was public enough that anyone could come across an article, TV show, or radio program about it. Some women had also been confronted with the issue when asked by acquaintances whether they would be willing to carry a child for them. Raya Antonovna, for instance, a thirty-year-old woman from Saratov Oblast in southwestern Russia, had been approached by an "elderly" woman at her husband's workplace a few years previously but declined, because at the time the couple did not need the money and they also feared the awkward situation such an arrangement might create.[4]

The concrete idea of becoming a surrogate was often sparked by specific advertisements found in women's or job magazines, or on social media platforms such as Vkontakte or Odnoklassniki (which are similar to Facebook). As previously indicated, adverts could also be posted on online platforms such as Meddesk, Probirka, or Ostrov Kenguru. These were distributed either by intended parents and surrogates themselves, by a clinic or agency, or by one of the many private agents. They reflected the two types of possible arrangements: mediated or direct. The first were arrangements made through agencies. They were often standardized in form, which allowed for a fairly quick matching process and for outsourcing the control of the surrogate to an agency, which monitored the pregnancy, regularly updated the intended parents, and took care of or assisted in the bureaucratic and legal paperwork. While some mediated arrangements were completely anonymous, otherwise contact between the two parties was usually restricted. Direct arrangements, in contrast, allowed for intended parents and surrogates to have closer contact as well as more say in terms of conditions, payments, and forms of contact. One of the surrogates I spoke with compared the search for such arrangements with a physical marketplace:

> You see tomatoes that you like, you go there, ask whether they can cut them open for you, so you can see what they look like inside, whether you want these tomatoes. With surrogacy, it's the same. I offer my services and they (i.e., the intended parents) come and ask about my health, my [medical] analyses. They like it or they don't like it. That's it. They take it or they don't take it.

Navigating such a marketplace required more time, patience, and nerve than when agencies took on the "matching" process. It was emotionally strenuous, as both parties were confronted with a vast array of uncertainties, and often felt alone and exposed. On the online platforms, these feelings gave rise to heated discussions between intended mothers and surrogacy candidates about fair payments and the limits of exploitation. Much research has captured the profound ambivalence of those who struggle to make ends meet under capitalism in Russia. Jennifer Patico, for instance, shows how Russian schoolteachers, celebrated in Soviet times but who encountered material and status loss in the 1990s and early 2000s, became "both eager consumers and vociferous critics of [or sellers in] the Russian market economy" (2005, 482). Likewise, the participants of compensated dating studied by Swader and Vorobeva (2015, 324) regularly claimed to be "exploited" by the other party, while actively engaging in and profiting from such processes of self-/commodification. This sense of ambivalence was also present among those who participated in surrogacy arrangements. Such arrangements were facilitated through marketization and, yet, it was this marketization that many criticized. This was evident in the response I received to an interview request from an intended mother whose anonymous announcement about searching for an egg donor I had read online:

> All of my information is about me—this is my private life and I don't plan to tell anyone about it just like that. How much can you pay for this information? No donor programs are free of charge, and surrogate mothers demand a horrendous salary. Why should we, bio-parents (*bioroditeli*), provide information for free? Nobody does anything for free for us.

The woman's answer clearly underlined her sense of vulnerability in the face of the financial burden infertility treatments brought with them—vulnerability that made her feel at the mercy of the market and of surrogates who demanded a "horrendous salary." She was not willing to give out information for free, while everyone else squeezed profit from her.

Surrogate Raya Antonovna was verbally attacked by intended mothers for this same reason. After she published an announcement offering her services, several intended mothers complained that requesting ₽800,000 (roughly US$17,000) as a salary was too much and accused her of only being interested in the money—a common reproach made toward surrogates, as documented by Natalia Khvorostyanov and Daphna Yeshua-Katz (2020) in their analysis of the Russian online forums. "Well excuse me, I'm not doing this for free," Raya would typically respond to such an accusation—"I will not risk my health for nothing." She said that some intended mothers questioned the legitimacy of this sum, because she had "no experience." It made her very upset that surrogates were often divided into "the experienced" and "the idiots." "What is there to experience? Carrying a child? I have had this experience twice!" Raya stated, adding that her two children were fairly big, that she had "quite some hips" and could therefore give birth without any problems. But among the fifteen to twenty such responses she received within a day, there were also many that were entirely neutral or that comprised "entire memoires that take you half an hour to read and make you cry."

Most of the adverts intended parents—or rather intended mothers—posted online were, however, fairly uniform and concise. This was the case for Vera Romanovna's advert. When I met her for coffee in a Moscow shopping mall, she had only recently started her search for a suitable surrogate, at the age of forty-four. Two weeks before our interview, Vera had put her first announcement online:

> We're looking for a responsible surrogate mother (*surr-mamochka*) for a fresh protocol (i.e., an IVF procedure with fresh rather than frozen gametes) at the end of January.
> No experience necessary!
> If you have the analyses, we are willing to introduce you immediately to our doctor. This needs to be done in December 2014!!
> Blood +, and the usual requests.[5]
> In the first e-mail include all information and your demanded salary.
> We will give preference to those who are willing to move here for the entire period (separate one-room rented apartment).
> We are willing to pay the average market price.
> Strictly without intermediaries!!!!!
> Family couple from Moscow.

As Vera's post illustrates, such adverts were often written in a staccato tone, focusing on medical and organizational aspects. Such expressions as "the usual requests" point to the fact that some degree of knowledge was required to fully understand the adverts. These requests usually meant that surrogacy candidates should be between twenty and thirty-five years old, have a child of their own, and not have any "harmful habits" (*vrednye privychki*). Vera's use of "analyses" referred to the preliminary medical tests that determined a specific woman's suitability for an IVF procedure. Intended parents often requested such analyses in advance, in order to save time. From the perspective of the surrogates-to-be this was a disadvantage in monetary terms, as they had to pay for these out of their own pocket and were only (partly) refunded if they entered an arrangement with a specific couple.

Following her post, Vera was flooded with offers from prospective surrogates. At the time of our interview, she had already written at least six hundred responses and had dedicated the preceding weeks entirely to this issue. She was supported by a friend who had gone through surrogacy herself and who gave her advice on how to handle the numerous candidates. From this friend—Vera called her "my instructor"—she had learned how to write announcements, how to talk to surrogates, and what to focus on in negotiations. They spoke once or twice a day. According to this "instructor," she should always have two to three candidates in hand, because one never knew whether they would be suitable in medical terms or whether they might change their mind at the last minute. Similarly to surrogate manager Natasha Sergeyevna, Vera Romanovna also complained about how unreliable the women were. Often, she would have already had frequent exchanges with someone when she would suddenly stop hearing from them. This seemed to be a common issue. With both sides needing to enter into negotiations with various people at the same time, it was not surprising that surrogates complained about exactly the same problem. Sveta Valentinovna, for instance, a twenty-seven-year-old married woman from Volgodonsk, said that she had clearly mentioned that she was Rh negative in her announcement, assuming that intended parents who contacted her were aware of this. Numerous times, however, conditions had already been agreed upon with the intended parents when they suddenly "discovered" her negative rhesus factor and consequently turned her down—a fact she found extremely irritating.

When I asked Sveta what her ideal arrangement would be, she told me about a collaboration she had considered with a wealthy Russian businessman living in Boston. He had two grown-up children with his ex-wife but now wanted one more child on his own. The man would not have needed to fly over to Russia, as his sperm cells were already frozen in a clinic in Moscow, and the egg cells would have been provided by a female friend, who was a lawyer and would have also taken care of the legal part of the arrangement. "From all the people that have written, this would really be the ideal option," Sveta said, because this man would clearly not have intervened too much in the pregnancy. I wondered whether I had heard of the man before. Upon visiting the same clinic a few months earlier, the director told me about being in contact with a "rich businessman," a Russian living in the United States, who was willing to pay twice the amount for the surrogacy program. While the director generally did not work with single men—assuming them to be incapable of rearing a child—he took on this case, concluding that a rich man would have enough money to find a good solution. If this was the same man as in Sveta's case, then the planned solution for the child's first year was to leave it in Moscow with a nanny. Such arrangements were not common, but from time to time I stumbled across announcements suggesting similar ideas. Sveta had also received requests to give birth and then look after the child herself for a year, or requests from single men who were looking for a surrogate who would be willing to also provide the egg cells (which is illegal in Russia and Ukraine)—offers she declined, assuming that the child would feel like *her* child.

This virtual marketplace has, of course, not existed always and everywhere. Rita Tikhonovna, for instance, had great difficulty in finding a surrogate when she was still living in her home country, Uzbekistan, a country that was not covered by the existing forums. She resorted to carefully asking around as to whether anyone knew of any women in a bad financial situation, who might be willing to take such a step. This was tricky, because her quest took place in secret and because surrogacy was not a known topic in Central Asia in the 2000s. Many of the women she approached had never heard of it. Time and again, Rita had to explain "what and how and why. I was conducting some kind of *likbez*," she said and laughed, referring to the abbreviated name for the Soviet programs for tackling illiteracy in the 1920s and 1930s (which were called *likvidatsiya bezgramotnosti u naseleniya*). Also for Rita herself it was difficult to find out how the whole process of surrogacy worked. Things became easier when she and her husband had moved to Moscow a few years previously and she continued her search on online platforms. Before finding her current surrogate, Rita had been in contact with around seventy candidates.[6] She recalled the notebook in which she kept track of all the women: every potential surrogate had one page, so that she could make easy comparisons.

Masha Arkadyevna also remembered what it was like in the 2000s, at a time before online platforms and big agencies that facilitated the matching process existed. After having worked as a surrogate herself twice—in 2003 and 2007—she had gained so much insight that she continued supporting surrogates and intended parents in their quests. She first did so on a voluntary basis but soon realized that she could not keep up with the demand and eventually founded her own small agency in southern Russia. It was a family business, in which her son and daughter actively helped out. The agency offered matching and—if the intended parents wanted—also accompaniment of the surrogates throughout the pregnancy. Masha also promoted her services on online platforms, and it was after reading the following announcement that I had contacted her:

> Dear BIO (i.e., intended parents), I offer my services in the selection of surrogate mothers, for a very attractive and modest price. At the moment we have six women ready to be wonderful surrogate mothers (*surr-mamochki*) for you, all young and healthy, with their own wonderful children. Their attitude is decent (*adekvatny*) and serious; every one of them has her own requested salary ranging from 600,000 to 800,000 rubles. They are waiting for their BIO, who should be responsible, decent (*poryadochny*), caring, and they should keep their word and honor agreements, oral or written. Call, write, I answer everyone... All of us are parents ourselves and we have a responsible attitude.

The advertisement reflects the way Masha's agency worked: In contrast to big agencies that only offered standardized conditions and salaries, Masha understood her position rather as facilitating arrangements, in which surrogates had a certain liberty in deciding on the conditions and payments they were willing to work for. Unlike many other agency advertisements, hers also emphasized the responsibility of intended parents, not only in terms of reliability but also in terms of care—possibly a result of her own experiences as a surrogate.

Besides the different kinds of agencies that operated in the field of surrogacy, there were also numerous private agents who were involved in brokering in a more "freelance" way and who were, like Masha, themselves sometimes former surrogates. I refer to this group as "private" agents. They often worked on their own and focused on merely setting surrogates up with particular intended parents, clinics, or agencies. This was a temporary occupation that individuals engaged in. Such brokering took a different form from the way it is practiced, for instance, in India, where private agents are very common. While they are also often former surrogates, they usually work through word-of-mouth in their neighborhoods and communities, often also among their kin (Deomampo 2016; Pande 2014; Rudrappa 2016a). In Russia and Ukraine, private agents mainly recruited in the virtual space, on social media and online platforms. Women interested in becoming surrogates could discuss preliminary questions with them, then they would refer and, at times, accompany the women to a specific clinic. Sometimes they worked for numerous clinics with differing payment schemes, recruitment procedures, and standards of medical treatment. This allowed private agents to present potential surrogates with various options. Usually, their involvement ended once the surrogacy candidates were accepted or rejected by the clinics they collaborated with, and thus they did not accompany them throughout the process. The commission they received was often subtracted from the salary that the respective surrogates would be paid. One of the women I spoke with, for instance, received ₽120,000 (US$2,500) less than most other surrogates at the same clinic, because she had gone through a private agent from her hometown in Ukraine.

Considering the fact that the women were interested in participating in surrogacy for financial reasons, I was surprised that many responded to the first advertisement they found—a finding echoed in Alexandra Kurlenkova's research into egg providers in Moscow (2018, 186). However, several had investigated their options more thoroughly through online ratings or payment comparison. Some, like Masha Arkadyevna and Zhenya Pavlovna, had even visited numerous agencies and clinics to get a good overview, as some offered different salaries for different women. One clinic, for instance, set payments according to nationality: women from Central Asia would receive ₽600,000 (US$12,500), women from Ukraine ₽700,000 (US$14,500), and those from Russia ₽800,000 (US$16,500)—a ranking that also reflected racialized imaginaries about how trustworthy and, thus, desirable surrogates from these regions were (Weis 2021a, 46–52). Elsewhere, payments varied according to whether women were above or below the age of thirty. And frequently "experience" also played a role, and women who had already been surrogates before would receive a higher salary. Such "price lists"—as Katya Yefimovna termed the differences in salary—reflected a higher valuation given to women of Russian nationality (assuming they were more healthy but also more demanding in financial terms), to young women (because they had higher fertility), and to experienced surrogates (who had proven their fertility and knew what to expect).

As the "price lists" reflect, women were also prepared to cross borders to become a surrogate. Like Katya Yefimovna, many of the surrogates and egg providers working in Moscow were from other post-Soviet countries. Most were Ukrainians, many from Belarus, and some from Central Asian countries.[7] The doctors and agents in my research estimated that this was the case for around 30–40 percent of the surrogates. They came to Russia either because surrogacy was not legal or regulated in their countries or because—and this was the more common reason—surrogacy salaries in Moscow were much higher than the total of approximately US$11,000 in Ukraine. The high salary in the Russian reproductive hubs also attracted potential surrogates from all over Russia. One of the surrogates in my research regularly traveled to Moscow from the Russian east by train, which took her around seventy-two hours one way. Mobility thus plays a crucial role for surrogates to turn their "reproductive capital" into "economic capital" (Weis 2021a).

"More Miracle than Medicine"

IVF treatments are uncertain medical procedures, and despite the large amount of hormonal medication women take, even doctors often cannot explain why some embryo transfers result in pregnancies while others do not and why some pregnancies result in birth while others result in a spontaneous abortion. This element of chance is highly stressful and frustrating for surrogates and intended parents alike. Zhenya Pavlovna, for instance, complained about other surrogates who did not stick to the rules and nevertheless got pregnant on their first attempt:

> For instance, we should eat healthy food but they eat whatever they want. [...] we should not take a bath and they take a bath. They say we should keep from strenuous activities and they don't and nevertheless they get pregnant! And you protect yourself like a crystal vase [...] and it doesn't work out.

She found it "insulting" (*obidno*) that her first embryo transfer had failed but consoled herself with the fact that the whole IVF process appeared to her to be "more miracle than medicine" anyway. Both surrogates and intended parents lived with the constant fear that something might—for unknown reasons—go wrong during the pregnancy. Citing a Russian proverb, Zhenya said that you should not divide up the skin of a bear that you have not yet even killed (*nye delit' shkuru neubitogo medvedya*). She stressed that a positive pregnancy result was not yet cause for celebration—it might be an ectopic pregnancy or the fetus could suddenly stop growing. And you should not even feel relieved in the fourth or fifth month of pregnancy. Only once the child had been born and the money paid could you be sure that everything had gone well. This uncertainty also caused some women to stop trusting their own bodily sensations. One of the surrogates said that she was very nervous after her first embryo transfer and wanted to get pregnant so badly that she experienced all the signs of pregnancy in the first two weeks, such as morning sickness and swollen breasts. This made it even harder for her to come to terms with the fact that the pregnancy test turned out to be negative. After the second attempt, she tried to be calmer: "I just waited for the results," she told me with a smile. "I am just waiting for whatever happens next." Intended mothers were confronted with similar challenges. Rita Tikhonovna said she was trying to think just about the here and now, and not get her hopes up about what *might* be. When we got to know each other, the woman carrying her baby was in the fourth month of pregnancy, but having lost her own child upon delivery, Rita had good reason to remain cautious.

The uncertainty of when a pregnancy would finally set in had particularly troubled Ksenia Demyanovna, whose story best exemplifies how surrogates manage their lives and options in light of unknown outcomes. After her mother, who, like Ksenia, had also been a single parent, had died of cancer a few years previously, she was taking care of not only her own daughter but also her younger sister—a great emotional and financial burden. When I got to know her, Ksenia was only twenty-one and had already spent nine months at the clinic trying to become a surrogate. While most women in my research had become pregnant within half a year at the latest, it had taken this time alone until she had the first embryo transfer, which was not successful. She felt like she was "on the backburner," because every time she came to the clinic, some kind of "problem" was discovered. First, she had polyps and needed a hysteroscopy—which a significant number of surrogates had to undergo—then there were other issues that she did not understand but that delayed the possibility of an embryo transfer. Ksenia had been on and off hormone treatment throughout these months and was tired of traveling to Moscow, which was a thirteen-hour train ride from her hometown, Ulyanovsk, a city on the shores of the Volga River. She usually came on the night train, went directly to the clinic for a few hours, and then got the next possible train back home. "I run from work to the train station to come to Moscow and do all the things here, then from Moscow I travel back again, run as fast as I can home to change clothes and run to work. I can never relax, you know? I'm so tired of this," she said. Ksenia had lost all her energy and was extremely frustrated. She kept asking herself: "Why isn't it working? Why doesn't it (i.e., the embryo) lodge? I don't understand this. What does this mean?" She suggested that it might be fate, that she might not be supposed to become a surrogate, that "it is not to be." Many times she had gone to a fortune-teller, who had predicted that she would have a second child. Ksenia was wondering who this second child might be: whether the fortune-teller was referring to a surrogate child or to her own; and whether the fact that she had not yet become pregnant was a sign that she should instead try for a second child for herself.

Similar to Ksenia Demyanovna, numerous other surrogates and intended parents spoke about the medical uncertainties by evoking a higher power. This is not uncommon in the context of IVF treatments and often reflects the limits of medical expertise and control (Bärnreuther 2021). In her work on Ecuador, Elizabeth Roberts (2006), for instance, shows that clinic employees tended to evoke God's influence on the success of IVF attempts particularly in such moments as the fertilization or embryo transfer, when they lacked control themselves. Similarly, Aditya Bharadwaj (2006) argues that Indian clinicians and patients make sense of unsuccessful treatments by pointing out the "incompleteness" of Western science and technology and "enchanting" the process of IVF by calling on spiritual and cosmological explanations for the "why questions." Like the Indian couples who, after treatment, were told that "their case now rested with a higher court of appeal" that would decide on the outcome of the treatment (456), Russian intended mother Vera Romanovna joked that she had no influence over the results of IVF and that it all depended on what the stars and the "heavenly office" (*nyebyesnaya kantselyariya*) decided.

Surrogate Lyuba Dmitriyevna also told me about all sorts of "traditions"—as she called them—that one should follow in order to get pregnant. According to one such tradition, you should request a *positive* pregnancy test at a pharmacy on the day before the embryo transfer. "You have to say it exactly like that in order for it to work," she said with a smile. Then you needed to write the words "get pregnant" on a small jar and put it underneath your bed. After the transfer, you should pee into the jar and then do the pregnancy test. Another tradition suggested bringing a red towel to the embryo transfer and putting it underneath your lower back while lying down in the recovery room after the procedure. Lyuba had not followed any of these recommendations herself, she said laughing, but had read about them with great interest on the online forums. Such popular beliefs and vernacular religious discourses are widespread in Russia and often exist alongside or fused with Orthodox practices (Panchenko 2012).

Many of my interlocutors referred to spiritual and religious powers in ways that left whether or not they believed in them open. As such, despite pondering the fortune-teller's statements, Ksenia Demyanovna did not seriously consider giving up on surrogacy. When I accompanied her to the second embryo transfer, she presented me with her new plans: If she did not get pregnant this time, she would take a month off from all the medication and just rest. Then she would become a donor to at least earn some money to get by, then rest for another month before becoming fully involved in doing surrogacy (*plotno zanimat' surrogatnym*) again, but this time in a direct arrangement. "I will try till the end, even if it takes fifty-five transfers," Ksenia stressed. Considering her lack of success in this endeavor to date, her determination was remarkable. But by then she was already too curious about what the process would be like, and she had already invested too much time, energy, and emotion to give up now—Ksenia wanted all this effort to pay off. I was also startled by her new idea of selling her eggs—a few weeks previously, she had said she was afraid of the hormonal stimulation and she could not live with knowing that "somewhere a part of me is walking around." But she seemed to have changed her mind after finding an agent online, who suggested becoming an egg provider in Spain or India. "She pays for the journey plus 60,000 rubles for the donation, and I can take a few days of holiday there," Ksenia said approvingly. The prospect of becoming a "travelling donor" (Kroløkke 2015; Pande and Moll 2018) and enjoying a holiday abroad resonated with her, but I assume that her change of heart was also linked to the fact that she needed the money and could no longer wait. The Altra Vita IVF Clinic covered all her travel costs to and from Moscow, but the traveling, in combination with not knowing when and if a pregnancy would set in, made it challenging for her to secure a steady income during this time.

Ksenia needed to juggle the few options available to her and have several plans to hand, following one of the main principles of "practical realism": "When life is experienced as constantly changing and unpredictable, being ready to cope with unpredictability by leaving several life options open takes center stage" (Utrata 2015, 118). Since egg provision usually requires more hormonal medication than surrogacy, many women shied away from it, and Ksenia was initially no exception. However, during the long time that she had been trying to become pregnant she had given up on the idea of sparing her body the hormones, and the option of selling her eggs no longer seemed so bad, even if it demanded an emotional or moral compromise.[8]

Like a Crystal Vase

The degree of medical uncertainty made it all the more important to have a tight grip on all those aspects of a surrogate pregnancy that *could* be controlled. This control was directed mostly toward the surrogate and her body. A particularly critical phase in this regard were the first twelve weeks of pregnancy, when the risk of losing the embryo or fetus was greatest. From the embryo transfer onward—as previously indicated—surrogates were instructed to think about their bodies as a "crystal vase," a metaphor that underlined the fragility of the embryo, which could suffer harm if one were to make a wrong move. This was exemplified in a particularly delicate situation during one of surrogate Alevtina Leontyevna's ultrasound, when the doctor became angry and implied that she had behaved in an irresponsible way. With a strict tone, the doctor said, "This is only the beginning! The first twelve weeks are the riskiest and you are only in the fifth. It's all your responsibility!" She took the woman by the shoulders and continued: "Jumping, running, the wrong food—this all has consequences." The doctor reminded her that one mistake was enough to lose the embryo and that she had better "get her priorities straight." She later whispered to me with a smile: "I have to educate (*vospitivat'*) them."

The situation illustrated the amount of pressure put on surrogates to "educate" them about what their priorities should be. Many surrogates emphasized that they were even *more* responsible and *more* careful than during their own pregnancies. During one of my visits in the surrogate flats, a conversation emerged that revealed the insecurity such intimidating "education" could provoke. One of the women mentioned feeling "guilty" for having run to catch a bus and another said—though half-jokingly—that she hoped the small mineral water she had drunk would not affect the embryo, because they were told not to drink anything carbonated. When I asked her whether there were many such rules, she said no, but the situation in the surrogates' flats indicated that there was a certain amount of confusion about what the rules were. Many women seemed compelled to comply with all the guidance—whether or not they deemed it sensible—so that they could not be blamed if something went wrong. Masha Arkadyevna, for instance, the surrogate-turned-agent, told me about her anxiety when finding out that her pregnancy result was negative: "I was really, I don't know, there was so much going on in my soul. I was crying; I became hysterical. I just didn't understand how this could happen." She did not know how to explain to "her" couple that it was not her fault, that she had done everything exactly the way she was supposed to. When her second attempt proved successful, she was incredibly relieved and happy, possibly happier than when she found out about her own pregnancy, Masha said with a laugh. Her comments reflect how uncertainty about pregnancy outcomes triggers fears of being or being made responsible. It is not uncommon that surrogates are highly disappointed when transfers fail or medical problems emerge during their pregnancies. Not having encountered fertility issues during their "own" pregnancies, they do not anticipate complications and feel unsettled and guilty if these arise (Jacobson 2016; Mitra and Schicktanz 2016; Teman 2010; Toledano and Zeiler 2017; Ziff 2020).

Anxiety about pregnancy outcomes was exacerbated by the fact that payment was tied to "success." The amount and the timing of payments were established by the contract. Regular monthly payments either started once a pregnancy was confirmed through a test, at around two weeks after the embryo transfer, or after the first ultrasound confirming the pregnancy, in the sixth week of pregnancy. At Altra Vita, surrogates received ₽3,000 (US$60) per week in the first two weeks and from then on ₽20,000 (US$420) per month. Some agencies and clinics established that surrogates living in their flats received a smaller amount per month and food products instead. Twin pregnancies at Altra Vita were compensated with an additional ₽300,000 (US$6,300) and a C-section with an additional ₽100,000 (US$2,100). Sometimes surrogates received a one-time payment for maternity clothes or a bonus payment for "good behavior"—an undefined term that most probably referred to the surrogates' compliance with the medical regime and the intended parents' wishes. The main payment was referred to as a "salary" (*gonorar*) or "compensation" (*voznagrazhdyeniye*) and was paid upon the surrogate signing away her maternal rights after delivery. As previously indicated, in Moscow this payment could range from ₽600,000 to ₽1 million (US$12,500–21,000), with Altra Vita paying the latter sum. One of the contracts I read stated that this sum would be paid for the birth of a "healthy" child, but without specifying what this meant. I assume that the birth of an "unhealthy" child would result in investigating whether or not the surrogate's behavior had contributed to the child's status in terms of health and dis/ability. The same contract stipulated that if the surrogate's behavior was responsible for a miscarriage, if she terminated the pregnancy, or if she refused to relinquish the child, she would have to return all expenses (e.g., medical or transport expenses) and pay a sanction of ₽1.4 million (US$29,000). Moreover, she would only receive half the compensation if the fetus died after the thirty-sixth week of pregnancy or during or immediately after delivery, without her fault. This meant that surrogates risked financial loss even if they did not contribute to a negative pregnancy outcome—a practice also common in surrogacy arrangements in India (Deomampo 2016; Moreno 2016; Vora and Iyengar 2017). Critically commenting on this practice, Daisy Deomampo notes that payment in such contracts is explicitly linked to the surrogate "bodies' performance" as well as to the "idea that surrogates are being paid for a 'product' of determinable quality"—an aspect that considerably stressed the surrogates, as they had limited control over the "performance" of their bodies or the "products" they were supposed to deliver (2016, 186). To my knowledge, the "products" of the women in my research were all alive and healthy when they were born. I only know of one woman whose pregnancy was terminated after the twelfth week, because a "genetic problem" was diagnosed, as one of the other surrogates told me. I do not know what compensation she received in this case, since her contract only regulated medically indicated terminations after the sixteenth week of pregnancy (for which the surrogate would receive ₽150,000 as compensation)—a sign that contracts were not detailed enough, leaving open what would happen in undesirable situations. It was, however, stipulated in the contract that surrogates needed to agree to a medically indicated termination as well as to prenatal screenings and tests, including amniocentesis. In addition, the contract specified that she needed to agree to a selective reduction should the embryo transfer result in a pregnancy with more than two fetuses.

Despite the fact that clinic employees at Altra Vita stated that all women had the same contract, surrogates told me they risked monetary sanctions when talking to each other or anybody else about their contracts. This was a common prohibition in clinics and agencies, and was probably a measure to suppress the possibility of collective resistance by keeping surrogates isolated. Such a payment scheme, and the constant threat of monetary sanctions, were, in themselves, a control device that made sure surrogates structured their lives around the metaphoric crystal vase. Paying only small amounts of money at a time, the agency and intended parents could make sure that they would not lose too much money in the event of a pregnancy loss, while surrogates were motivated to stick to the strict rules of the contract. At the same time, the prospect of gaining an additional bonus for "good behavior" functioned as an incentive to comply with the rules and to think twice about making claims or demands. Moreover, paying the salary upon childbirth avoided the risk of surrogates not wanting to hand over the child—the intended parents' greatest fear.

Relief and Confinement in the Surrogate Flats

Another way of ensuring control over the surrogate body was by housing the surrogates in clinic accommodation. Such shared housing is also typical in India, not least because surrogates are usually required to spend their entire pregnancies away from home. Amrita Pande (2010), for instance, describes the all-encompassing nature of the "hostels" she visited during her fieldwork, where women shared meals, prayers, educational classes, but also their stories, struggles, and experiences. These spaces, while being limiting and controlling, could also become spaces of community, support, and resistance.

In Russia and Ukraine, some agencies and clinics also offered housing—some had several shared flats within Moscow, others entire houses that were often located on the edge of the city—but they were much less encompassing and only seldom created a sense of community. Altra Vita's six "surrogate flats" were situated in two prefabricated buildings near to the clinic itself. Surrogates who did not already live in Moscow were obliged to stay in the clinic's flats and under its control for at least two weeks after the embryo transfer, until the pregnancy test could be taken. If this test was positive, they stayed for another three to five weeks before they could return home. In the following months they traveled to the capital for medical checkups every week or two, and later only once a month. Around the thirtieth or thirty-second week, they had to move back to Moscow until giving birth. The flats mainly housed surrogates but sometimes also egg providers and in rare cases regular patients who had to stay the night. There was one flat for short-term visitors that consisted of a kitchen and two rooms, offering space for a maximum of six women. The flat was sparsely furnished but always orderly and clean—thanks not least to the numerous instructions on the kitchen walls reminding women to wash their dishes immediately after eating or to take all their food with them when they left. Because turnover was high, the women generally did not develop close bonds with each other and often appeared quite isolated. They usually spent considerable time reading and texting on their mobile phones and showed little interest in interacting with the others. Sometimes minor tensions arose between surrogates and egg donors or between women from Russia and those from Ukraine, due to the ongoing military conflict. At other times, however, women found themselves sharing the flat for several weeks and formed friendships, some of which went beyond their shared time in Moscow.

The other flats accommodated one or two people, usually surrogates whose intended parents paid the rent for them to live in Moscow during the entire pregnancy. During my time at the clinic, this was only the case for Lena Mironovna and Katya Yefimovna, whom I accompanied throughout their pregnancies until they gave birth in summer 2015. Despite living in Moscow for nine months, both hardly moved around the city. The capital was overwhelming for many surrogates who came from smaller cities or towns. The fear of sudden pregnancy complications also contributed to most women's wish to stay close by the clinic. In a sense, the flats could be described, following Miriam Ticktin, as a waiting room—a "peculiar sort of place, a space of liminality, suspended time, even containment" (2013, n.p.). The surrogates were dislocated from their usual surroundings and routines and had to set up their homes in new, temporary places. They found themselves waiting, in a "situation where what is hoped for or anxiously anticipated has not yet been actualized" (Bandak and Janeja 2018, 1) and where doubt, uncertainty, and hope coexisted (5). The women who moved to Moscow for the duration of their pregnancies or for the last two months seemed to surrender their lives to the everyday dullness of pregnant and (monitored) waiting (see also Deomampo 2013a).

Clinic staff made weekly visits to check the content of the fridges and the cleanliness of the flats. "Usually we try to do it unexpectedly," one doctor told me, laughing, "we just call half an hour before we come, so that she doesn't have an opportunity to prepare or hide anything." These visits were gradually replaced by cameras that were installed in each flat's hallway. The cameras surveilled not only the surrogates but also all visitors. Lena Mironovna once received an angry telephone call from one of the surrogate managers for they had seen me on the camera recording and had thought I was a man. Men—unless they were husbands—were not allowed to enter the surrogates' apartments. While I was only accidentally targeted in this example, the cameras also came to control my movements once my presence near the clinic was no longer desired. The possibility of clinic accommodation therefore represented relief and confinement at the same time. On the one hand, many surrogates welcomed the opportunity to move there to escape nosy neighbors and friends, or to be absolved from family and household obligations for a while. But, on the other hand, the flats enabled the clinic to take control of the surrogate bodies.

Several women felt disturbed by this form of surveillance, stating that they were "not birds in a cage" and did not need constant threats, as they understood very well what they should and should not do. Others passively surrendered, claiming that they had nothing to hide or did not care. Katya Yefimovna even suggested that more control was necessary, because some of the surrogates behaved in highly irresponsible ways. However, while she had many bad things to say about other surrogates, she also had to endure the weekly surprise visits of the self-proclaimed "queen of the flats," as Katya referred to the clinic employee responsible for conducting the controls. Time and again such visits made her feel that the place she lived in for nine months was not *her* place and could therefore be intruded upon any time.

The clinic's infringement of Katya's privacy culminated in the week I came to the clinic with Sarah Hildebrand, a Swiss photographer I was collaborating with on a joint book and exhibition project with the title *hope* (Hildebrand et al. 2018; Siegl 2018c). We had agreed with the director that Sarah could take pictures in the clinic as well as in some of the surrogates' flats. Concerning the latter, Sarah's intention was to capture traces of the surrogates' everyday lives in the flats themselves and the objects there. Katya had agreed that we could visit her with the camera but had also warned me that we would not be able to capture any traces of her, as her "soul" (*dusha*) was certainly not in this flat, and not even in Moscow (Siegl 2018b). Unfortunately, the day we were assigned by the clinic to take pictures in the flats was one of the few when she was out, as she needed to have laboratory tests. The flat manager suggested we go anyway. "Why does it matter if Katya is at home or not?" she asked me with a forced smile, and then added that it was not Katya's flat but the clinic's and that we were not allowed to take pictures of "their" surrogates anyway. In order to guarantee this, she would accompany us and answer all questions we might have about the flat and, yes, also about Katya's personal belongings.[9] I was taken aback by the way the clinic claimed the surrogates' bodies as theirs and how the flat manager professed to be able to talk about Katya's belongings. Both these aspects suggested that the surrogates were often not seen as individuals with their own unique personalities and biographies.

Managing Uncertainties

Commercial surrogacy constitutes a thriving market populated by a vast array of actors who operate across virtual and real worlds, move within and beyond national borders, and try to realize their needs and desires between the doable and its moral boundaries. They come together in a carefully orchestrated "choreography" (Thompson 2005), from which some hope to emerge as parents and others as women who can escape their dire financial situation. In a labor market and a social system that discriminates against women, particularly single mothers, prospective surrogates tried to turn their reproductive capacity into economic value (Cooper and Waldby 2014, 83–87). Intended mothers, on the other hand, tried to mobilize their economic capital in order to overcome the reproductive constraints of their own bodies. Both groups of women entered a new realm of uncertainty and vulnerability, in which terms of cooperation had to be fiercely negotiated or relegated to the organizational authority of agencies. Not being able to anticipate which arrangements would result in a contract and which embryo transfers in a pregnancy, women often had to juggle several potential commitments simultaneously. In this process, they often lost a lot of time and experienced a great deal of stress.

Being an uncertain endeavor, surrogacy arrangements called for various measures of control that promised to increase security. These measures were directed at the surrogates, who were "educated" to understand their bodies as "crystal vases" containing the embryo—a metaphor that came to shape their everyday lives in significant ways. The timed payments, constant threat of monetary sanctions, and the surveillance in the surrogate flats accompanied the "education" in order to ensure maximum compliance. As the situation with the flat manager indicates, these were also ways of "incorporating" the surrogate body into the clinic—as if by signing the contract, ownership of the surrogate body had been transferred to the clinic. This dynamic is furthered by the way the surrogate's body is understood not only as a crystal vase but also as a mechanical entity that can be worked upon and manipulated by medical professionals.

However, the power of the clinic was not total, and every now and again surrogates engaged in small practices of rebellion, such as reducing the prescribed hormonal medication during the "preparation" or smoking a forbidden cigarette after a failed embryo transfer. Moreover, most women were happy to speak to me about their contracts, even though they risked sanctions; and several continued meeting up with me after I had been dismissed from the clinic, arguing that they would not allow the clinic to intervene in their lives to such an extent. Lena Mironovna's husband had even researched the type of cameras the clinic had installed and concluded that the quality was so bad that I could easily come for a visit if I walked through the entrance hall fast enough. Lena and her husband in particular celebrated these small acts of resistance, finding creative ways of hiding alcohol or getting rid of the cigarette smell when the flat manager came on her inspection visits. It was only her husband, though, who smoked and consumed alcohol—the stakes for Lena were too high, and like most other surrogates, she strictly followed the "regime" (*rezhim*) the clinic imposed on her.

4
DOING IT BUSINESS-STYLE

"We like to say that she should be a decent (*adekvatnaya*) woman." Doctor Natalya Nikolayevna set out to answer my question about how she would describe the perfect surrogate. Elaborating further, she added:

> Such a woman is disciplined and regards the [surrogacy] program as her work [...], such that she will strictly fulfil everything without asking any unnecessary (*lishniye*) questions [...] and that she treats this as her workplace, that she understands that this is work and not an opportunity to live well on someone else's money. Well, just a worker's attitude and that's it (laughs). We don't ask anything else from her.

The doctor's words are emblematic of the way professionals and intended parents characterized the perfect surrogate as a worker. This kind of worker should be disciplined, obedient, and should fulfil all demands without causing delays or problems. She should be *adekvatnaya*, which—when describing a person—translates as decent, trustworthy, orderly, and with good manners. The term has a strong moral component, indicating that being a good surrogate worker is not merely a question of attitude but also of moral integrity. Conceptualizing surrogacy as work, doctors, intermediaries, and intended parents not only accepted but also welcomed surrogates' financial motives. As previously indicated, this crucially distinguishes the Russian and Ukrainian context from other countries in which surrogacy has been studied, most notably from the United States. To recall: Surrogacy in the United States is clearly framed in terms of gift-giving, and clinics reject surrogacy candidates who foreground financial motives or obviously act out of economic necessity (Berend 2016; Jacobson 2016; Ragoné 1994; Smietana 2017b). Market players thus largely obscure the "labor" involved and the income made (Jacobson 2016, 38). For instance, while agencies do frame surrogacy as work, they emphasize that good workers are those who seem like they would become surrogates even without the financial compensation: "Good workers put up with a lot—because they care" (40). Likewise, my research participants from Spain, Germany, and Austria emphasized the importance of altruistic motives and tended to regard the economic as "polluting" the sphere of intimacy (Zelizer 2013). Such views and practices are embedded in cultural settings, in which the intimate commercial use of one's body is heavily problematized, and surrogacy is commonly criticized as exploiting poor women's reproductive labor.

In Russia and Ukraine, these concerns are not central to debates about the morality of surrogacy. Rather, as the previous chapters have shown, the moral economy of surrogacy in Russia and Ukraine is shaped around the intended parents' vulnerability and their need for distance and secrecy. Increasing their security and power within the surrogacy process is paramount from the perspective of the surrogacy industry, in which the parents are the paying clients. Their prioritization—as I will show in the following—is eased by the acceptance of an instrumental and consumption-oriented approach to commercial intimacies such as surrogacy.

The need for secrecy throughout the surrogacy program often translates into the need to cut ties and erase traces after the completion of the program. This anticipated outcome plays a crucial role in the way surrogacy is understood and organized as work and the surrogate as a financially motivated worker: whereas a gift relationship creates ongoing bonds of reciprocity, a neat economic relationship ends after the exchange of money and baby. In order for this relationship and the resulting exchange to run smoothly, a number of mechanisms and practical measures have to be implemented, starting from the recruitment process. These revolve around detaching the child from the surrogate, with whose body and care it is so intimately linked. This detachment is accomplished through efforts to erase the gift surrogacy might entail. On a discursive level, this is achieved by erasing the surrogates' active labor and their subjectivities. They are turned into mechanical workers and marginal strangers—a dynamic that allows the commoditization of a relationship that is regarded as "protected" from such commoditization (Appadurai 1986, 15). This is not in opposition to the above-mentioned acceptance of commercial intimacies. Rather, in the case of surrogacy, the acceptance is linked to the need for surrogacy to be an economic relationship. In other words, many of my Russian and Ukrainian research participants regarded surrogacy as ethical only if it was a purely economic exchange and if the surrogate had a "worker's attitude," as Dr. Natalya Nikolayevna stated.

Efforts to detach the child from the surrogate's body were all the more necessary, because the surrogate was perceived as risky, "hormonated," and capricious—characteristics that might endanger detachment. Consequently, the surrogate's body needed to be tightly controlled, and this was achieved by the material incentive a surrogacy program provided and the many financial sanctions that surrogacy contracts entailed.

In this chapter, I explore these aspects by investigating what *kind* of work surrogacy is framed as, what *kind* of worker a good surrogate is supposed to be, and how these framings are circulated by market actors. I will come to argue that—under the conditions described in part 1 of this book—"doing it business-style," as one of the intended mothers phrased it, is presented as a morally necessary approach to surrogacy. My focus in the following is on discourses *about* the surrogates and their work, as I am here interested in how market actors in the more powerful positions shape the possible relationships that can evolve in surrogacy. I thus draw mainly on interviews with Russian and Ukrainian intended parents, agents, and doctors; the following chapter will then center on how the surrogates engaged with the discourses about them and how they shaped their own understandings of surrogacy.

Recruiting the Perfect Surrogate Worker

According to surrogate manager Natasha Sergeyevna, 70–80 percent of the surrogacy candidates were rejected by the clinic, 20 percent of them for psychological reasons. Considering different statements by clinics and agencies, only between 10 and 50 percent of all surrogacy candidates make it through the tests. Such numbers need to be treated with caution, because agencies and clinics use them to proclaim their "seriousness" and "professionalism," and thus legitimacy. In fact, during my time at the Altra Vita IVF Clinic, most women passed the examinations administered by psychologist Aleksandra Denisovna. She had a small consultation room in the clinic, consisting of an examination bed, two chairs, a table with a computer, and on the wall one of the numerous paintings displayed at the clinic—this one of a naked woman swimming amid thousands of tiny sperm cells. "What I do is an anamnesis," Aleksandra Denisovna explained in response to my question regarding how she evaluated whether someone was suitable to become a surrogate. "I make a record of her biography. How was her childhood? Were there any traumas? Infections? How was school? What is her character like? Her marital status? Children? Work? Alcohol, cigarettes, drugs? Surroundings—friends and family? Atmosphere at home?" She listed a seemingly endless number of aspects. Then she told me about the tests that evaluated the nervous system and how the body reacted to stress. She also made sure that the potential surrogate was not "mentally retarded" (*umstvenno otstal'naya*): "The intellectual level is important, because if it's too low, then they don't understand how many tablets they have to take," she explained. Examinations lasted between one and two hours, depending on whether Aleksandra Denisovna followed the standard procedure or whether the specific intended parents had particular wishes, for example that the surrogate should be a calm person. Furthermore, the tests were concerned with distinguishing between those women who "really understood what surrogacy is about" and those who had "an inclination toward adventurous and spontaneous behavior," a trait that could be dangerous in surrogacy. When I asked how she could recognize such traits, Aleksandra Denisovna tilted her head backward and crossed her arms: "This is what I studied for ten years. I have my methods." She could tell a great deal about any person from the moment he or she stepped into her consultation room—a statement that made me feel slightly uncomfortable—but by referring to her methods as a "professional secret," Aleksandra Denisovna indicated that she did not want to go into further detail. It was only from the surrogate workers themselves that I learned about them having to paint pictures, list the colors of the Russian flag, name the president of the United States of America, or put commas into a sentence. "They just check that you're not a total idiot," Lena Mironovna said with a wink, mocking the procedures but also worrying that she might not have spelled George W. Bush's name correctly. I had to smile at the way some surrogates ridiculed these tests retrospectively, particularly because many were nervous before taking them, not knowing what to expect or what they would find out about themselves, and also because I noticed that they were somewhat proud to have "made it" (see also Teman 2010).

Some agencies even went to such lengths as using lie detectors when conducting the psychological examinations. According to Konstantin Pavlovich, representative of one of Russia's biggest agencies, this was a great advantage for intended parents. We had met for lunch in a small and entirely empty Asian restaurant in Moscow's city center, where he seemed to be a regular. The agency he worked for had a database of around twenty—sometimes up to fifty—women who had already been examined and were ready to start a surrogacy program at any time. The intended parents could choose their surrogate based on dossiers they received, containing information about place of birth, place of residence, age, marital status, number of children, nationality, ethnicity, education, and occupation. Konstantin Pavlovich did not understand how it was possible, or even desirable, for anyone to make decisions based on these factors. Furthermore, intended parents would not meet their surrogates anyway, so he regarded the whole procedure as entirely pointless:

> We guarantee that all our surrogate mothers are *healthy* and psychologically stable. They will fulfil all their responsibilities. They are all 5+ (i.e., the best mark in Russia). So how can you select a surrogate mother by looking at a questionnaire? . . . It's like when you stand in a shop in front of various fridges, all the same brand. . . . How do you choose? . . . Let's be honest. The surrogate mother—she is an incubator. . . . She is a living being, of course, but I'm speaking about the child-bearing aspect. Only one thing is needed from her: that she is in good health, that she is capable of carrying a child, and that she is a responsible mother, that she doesn't do things that are, let's say, not allowed for pregnant women. That's all we ask for.

This quote is particularly intriguing when considering that Konstantin Pavlovich was the agency's public relations manager—a position in which, I would assume, he deliberately and carefully chose his words in order to promote his agency's interests. What struck me most were the metaphors he drew on: the incubator and the fridge. Both imply that the body is analogous to a machine, which is another very common metaphor in relation to the female body, particularly in the context of pregnancy and childbirth. Metaphorical language is often meant to make something sound familiar and thus to normalize it (De Lacey 2002, 45). As such, Konstantin Pavlovich's analogies could be understood as a way to portray surrogacy as an easy and harmless kind of work for the surrogate: being a machine, the body can easily be adapted to the task at hand. Moreover, it separates and disentangles the person from the body.

Konstantin Pavlovich's quote is exemplary of how in the context of commercial bodily labor "metaphorical thinking rapidly depersonalizes, desubjectifies, and thus dehumanizes the body and its parts" (Sharp 2000, 315). Speaking of gestational surrogacy, he not only drew on the by now common image of the incubator but also went a step further with his image of the fridge. While the incubator seems to reflect at least some sort of agency, because of its warm, nurturing, and enabling attributes (in the sense of enabling a human being to grow), the fridge is cold and only stores its contents. Comparing surrogates to fridges from the same brand, Konstantin Pavlovich implied that they were superficially all the same and only special knowledge revealed the differences between them. While intended parents were, according to him, usually concerned with the wrong issues—having a blue-eyed surrogate or a woman with a perfect figure—he emphasized that the agency knew what counted, how to "deal" with surrogates and "how to talk to them," as if to suggest that these women were a very specific category of people. Employing psychological examinations and expertise, the agency could "pick the right ones," those who had the right understanding about surrogacy.

The "right understanding" was an expression I frequently encountered during fieldwork. As indicated by doctor Natalya Nikolayevna at the outset of this chapter, this notion often referred to the conception of surrogacy as work. At the same time, however, this work was continuously devalued—it seemed not to be recognized as "real" work but as involving "subjects giving clinics access to the productivity of their in vivo biology" (Waldby and Cooper 2008, 59). This access was provided by a number of "second-order tasks" that merely required a woman's "compliance with often-complex medical regimes of dosing, testing, appointments and self-monitoring" (59). In Melinda Cooper and Catherine Waldby's explorations of what they call "clinical labor," the authors argue that the labor involved in the context of surrogacy—but also in the context of the provision of bodily substances, such as gametes, or the participation in clinical trials—thus often goes unrecognized. Not (fully) recognizing this labor facilitates other market actors' extraction of biovalue from the re/productive body, enhancing their own profits.

Discourses and metaphors that describe the surrogate body as a passive vessel clearly reflect this element of "giving access." Such metaphors construct the surrogate's womb as a mere rental space, through which the "intellectual, mental, and emotional energy" that women invest when "converting pregnancy from a meaningful, nonalienable event into wage labor" remains unrecognized (Rudrappa 2016a, 105). The surrogate body is rather rendered a site of production, while the child emerges as the "product of a mechanical process" (Davis-Floyd 1994, 1127). Consequently, this body is mainly seen as being worked upon by others: following Emily Martin (2001, 54–67), the doctors could be seen as the mechanics or even factory owners or supervisors, and the women as merely the workers following the instructions. This latter aspect was particularly prominent in my interview with another doctor, Anton Feodorovich:

> If you tell a surrogate mother she needs to do *this*, then she will do it. If you say "take a step to the left," she will take a step to the left. If you say, for example, "sneeze twice," she will do so. They are very obedient (*poslushniye*) and conscientious (*stradatel'niye*).

Anton Feodorovich's words suggested that even if one were to make completely pointless demands, the surrogate should and would fulfil these without questioning. More so, again alluding to the metaphor of the body as machine, the doctor stressed that a surrogate could even sneeze on request—a bodily reaction that cannot usually be initiated deliberately. Thus the "mechanic" could take full control of the surrogate body, as the surrogate herself did not reflect on requests and demands.

The surrogates' marginal role was further emphasized by two intermediaries, who asserted that they are "just one element in the cure for infertility" (Sergej Petrovich) and that they "absolutely understand that this is really not their story (*sovsem nye ikh istoriya*)" (Anastasia Anatolyevna). Both statements stripped the surrogates of their personhood and reduced them to one of the many things that needed to be coordinated in the course of the program. Being an "element" rather than a "person," the surrogate body is again inscribed as the passive site of production, while the surrogates and their active labor are erased. This was part of the "worker's attitude," as Sergej Petrovich phrased it, which the surrogates had to accept.

In some of the agents' and doctors' accounts, a certain tension appeared between the various requirements a surrogate should fulfil—for instance, when Konstantin Pavlovich stated above that "only one thing" is needed from the surrogate but then goes on to list several criteria for the selection of surrogates. This tension was also apparent in the interview with Ukrainian agent Sergej Petrovich. After stating that a "worker's attitude" was "all we ask for," he listed a number of other factors he deemed important: a surrogate should be a woman who generally liked children and enjoyed being pregnant, because she should feel "motherly care" toward the child, even though she knew that she was just a nanny and not a mother. She should "invest her soul" and "do her work with pleasure," but at the same time she should not be "emotional" (*emotsional'no*) but "calm" (*spokojniye*). In Russian, the word *emotsional'no* often implies an excess of emotion, and what Sergej Petrovich was referring to was anxiousness and stress or the possibility of getting attached to the child. The agent's descriptions sounded like he was searching for what in German could be termed an *eierlegende Wollmilchsau*. This fantasy animal combines the qualities of a hen, a sheep, a cow, and a pig. The expression is used for a person or a thing that "fulfils all needs and all demands" and usually signifies that these are incompatible—just as the image of the surrogate as "element" stood in curious contrast to the image of the surrogate as a nanny who "invested her soul."

Sergej Petrovich's list of desirable traits can also be read as analogous to Amrita Pande's (2010) concept of the Indian surrogate as "mother-worker" subject. Pande examines how this subject is produced through disciplinary measures and counseling in Indian fertility clinics and surrogate "hostels." In these spaces, the surrogates are trained into an understanding of being "just the womb" but nevertheless not regarding surrogacy as work but rather as a God-given gift—an opportunity God gave them, so that they could financially support their own families. This framing ensured that surrogates would be humble and compliant rather than "greedy" and demanding. The surrogate should therefore be a "mother-worker": "a subject similar to a trained factory worker but one who is simultaneously a virtuous mother," thus being "cheap, docile, selfless, and nurturing" at the same time (970). The image of the "mother-worker" resonated with the Russian and Ukrainian context in a double sense: it overlapped with ideas of the perfect surrogate who worked with pleasure and "soul," while subjecting herself to the dehumanizing image of a clinical laborer; furthermore, it reflected the Soviet ideal of the working mother, who—miraculously—managed to combine a full-time job with childcare and household responsibilities (Utrata 2015).

However, in contrast to the factory worker, the surrogate "embodies the means of production" (Cooper and Waldby 2014, 60). Pande has therefore referred to surrogacy as a form of "embodied labor," in which "the body is the ultimate site of labor, where the resources, the skills, and the ultimate product are directed primarily from the body of the laborer" (2014, 106). The requirements for such labor are almost exclusively linked to the surrogate's body. This also means that agents and doctors can reduce them to this body, describing the surrogates as uniform and interchangeable. However, their status changes once pregnancy sets in. From then on, the surrogates cannot be replaced, which gives them a certain position of power and legitimizes all the more a strict system of control (see also Rudrappa 2016a, 154).

Dangerous, Capricious, Unpredictable

From the moment of conception onward, the surrogates were imagined as inhabiting a risky body (Deomampo 2016; Hovav 2020; Mitra 2017) that accommodated something very precious: a genetically unrelated child for whom somebody else was paying a large amount of money. In the context of my research, the riskiness of the surrogate's body was connected to several kinds of uncertainties. I discussed the range of medical uncertainties in the previous chapter. A further significant uncertainty was caused by the fear that the surrogate might develop an affective bond with the child she carried and thus might not want to give it away—a fear that was nurtured by the image of the pregnant body as being saturated with affect. The third aspect related to the surrogate's potential entrepreneurial spirit. In this regard the image of the surrogate as worker was ambivalent, since it entailed the risk that surrogates could be concerned too much with their own profit and could thus act in undesirable ways. Horror stories about such "greedy women" circulated widely in the field of surrogacy, and some of the Russian and foreign intended parents looking for a direct arrangement had been confronted with cases of fraud. The less extreme stories included the German couple Stefan and Teresa Wagner paying a woman in the United States for a plane ticket to Germany before she broke off contact, or Russian intended mother Galya Yanovna paying a potential surrogate for a train ticket to Moscow and then never hearing from her again. The latter woman had already gained a bad reputation on online platforms, where there were entire threads about her and other untrustworthy women. Discussions were often accompanied by a scan of their passports and photographs, and some agencies even published "blacklists" online. One of the foreign couples I interviewed was confronted with a case of more serious fraud, when tricked by a Polish woman who had for six months pretended to be carrying their baby. She had faked examination results, medical documents, and ultrasound pictures, but for a number of reasons the intended parents were eventually able to work out her tactics. The woman must have been very active, because Juan Romero, one of the Spanish intended fathers in my research, had also been in contact with her, through one of the transnational websites on which intended parents and prospective surrogates worldwide could search for arrangements. Such stories led Juan Romero to argue that—contrary to common assumptions—it was not the "poor surrogates" but the intended parents who were the "weakest link" in the process of surrogacy. This view was shared by most intended parents and professionals. Galya Yanovna, for instance, mentioned that the law protected the surrogate but in no way the parent. While the law did not protect either side adequately, the statement reflected her own feeling of vulnerability. What she hinted at by emphasizing the surrogate's legal protection was that according to the Russian Family Code (1995), the surrogate was considered the legal mother to the child until she signed over her maternal rights after delivery. This passage in the legislation caused much anxiety for intended parents and professionals, because they had to live with the constant fear that surrogates might change their mind and want to keep the child or refuse to relinquish it in order to blackmail the parents into additional payments.[1]

Even the two agency owners who had previously been surrogates themselves had reservations about other surrogates. When I asked them whether they would resort to surrogacy in the event of infertility, both of them were hesitant. Masha Arkadyevna, a Ukrainian agent who had participated in two surrogacy programs—one in Moscow and one in Poland—first said she would adopt, then reconsidered and stated she would hire a surrogate but only if this woman would live with her, "so that I can see what kind of life she leads." Diliara Eduardovna, from the city of Krasnodar in southern Russia and also a two-time surrogate, had a similar opinion. "I don't know—this is a really difficult question," she stated, and went on to say that you would need to really trust a person and "there are some surrogates, you can't imagine." She recalled the story of an intended mother from Moscow who went to visit her pregnant surrogate and found her drunk and surrounded by cigarette butts. "To entrust some girl with my pregnancy—I would be afraid to do this." Diliara had had bad experiences, particularly with Ukrainian women. "I don't know, they behave in incomprehensible ways," she said. "The contract states *this* amount of salary and then, after birth, they demand a different sum. And based on that, they won't give away the child." She went on to tell me about a friend's surrogate, who had been hiding for three months in Ukraine, refusing to give her the child until her salary was increased in line with current inflation. For these reasons, Diliara had stopped working with women from Ukraine—she simply could not "take on this responsibility." In her opinion, the intended parents did not "deserve" a surrogate who "drained their blood." Ukrainian women seemed to occupy an intriguing position in Russian discussions about surrogacy, having a diverse set of partly contradictory characteristics attributed to them. According to intermediaries and doctors, however, cases of serious blackmail were not common. Rather, surrogates often asked for smaller things, for instance for additional money because their washing machine or phone had broken down.

In relation to issues of trust and risk, a surrogate's "experience" was also regularly mentioned by doctors, agents, and intended parents, albeit in ambivalent ways. For them, the advantage of surrogates "with experience" (*s opytom*) was that they already knew the process and that—ideally—they had proven to be good and obedient women, who did not cause difficulties after delivery. On the other hand, the exact same aspects could turn into disadvantages. This was the case when women viewed their experience as some kind of "high qualification" that made them "experts," as one agent said, while sticking her nose in the air to hint at the excessive self-esteem such a woman might have. For the intended mothers, "experience" could be a delicate issue as well. Galya Yanovna, for instance, initially wanted an experienced surrogate but could not afford the high salary. With hindsight, she deemed this aspect completely unimportant—after all, you could teach "any normal and decent (*adekvatnyj*) person" to take the right medication at the right time. In addition, she expressed the fear that such surrogates might exploit their experience, implying that they could assume an even more powerful role in the process of surrogacy as a result. The benefits of experience, then, seemed to relate primarily to the fact that such a surrogate had been "proven" to have a reliable uterus and to be a good worker, while the expertise such a surrogate might have acquired was regarded as a potentially dangerous asset.

The intended parents' fears were coupled with a powerful discourse about the hormonal bodies of pregnant women that might affectively bind them to the fetus. Olessia Valeryevna recounted a situation in which her husband nearly caused a car accident. When driving the surrogate back home after a medical examination that had revealed that they were expecting a girl, the surrogate mentioned that she had always wanted to have a baby girl. Olessia's husband was so shocked that he almost lost control of the car. Galya was also so afraid that her surrogate would "change her mind" that she tried to talk the doctor into inducing labor a few weeks early—which he refused to do. The intended mothers were constantly worried about their surrogates' behavior, even though they or their husbands were in frequent and good contact with the surrogate throughout the pregnancy.

Hormones were regarded as dangerous not only because they connected "mother" and baby but also because they were thought to make surrogates overly "capricious." The Russian term *kapriznyj* was often used when speaking about surrogates. It denotes being unpredictable, unreasonable, somehow out of control, and behaving in inappropriate ways, and thus has negative and disrespectful connotations. Illustrating what she meant by *kapriznyj*, Kyiv-based agent Larissa Osipovna explained that the hormone medicine could make the surrogate "very emotional—she cries, she laughs, she has fears, she has doubts and everything." Women could, consequently, behave in "not such good ways," for instance asking for additional money. Doctors, agents, intended parents, and surrogates joined hands in upholding this discourse about the hormonal body. Some surrogates embraced "hormone-talk" because it enabled them to make sense of their bodies' affective responses and of what they perceived as the "emotional rollercoaster" of surrogate pregnancy.

Some women also opposed the image of the capricious surrogate. Polina Davidovna, for instance, a surrogacy candidate from the Russian city of Penza, claimed: "We are not capricious, as Natasha Sergeyevna says, we just offer our point of view, we ask for additional help. If they (i.e., the parents) don't want to help, then fine, but we should be allowed to ask." She was the only surrogacy candidate during my time at Altra Vita who openly resisted being reduced to an irrational body and started expressing her wishes and expectations toward the clinic. From their perspective, she was probably not seen as the *adekvatnaya* and easily controllable woman they were looking for, and it would not surprise me if this was why—after her first embryo transfer failed—I never saw her again.

Polina took the view that pregnant women should have certain privileges and that if couples opted for surrogacy, they needed to take on more responsibility for the women who carried their children. Among other things, she was very unhappy about the food the surrogates received from the clinic. "I am *very* picky about food," she stated. "I will not eat just anything that falls into my hands." While vehemently rejecting the notion that surrogates were generally irrational, she supported the idea that pregnant bodies could express irrational cravings. She emphasized that "pregnant women have their own tastes—suddenly, in the middle of the night, they want strawberries! Or pickled gherkins! Or fish!" Such cravings were a common topic of discussion. Intended mother Vera Romanovna told me how her friend—the "instructor"—had spent entire nights cooking special soups and then driving across the city to satisfy her surrogate's culinary desires—which were often thought to reflect those of the child. While some intended mothers perceived these moments as opportunities to participate in the pregnancy, others devalued such behavior as unnecessary "capriciousness."

The adjective *kapriznyj* is a word that in everyday language is commonly attributed to children, and various discourses and practices in the field of surrogacy reflected that surrogates were often infantilized—for instance by the frequent use of the diminutive *surr-mamochka* rather than *surr-mama* or by speaking of them as *devochki* (the term for little girls) rather than *devushki* (the term for young women). Moreover, agency and clinic staff often took the liberty of commenting on some surrogates' and egg sellers' maturity in relation to how they spent their salary. One of the doctors said this question depended on the "level of intelligence," and with a laugh he told me about one woman who had sold her eggs to get hair extensions. And Natasha Sergeyevna shook her head at Katya Yefimovna, who—after completing the surrogacy program—decided to buy a golden retriever. Investing the money earned from surrogacy into housing, education, or medical expenses was regarded as a more responsible form of spending.

Agencies as Buffer and Protection

The constant worries and fears about capricious, entrepreneurial, abusive, overly affective surrogates were heavily circulated and instrumentalized by agencies. Often, agency websites contained passages on the dangers of direct arrangements. Similarly, in my interviews agency staff usually judged close contact between both sides as not only dangerous but also "bad" or "unnecessary." Agencies based their legitimacy on such narratives, foregrounding their expertise in selecting the "right" surrogates and protecting both sides from each other. They thus significantly shaped a moral economy that established tight control of the surrogates as a moral practice, while capitalizing on claims that they could reduce the risks and uncertainties associated with surrogacy and the surrogate. They did so not only by performing the elaborate psychological examinations mentioned above but also by restricting and mediating contact between the two parties. In mediated arrangements, agencies therefore play a crucial role in shaping the possible relationships between intended parents and surrogates. This has been particularly well documented in the case of transnational arrangements, in which the two parties often lack a common language of communication, which increases the dependence on intermediaries (Deomampo 2016; Lustenberger 2016; Majumdar 2017; Whittaker 2019).

The agencies I encountered often presented themselves as a "buffer" and "protection" for both sides but slightly more for the intended parents, because they were "psychologically in the weaker position" (Konstantin Pavlovich) and because they were the paying clients—a factor that was, however, often not explicitly mentioned. Masha Arkadyevna, the former surrogate and now agency owner, stressed that

> With us, the surrogates are under control from A to Z. [. . .] When the pregnancy sets in, we literally put them in the car and drive them to the doctor's and then drive them back home. Because there is always this, you know, "You have to go to the doctor today"—"Oh, I overslept," or "I'm not in the mood," or "Let's do it tomorrow." So there are constantly these nuances. [. . .] Basically, you just have to take every girl by the hand. So we don't ask, "Are you responsible?"; we just take them."

Hinting at the "capricious" character of pregnant women, Masha's quote exemplifies the all-encompassing control the agencies exercised over the surrogate body, coupling it to an image of surrogates as little girls who had to be taken by the hand. She cast these women (and their pregnancies) as "risky," since one never knew whether they would reliably take their medication or go to the doctor's appointments. This was also reflected in my interviews with Spanish agencies that cooperated with clinics in Russia and Ukraine. Ricardo Delmonte, for instance, got very upset about intended parents who wanted to complete the process without an agency, so in a direct, nonsupervised arrangement: "A woman who is pregnant and *over-hormonated* (*sobre-hormonada*) is *carrying* an embryo that is *not hers*. [. . .] Forget it! Doing this freestyle is crazy!" he said, hitting his office table. Then he continued:

> It's *crazy* (laughs). Because this woman can do whatever, you never know what kind of nonsense (*barbaridad*) she will come up with. This is a situation in which there needs to be constant control, support, accompaniment, and *monitoring* [by an agency]. You can't give a woman so many hormones (*sobre-hormonar*) then say "Bye, I'm *leaving*. I'll give you a *call*." (laughs) This is really crazy.

I was surprised that Spanish intermediaries such as Ricardo Delmonte made similar statements about the supposedly unpredictable surrogates as their Russian and Ukrainian counterparts. The former were eager to emphasize how "affectionate" and "wonderful" the surrogates were, but then suddenly associated these women with rather different characteristics when it came to the issue of how to regulate contact—a dynamic I also encountered in my interview with another Spanish intermediary. Álvaro Fuentes emphasized that they could not allow direct communication, "because you never know what this person is capable of doing (*hasta donde puede llegar*)." While he did support that the two parties should know each other, contact should only take place "under the watchful eye of caretakers (*cuidadores*)," who would "ensure that things take place in an orderly way, so that this person cannot gain immediate access [to the intended parents]." He implied that "this person" might abuse any brief moment of inattention for her own purposes. The surrogate could commit some kind of "nonsense" at any point, because "you never know what this person is capable of doing," and because "the parents feel vulnerable," as Álvaro Fuentes added. Therefore, he stressed, control and mediated contact were absolutely necessary.

Restricting contact was an important measure not only during the pregnancy but also afterward. For this reason, Konstantin Pavlovich's agency recommended no contact at all:

> You know, life can be quite long.... We are sure our surrogate mothers understand that they are doing a good deed, that they give great happiness to these parents, and that for this hard task they receive well-deserved compensation that they could not earn through any other activity. But what about in three years? What will cross her mind? There are no guarantees. And we can't guarantee that in three years she won't stand on your porch and say: "Let me see my child." We can't guarantee that she won't suddenly develop motherly feelings or that she won't blackmail the parents because she ran out of money again.... To avoid these things the surrogate mother doesn't know whose baby she's carrying and the parents don't know who their surrogate mother is. When the program finishes, they both receive what they wanted from each other and they can go their separate ways again.

Konstantin Pavlovich's quote also reflects how agencies cast their role as crucial in protecting the intended parents from the unpredictable consequences of direct contact that might set in even years after the program has been completed. Even though at that point former surrogates were surely no longer "over-hormonated," Konstantin Pavlovich still constructed them as unpredictable and opportunistic, suggesting no or only mediated contact. But intended parents also needed to be protected from less serious situations. Agent Larissa Osipovna explained that when she was approached by the kind of "very emotional" woman who behaved in "not such good ways" by asking for additional money, food products, and the like, she usually told the client: "Look, her behavior is a bit inappropriate because she is pregnant, but don't worry, we will handle it." Or she did not tell them at all, because "they are stressed enough" anyway. Another Ukrainian agent, Anastasia Anatolyevna, articulated a similar issue when mentioning that "hormonal outbursts" were to be expected from a pregnant surrogate: "She can be really worried for some reason and get wound up and then two hours later she can say: 'Oh, sorry, something happened with me (laughs); I don't know, I had a hormonal fit.'" Intended parents would get too emotionally drawn in by such outbursts, but as an agency it was easier to deal with these situations. Agencies "take out these emotional elements," one of the agents said, by positioning themselves between the entrepreneurial and hormonal surrogates, and the emotionally strained and vulnerable intended parents.

Agencies had different takes on how much contact to recommend. While Konstantin Pavlovich's agency seemed rather strict in their no-contact rule, others allowed contact but recommended it only once the critical phase of the first twelve weeks had passed. They suggested that there was no point in getting to know each other earlier, because it was uncertain whether things would work out well. One of the Spanish agents, Lorenzo Rivera, said that it was easier this way, because once both sides knew each other, affection (*cariño*) might develop and then the process of changing the surrogate would be more "painful" (see also Rudrappa 2016a, 138–39). This approach to handling contact was also reflected in the wishes of some intended parents. Spanish intended mother Marta Pérez, for instance, being at the beginning of the surrogacy process, said that she had so far not met her Ukrainian surrogate, "because there hasn't been a pregnancy yet, so logically there is no reason to do it, you know?" Marta deemed it "logical" that both sides would only meet once their "collaboration" was confirmed, rather than merely anticipated.

Protecting the intended parents from the surrogate meant that the former could usually choose and regulate the amount of contact they wanted, while the latter had to accept their decisions. In one of the agencies, for instance, intended parents were given the chance to get to know the surrogate surreptitiously, as the agent told me with a complicit smile. When the surrogate came to the clinic, she could point her out for the parents, without her noticing. For around 30 percent of the intended parents this was a soothing option, because they did not want to officially meet the surrogate but just reassure themselves that she was not some "clochard" from the street. The agent added that most parents, though, were just interested in the "result" (the child) and not whether the surrogate was "fat, thin, intelligent, stupid, or where she comes from." They did not want to see the surrogate, because then they would always have her image in their head.

Agents actively contributed to a victim discourse based on the vulnerable position of intended parents, particularly the mother. As one of the lawyers, Maksim Antonov, explained:

> These women (i.e., intended mothers) come here physically and psychologically exhausted. They have been through a lot of suffering, many failed attempts at getting pregnant. Of course it is not so easy for them to see a young and blooming woman bearing their children. [...] She is like a direct competitor.

This competitive situation could also be one reason for the absence of surrogates in the intended mothers' accounts. As Sharmila Rudrappa (2016a) has shown in her research on surrogacy in India, the position of the surrogate was threatening to the intended parents and their claim to the child—she thus had to remain a "nonperson." Understanding the surrogate as only one of many "elements in the cure for infertility," as Ukrainian agent Sergej Petrovich said, it became less important what kind of person she might be or what kind of relationship one might want to have with her. My interviews with surrogacy agents also underlined how they normalized the distant or absent relationship between intended parents and surrogate by referring to the aspect of vulnerability as well as by claiming that this corresponded to the intended parents' wishes. One agency employee, for instance, stated that foreign parents had the opportunity to talk to their surrogates via Skype but that "nobody wanted that." Most parents only met the surrogate when picking up their child from the birth clinic. When I asked whether parents were not curious to know more, she said: "Well, they *know* all the basic information. And they see a photo in the database. So I guess that's enough for them."

In arrangements where both parties had direct contact, the weak position intended parents saw themselves in could also make them overprotective or overcontrolling, wanting to intervene too much in the surrogates' daily lives. Many surrogates were well aware of these dangers, and some had already had bad experiences. One of the women told me about a private arrangement with an intended mother who wanted her to stay in her flat in Moscow for the period between the embryo transfer and the pregnancy test. During these two weeks, she had not been allowed to leave the bed, not even in order to go to the bathroom, because the intended mother feared that the embryo might slide out of the surrogate's womb. Most of the women who worked through agencies stated that they were afraid of private arrangements for exactly these reasons.

Agencies not only shaped a discourse that constructed (close) contact as potentially harmful for both sides but often presented this as the surrogates' and intended parents' own wish. Larissa Osipovna, for instance, summarized the attitude of most surrogates as: "I am doing this job for you and I'll take care of the baby in my belly but then I will give it to you, you give me the compensation, and we are done." While this statement certainly corresponded to the attitude of some surrogates, agencies actively created and nurtured this wish. This was particularly well illustrated when Konstantin Pavlovich explained how most intended parents initially wished to meet the surrogates, but he would explain why contact was not recommended and "usually, after that they no longer want to." Several surrogates told me that they only met their intended parents upon giving birth and that these moments revealed that both sides had wanted to "share" the pregnancy with each other but that the intended parents were discouraged by the agency. Considering this, I developed a certain caution regarding agency statements about what kind of contact intended parents and surrogates usually wanted with each other, especially after two women working in the same agency made very different statements: while Larissa Osipovna told me that there was usually no contact between the surrogates and the intended parents, another employee mentioned that relationships could be so intimate that the two women sometimes even asked to stay in the same room after the delivery of the child. Larissa Osipovna's claim could be seen as an attempt to legitimize the more anonymous form of surrogacy by presenting it as a reflection of the intended parents' and the surrogates' wishes. Shaping contact in such a way facilitated the work of agencies and clinics. They could monopolize information and strengthen their own position by circulating fears and referring to their authority as neutral and experienced entities in a reproductive marketplace, where hidden dangers were lurking in many places.

"The Best Motivation Is Money—for Both Sides"

Despite the fact that surrogacy agencies were very successful in constructing an image of themselves as indispensable, the Russian intended mothers and numerous surrogates in my research had opted for so-called direct surrogacy arrangements. These intended mothers either could not afford the expensive agencies, did not see their added value, or did not trust them. Two of them had initially been to an agency but then left again, because the agent tried to talk them into expensive procedures they did not want—conducting the IVF procedure in the Czech Republic or Spain, organizing the birth in an EU country, or hiring a U.S.-American surrogate. Trust was a big issue for the intended mothers. "How can I trust an agent? This is a complete stranger," said Alisa Serafimovna, now mother of three children. She considered it much better to accompany and control the surrogate herself. Agencies were firms for "big businessmen," who wanted a ready-made child. "But whether this will really be your child remains an open question": Alisa suggested that agencies wanted positive results and money and might take measures such as exchanging embryos "without batting an eyelid." "This is why I decided to take control, to look [for a surrogate] myself, and to be sure that it (i.e., the child) is really mine." Her fears were not entirely ungrounded, as was proven by the case of *Paradiso and Campanelli v. Italy*, which was brought to the European Court of Human Rights in 2012—the case of an Italian couple who lost custody over the child that a Russian surrogate had gestated for them but that turned out to be genetically unrelated to both of them.[2] Other intended mothers also voiced concerns about the moral integrity of private agencies and clinics in relation to genetic material. Olessia Valeryevna, who had completed a surrogacy program including an egg donation, told me that her clinic had offered her the remaining egg cells of a woman who had successfully undergone IVF treatment. She gratefully accepted, because using these highly promising oocytes meant she could increase her surrogate's chances of getting pregnant, while saving on the costs of an egg donation. Although even then she knew that this particular woman had in no way been consulted about the further use of her oocytes, Olessia had only much later realized how problematic this offer had been and was relieved that in the end the embryo transfers with the uninformed "donor's" oocytes did not result in a pregnancy.

Intended parents who opted for direct arrangements could not resort to the same measures as clinics and agencies when selecting and controlling surrogates. They did not have an institution backing them and had to rely much more on the surrogates' self-governance. In the cases of the Russian intended mothers I spoke with, this control was achieved primarily through the economically unequal position of the surrogates. Acknowledging that surrogacy was an emotionally challenging process for the gestating woman, Alisa stated that surrogates had to be "very strong" and "really have to know what they want"—and this should be money. While many doctors and agents also foregrounded the benefits of having financially motivated surrogates, the intended mothers were much more explicit that this was the single most important aspect when choosing a surrogate. "The best motivation is money—for both sides," Olessia stated: For the surrogate, because it would be easier for her to give away the child when she received something material in return, especially when she already had a concrete aim from the beginning. And for the intended parents, because they had the security that she would fulfil her duties and not get distracted by emotions:

> For me, it was important that this is a business project for her. [. . .]. Because help, so-called charity, when someone helps someone else— this is very dangerous. [. . .] Well, you never know what will happen

during pregnancy. One compact progesterone [pill]. Well. [. . .] You never know what will cross her mind. That means, a person who is generally, let's say, at the beginning, a strong altruist, you understand, suddenly these altruistic thoughts turn to the child.

Olessia seemed to suggest that if a woman was generally altruistic, then her feelings could easily shift and attach to the child. Pregnancy was an unpredictable state in her eyes, and there were no guarantees what a woman on progesterone might come up with, so it was better not to take the risk. Galya Yanovna implied similar dangers, when she mentioned that she could only be sure the surrogate would *not* want her child if it was clear that the latter perceived what she was doing as work and wanted money for that work.

Olessia's and Galya's statements reflected a conflation between altruism—or, so it seemed to me, the surrogate more generally having feelings—and wanting to keep the child. This conflation had another consequence, which became apparent in Alisa's account when she said that "when it is money that is in first place for the *surr-mamochka*, then the *bio-mama* is lucky." When there were other motivations, then "it is very difficult to take the child." She later repeated that "one really needs to motivate this with money," stating that she thought it would be easier that way for the surrogate—"that emotionally, in the soul there will be peace. I gave him away, but I got something in return." Alisa's words imply that giving the baby away is an emotionally difficult process and that the surrogate would feel better if she benefited materially. In addition, it became clear that she herself would also feel better. Mentioning that otherwise "it is very difficult to take the child," she suggested that she might feel like she was taking the child *away*. If the surrogate was mainly interested in the money, however, she could take the child, pay the money, and regard this compensation as concluding the relationship with no remaining obligations.

Overall, as opposed to most intermediaries and doctors, the intended mothers did not make surrogacy sound easy, and they seemed aware that the body was not a machine that could be manipulated in all sorts of ways. They recognized that surrogacy was an emotionally challenging endeavor and stressed that only women who were financially so dependent on the salary that they would not be able to get distracted by these emotional challenges could—and should—become surrogates. The intended mothers' mistrust of the surrogates translated into control through financial promises and grounding this control in the surrogates' precarious situation. This was also illustrated when Rita Tikhonovna recounted her quest for a surrogate worker. She was very articulate about Ukrainian women being the best and most "professional" surrogates. Rita praised them for fulfilling all demands without asking unnecessary questions.

They "*sold* themselves really well, so that you really wanted them," trying to convince the intended parents by adapting to any wishes. Unfortunately, they were also the most expensive surrogates, she said, and suggested that they had strategies for deliberately driving up the price—a statement that contradicted the observation the Russian surrogate Raya Antonovna had made that Ukrainians drove down prices by agreeing to "bad offers." Raya was originally one of Rita's candidates. They had met via Meddesk and had immediately become close friends. The embryo transfer, however, was not successful, and they had given up their mutual endeavor. Both spoke of each other in very affectionate terms. At the time of our interviews, they were still in close contact and regularly updated each other on their pregnancies. Rita's account of looking for a surrogate struck me as particularly intriguing, because of her tender way of speaking about Raya as a friend and equal, while simultaneously portraying surrogates in general in a highly derogatory way. This was evident in how she compared Ukrainian surrogates who knew "everything" about the surrogacy process and understood very well when to take which medications and to do which examinations with Russian surrogates:

> "Oh, I forgot to take the pills! Oh, I don't want to [take the pills]; they give me a headache." Yes, I understand that your head aches but this is your job. [. . .] you get paid for this. And here (i.e., in Russia), there appears to be a lot of "I forgot," "I don't want," "I won't." That is, it's like in kindergarten.

The notion of the kindergarten, again, infantilized the surrogates and emphasized their capricious and unreliable character. Framing surrogates' behavior in this way—their not wanting to take specific pills, because they caused a headache—could discredit it as either irrelevant or something they had to put up with for the salary rather than a health concern to be taken seriously.

Rita Tikhonovna would have preferred to work with a Ukrainian woman, but her husband was too concerned about the political situation in Ukraine at the time and Rita agreed that it might be too risky: "Well, I would be very worried that my belly is somewhere else and about what is happening to it," she said with a laugh, suggesting that this part of the surrogate's body had already become her property. What Rita described as "professional" seemed to instead reflect compliant behavior based on economic inequality. Ukrainian women had a more difficult position in the Russian surrogacy market, especially since the conflict between the two countries had broken out and an economic crisis hit their country. Rita said that "doing it business-style" was very comfortable for her, because "I know what I am paying for." And being the one who pays gave her the power to ensure that the surrogate would comply with her demands. After all, "it was her job." As previously mentioned, such an approach based on self-interest and economic inequality has become somewhat accepted in post-Soviet Russia, even when at the expense of others (Swader and Obelene 2015; Swader et al. 2013) whose abilities positioned them at the lower end of the power spectrum (see also Iarskaia-Smirnova and Romanov 2012; Trubina 2012; Walker 2012). The biopolitics of motherhood is thus inextricably bound to the rise of a bioeconomy that reflected—and to a certain degree "solved"—broader biopolitical concerns, not least by turning patients into consumers (Rose 2007; Schurr 2017). From this perspective, then, it was not surprising that Rita expected a surrogate to comply with her demands as she was the one who was paying.

Surrogates, particularly those in direct arrangements, often criticized such an "I pay, you do" attitude. Masha Arkadyevna, for instance, the surrogate-turned-agent, said that generally many things had changed since she entered the sphere of surrogacy in 2003. In those early days, relationships were more personal, while now carrying somebody else's child had much in common with working on an "assembly line"—a comparison that resonates with the way agents and doctors pictured surrogates as uniform, standardized workers.

Despite the fact that some surrogates had serious reservations about the way the reproductive market worked, time and again it was evident that the prospect of earning money made them compliant workers. One such instance was when I spoke with Lena Mironovna about her surrogacy contract. Having studied law herself, she explained that a closer inspection of the contract she had signed revealed a number of ambiguities. It was not always clear in the contract how "difficult situations" would be solved, but this was, according to Lena, generally a common way of handling such situations in Russia—"If there *is* a problem, we'll *talk* about the problem," she said and laughed. Things were usually not discussed in advance but only once the problem had surfaced. "They don't want to scare you unnecessarily in advance," she added—a statement that resonated with the complications I describe in chapter 7. Lena said she would like to change many things in the contract, but when I asked her whether she was concerned about the contract's ambiguities she shrugged her shoulders and said no—"I'm interested in the sum that's written there, that's all," she said with another laugh. I often encountered a kind of indifference in the surrogates' accounts about their contracts and working conditions. Some even clearly stated that they would comply with any and all demands, because they "had no choice." Such statements were mainly made by women working through agencies and clearly reflected their financially precarious status, as they realized they were not in a position to make big demands.

Cutting Ties, Erasing Traces

The conceptualization of surrogacy as work in Russia and Ukraine can only be understood by considering the broader context in which surrogacy is embedded. This context is marked by a certain normalization of economic inequalities and commodified intimacies, by an atmosphere of suspicion and fear, the imperative of motherhood, and a political climate of religious conservativism. This setting gives rise to the image of the vulnerable intended mother as opposed to the dangerous, entrepreneurial surrogate, who needs to be subjected to strict control. While the economic imbalance between surrogate and intended parents is apparent, it is the former who is perceived as more powerful in other ways—she is the one who is fertile and who can gestate a child (Ragoné 1994), who can therefore influence the development of the pregnancy. Worries about surrogates acting in inappropriate and selfish ways are nurtured by agencies that strongly advocate an anonymous form of surrogacy, in which the two sides do not know or have no direct contact with each other. In seeking maximum security in a process marked by manifold uncertainties, intended parents, agents, and doctors alike prefer surrogates who demonstrate a clear financial interest and who cannot afford to make demands, risk the pregnancy, or keep the child upon birth. The selection of surrogates and the entire surrogacy process are therefore organized in such a way as to contain them in a clinical setting and prevent emotional entanglements, making it easier to control the surrogate bodies. The excessive preoccupation with preventing emotional entanglements often led to conflating different kinds of emotions and affects, as my interviews with the intended mothers made clear; they suggested that a surrogate's altruistic feelings could easily attach to the child, making her not want to relinquish it. Agent Larissa Osipovna also stated that the only alternative to a "materialistic" approach would be that the surrogate developed feelings for the child and would then cry for "nights and nights because the baby is not with her." This conflation contributed to organizing surrogacy as if it were a sphere of pure economic exchange, free of affects and emotions. Besides enabling tighter control over the surrogate body, the "neat" business relationship had another, less emphasized, advantage from the perspective of the intended parents: as has been argued in relation to surrogacy arrangements elsewhere (Lustenberger 2016; Rudrappa 2016a), it enabled intended parents to eventually "close" the chapter of surrogacy, with no strings attached. Larissa Osipovna, again, found fitting words:

> When I give you the baby and I don't receive anything from you in exchange, how would you feel? . . . Just think about it. How would it feel? You will feel indebted. Always. . . . You will feel indebted. I don't

remember who said this or wrote this, but every favor should be returned. Otherwise you will feel like you owe something to that person.

Unintentionally evoking Marcel Mauss's famous elaboration on "the gift," Larissa Osipovna implied that the process of surrogacy could not come to an end if a feeling of indebtedness remained. "To give something is to give a part of oneself," Mauss (1966, 10) argued, and through this a lasting bond is created. Gifts are inextricably bound to their givers; they are "akin to persons" and thus constitute a "continual reminder of the need for reciprocation" (Tsing 2013, 22). To avoid such a reminder, the surrogacy process must be commodified. The agent's statement that one needed to "take out these emotional elements" can be read as reflecting Anna Tsing's claim that in order to alienate the "producer" from the "product" one needed to take "the gift out of the commodity" (21). This, she writes, is not an easy process and necessitates a kind of labor that is done over and over again. Educating surrogates and others into an understanding of surrogacy as a process of "giving access" to one's body can thus be seen as enabling this alienation, because the work it implies often remains unrecognized (Waldby and Cooper 2008, 59) and, thus, invisible. Also the anonymous form of surrogacy propagated by the agencies played an important role in the process of alienation—when intended parents and surrogates remained intimate strangers to each other, the contractual relationship could be upheld more easily. By reducing surrogacy to a form of mechanical work, the person and the personal become marginal, which was exemplified in the way agents and doctors spoke about the "perfect surrogate" in standardized terms, as only "an element in the cure for infertility." Payment could conclude the process and disrupt the otherwise ongoing commitment between the two parties—which primarily concerned the remaining commitment of the intended parents toward the surrogate. In the exchange, the baby and the money balanced each other out: "If the surrogate does it only because of the money, then yes, the baby and the money, the exchange, and that's it," one agent commented, using her hands to signal weighing exactly this balance. Commodities, as opposed to gifts, are "disengaged from their makers [. . .] and once exchanged, the exchange, and the steps that led to it, can be forgotten" (Tsing 2013, 22). The opportunity to "forget" was broadly welcomed by many intended parents—and surrogates—not just within Russia and Ukraine. Despite the fact that the foreign couples who traveled to these countries for surrogacy voiced the desire to move beyond a commercial relationship with the surrogate, the way agents stressed that the surrogates regarded what they were doing as "work" relieved the intended parents of the moral obligation to maintain contact after delivery. This point is also quite evident in research on surrogacy in India. Some of the U.S.-American couples interviewed by Rudrappa

(2016a), for instance, preferred surrogacy in India to the United States, because they wanted an arrangement that would not result in lasting relations; and the Israeli gay couples interviewed by Sibylle Lustenberger (2016) opted for India not least because they wanted to form a family in a "normative" way, not by including the surrogate in their kin network. Also the Russian intended mothers I spoke with wanted to form a traditional nuclear family. Furthermore, in a social setting that did not allow the surrogate to become part of their family biographies, it was almost a prerogative to cut ties between intended mothers and surrogates. To recall one of Olessia Valeryevna's statements: "This is a closed topic. And this is also why it was better to end the relationship with the surrogate mother. Because . . . how would I explain her to my child?" It was too risky for the intended parents to recognize the surrogates as more than mere workers.

The way surrogacy was conceptualized as paid work thus functioned as a tool of power to control the surrogate body and to draw a clear line after the surrogacy process. It facilitates "detaching" the surrogate *from* the child and "attaching" the parents *to* the child (Schurr and Militz 2018). Moreover, the framing of this work as mechanical or as merely "giving access" (Waldby and Cooper 2008, 59) meant that the surrogates' *active* contributions can be concealed and they can be—retrospectively—erased from the process, and any claims the surrogates might have are delegitimized by the exchange character of surrogacy. From the perspective of the intended parents, this tool of power is framed as an ethical instrument, as their social vulnerability restricts the kinds of relationships that can evolve between intended parents and surrogates. Not being able to integrate the surrogacy in the lives of the children, "doing it business-style" can be read as ethical labor performed to reproduce the norms of family-building as well as coming to terms with the multiple uncertainties surrogacy and infertility entail. "Quid pro quo" enables "closing" and forgetting the chapter of surrogacy after the long-desired child has been born.

5

TECHNOLOGIES OF ALIGNMENT

"More than half of the surrogates don't want to give away the child after birth, independent of what is written in the contract. Some even disappear with it. This woman carries the child for nine months, of course she develops a bond! That's only natural," Tatyana Vasilyevna, the embryologist-turned-gallerist explained to me when I interviewed her in her small art gallery in Moscow city center. Any "normal woman" would develop this kind of maternal instinct during the pregnancy, she continued. After all, it was women's nature to be nurturing and caring.

My own findings differed significantly from those of Tatyana Vasilyevna. While scandal stories quickly make their way into the media and the agencies' narratives, they remain the exception. Rather than reflecting the experiences of surrogate workers, I suggest that her words reveal powerful imaginaries that dominate public discourse about pregnancy in and beyond Russia. It is the imaginary of children as "happy objects" (Ahmed 2010), as objects to which happiness "sticks" in a way that would inevitably leave surrogates unhappy and desperate if this happiness were taken from them. Like Tatyana Vasilyevna, many people socialized in Western countries believe in the inevitable power of affective bonding between child and gestating woman. Women in particular tend to judge surrogacy by referring to their own experiences of pregnancy, suggesting that resistance to such a strong, "natural" feeling would unquestionably be emotionally damaging (Dow 2015, 15). However, feminists and other scholars from a wide range of disciplines have long "troubled" the supposedly natural qualities of human bodies and shown how these are socially produced and serve to justify specific (patriarchal) orders (Butler 2015; Fausto-Sterling 2000; Fine 2017;

Lock 2001; Roberts 2007). In line with this argument, Elly Teman (2008) makes a plea for acknowledging that the contingencies of bonding are related to social and economic factors such as poverty and life expectancy—reflecting different "reproductive strategies" (Scheper-Hughes 1985)—as well as to a conscious decision that women take. Teman insists on moving beyond supposedly natural categories and instead investigating how surrogates "maneuver within these cultural assumptions and preserve their social identities as 'normal' women and as 'good mothers' while involved in a process that threatens to cast them as 'other'" (2008, 1110).

Making this the aim of this chapter, I shift the focus from discourses and practices of external control (explored in the previous two chapters) to the ways in which surrogate workers engage in a form of internal control that I call "technologies of alignment." These form part of the "emotional labor" (Hochschild 2003) surrogates fulfill, and are expected to fulfill, in order to find the right balance between care and distance toward the child they carry, without "falling victim" to their hormonal bodies. Hochschild adds the dimension of emotional labor to other forms of labor that are performed for commercial reasons, such as physical and mental labor. She describes emotional labor as the conscious display of emotions oriented toward others and/or the "transmutation" of emotion work (the effort to actively change an emotion in degree or quality on the inside) into the commercial realm (Hochschild 2003, 19).[1] In the following, I focus on the second aspect. I explore how surrogates come to align their selves with the "feeling rules"—the often subtle social guidelines that influence how we want to feel or how we think we should feel (Hochschild 2003, 18)—of a moral economy of surrogacy that demands that they be effective but not affective workers.

Referring to the surrogates' emotional labor as "technologies of alignment," I lean on Foucault's notion of "technologies of the self," through which the subject "constitutes itself in an active fashion" (1997, 291) and conducts "a certain number of operations on their bodies and souls, thoughts, conduct, and way of being" (225) in order to reach a particular state. Technologies of alignment speak of the simultaneity of subjugation and freedom so prominent in Foucault's writing on subjectivity. His focus on how specific subjects come into being—rather than being simply "out there"—adds an important dimension to Hochschild's work, whose theories seem to imply an inner self that is authentic and entirely private.

Surrogacy research has shown that technologies of the self and emotional labor—even if not always named as such—are crucial elements in surrogacy and that they are highly dependent on how the practice itself and the role of the surrogate are understood and morally legitimized (e.g., Berend 2016; Jacobson 2016; Pande 2014; Vora 2009). Feeling rules can thus differ widely, depending on regionally and culturally specific norms and values. As the previous chapters have shown, in Russia and Ukraine, these feeling rules are primarily shaped by the imperative to be an effective rather affective worker, and for the surrogacy relationship to be an economic rather than emotional one. Taking this imperative into consideration, this chapter explores how surrogates negotiate and grapple with different social, medical, and surrogacy-internal "truths" about the pregnant body and shape their own understandings of their surrogate pregnancies, particularly at the critical moments of deciding for surrogacy and at the end of their pregnancies. I show how the women oscillate between different "modes of subjection" (Foucault 1990, 1997), strategically essentializing their bodies in order to make sense of their position and experience as surrogates and as "normal" women; their emotional labor can thus be seen as a form of ethical labor, as the surrogates are eager to emphasize that they are not immoral, "unnatural" women who sell their "own" children. Essentializing discourses, however, represent a double-edged sword: While offering soothing explanations in moments of affective turmoil, the same discourse is used as a powerful tool of control and conceals the inherent power disparities surrogacy entails by psychologizing and internalizing emotions and affects. Moreover, while the surrogates worked on "dis-emotionalizing" their pregnancies, trying to keep the economic and the intimate or affective apart, this separation could collapse in critical moments such as giving birth, as the accounts of Katya Yefimovna and Lena Mironovna will show.

The Emotional Labor of *Nastraivat'sya*

Many of the women in my research indicated that their decision to become a surrogate involved a process of inner *alignment*. They often used the Russian verb *nastraivat'sya*, synonymous with "getting" or "being prepared," when speaking about this process. According to the *Oxford Concise Russian Dictionary* the term can be translated as "to dispose oneself to" or "to make up one's mind" about something. But *nastraivat'sya* is also the passive or reflexive form of the verb *nastraivat'*, which can mean to "align," "at/tune," or "configure" something.[2] Thinking about surrogacy, the translation of "aligning oneself" seems most suitable as it implies the technical aspect of bringing oneself into the right mode to follow a clear line or path, as one of the doctors I interviewed indicated. Moreover, it is a term often used in business to describe strategies for achieving conformity among employees.

The surrogate workers described this process of alignment in very different terms. In fact, for some, it was not even a process but rather an effortless and technical moment, as became clear in the following statement by Zhenya Pavlovna:

"Even if I strongly oppose something, all I need is a certain push to change my mind. I can go beyond anything if the material incentive is high enough. You just need to prepare yourself emotionally. It happens on the inside. It's like a switch."

By referring to a "switch," she emphasized that "inside" she was adaptable to the circumstances of her life. Six years ago, she would have felt offended had somebody suggested she do surrogacy, but now—at twenty-nine years old—the situation had changed. The material incentive gave her the "certain push" she needed to flick the "switch" and agree to the embryo transfer that had been conducted a few hours before our conversation. Zhenya never had strong maternal feelings for her own two children and thus anticipated no emotional challenges in the surrogacy process. Other surrogates mentioned longer processes of reflection, at the end of which they came to "understand" what surrogacy was about, felt "emotionally prepared," and had "aligned themselves" properly. Their main concern in this respect was the question of whether they would be able to keep the necessary emotional distance from the child. Marina Nikitichna, for instance, a Moldavian woman living in Moscow with her husband and nine-year-old child, stated that it took her over a year to decide to become a surrogate: "At the beginning I was against surrogacy, of course. For me, a child is holy. How can you carry it and then *give it away*? It was difficult for me to understand that." She immediately rejected the clinic's offer to become a surrogate after having sold her eggs seven times. But the idea stayed with her, and over the course of a year she read articles, blogs, and online forums and came to *understand* what surrogacy was really about. The research made her realize that "the child is *not mine*, it's *chuzhoj*," that she would not be like a mother because she would not be genetically related to the child. In the context of such statements, women often used the Russian adjective *chuzhoj*, which can be translated as "alien," "strange," "other," "not of me," or "somebody else's" (terms that, however, do not fully grasp the meaning of the Russian expression).

Foregrounding a lack of genetic connection is not unique to the context I studied. In the United States, for instance, the move from traditional (where surrogates were also egg providers) to gestational surrogacy also marked the introduction of an emphasis on genetics (Jacobson 2016)—even though the notion of intent (i.e., of wanting a child and initiating a surrogacy program) remains central to how surrogates conceptualize the children as belonging to the intended parents and not to them (Berend 2016; Ziff 2020). In her research with traditional and gestational surrogates in the late 1980s and 1990s, Helena Ragoné (1994) even showed how women who were gestational and then traditional surrogates would shift from emphasizing genetics during their first pregnancy to intent during the second. This reflects a certain situational flexibility as to how belonging and kinship are constituted in the context of surrogacy. Despite this flexibility, however, an emphasis on nonrelatedness is crucial to U.S.-American surrogates, just as it was for the surrogates in my own research.

In Russia and Ukraine, where "grammars of kinship" (Gunnarsson Payne 2016) revolve around genetics, emphasizing that the child was *chuzhoj* allowed surrogates to repudiate the common accusation that they were mothers selling their own children. In Russia, this perception was not only linked to the widespread misunderstanding that surrogates were the genetic mothers of the children they carried but also to assumptions such as Tatyana Vasilyevna's cited at the beginning of this chapter—assumptions about the "quasi holy" link between woman and baby, thus making the surrogate carrier a bad woman or mother. Marina Nikitichna, however, emphasized that she was not giving away "her" child. Instead, she saw herself as a nanny—a reassuring metaphor she had encountered on a talk show. Having worked as a nanny before, she figured surrogacy was a comparable activity, except that she would be taking care of an unborn child, a child inside her. Intrigued by the long process of detailed research she went through, I suggested that it must have been a difficult decision. "No, I wouldn't say it was a difficult decision," she stated with a confident smile. "I just had to find the right words. I found the right words, right for myself, and then . . . I made the decision."

Metaphors such as the "nanny" seemed of central importance for the surrogates in "finding the right words" to describe their role in the process of surrogacy. As opposed to Indian and Thai surrogates who also did not regard themselves as mothers but claimed other forms of kinship due to shared bodily substances and gestation (Majumdar 2017; Pande 2009; Whittaker 2019), my research participants—surrogates and others—were very vocal about sharing absolutely *nothing* with the child and foregrounding its "otherness." Some actors went to great lengths to stress the unrelatedness of surrogate and child. The most striking comment in this regard was made by the representative of a Moscow-based agency who argued that women selling ice cream on the commuter train (*elyektrichka*) would feel similarly unrelated to their ice cream (cit. in Dushina et al. 2016, 69). Surrogate Zhenya Pavlovna stressed this unrelatedness by saying that the doctors had prescribed a type of medication that was usually taken by people who had received an organ transplant—that is, an alien element that the body would normally reject. The patient information leaflet stated that pregnant women should not take this medication, which made sense to Zhenya, because the embryo was not "hers" and because a surrogate pregnancy was an unnatural and artificial pregnancy. While I could not find out which drug she was specifically referring to, her statement made clear that she understood the embryo as completely other, as not part of her body in any way. In this regard, surrogate Lyuba Dmitriyevna's emphasis on the "otherness" of the child was also interesting, as she pointed out that she could be gestating for an "African" without knowing it. For this reason it was important for her to meet the parents before signing the contract, so she could make sure they were of "Russian ethnicity (*natsional'nost'*)." Her words suggested a certain ambivalence about the otherness of the child. Being an embryo when implanted within the body, its "anonymity" could also be threatening. It was important that the embryo was *chuzhoj*, but it should certainly not be *too* other.

While Zhenya Pavlovna and Marina Nikitichna made it sound easy to reach a state of alignment, the specific work on the self became more apparent in the way Yana Timurovna, a single mother from Volgograd who was seeking a "direct arrangement," explained how she managed to align herself to become a surrogate due to her dire financial situation:

> It is difficult, emotionally, you know, but I have aligned myself to realize that the child is not mine, that all this is, how can I say, well, just a means of earning money. So it's difficult and painful but somehow... Well, you know people are so strange, we rely so much on autosuggestion. I used autosuggestion to take this step. I told myself, "Yana, calm down. It's not your child, you are helping other people."

She implied that humans had the astonishing ability of deliberately reassigning social meanings, which helped in her process of alignment. Moreover, in her online research she found out that the Russian legislation (Medical Order No. 107, 2012) prescribed a "medical indication" for women who turned to surrogacy, thereby excluding those who were simply rich and did not want to spoil their figure, as Yana put it. For many surrogates, this was a crucial point: they wanted "deserving" parents (see also Jacobson 2016, 110). When I asked them what kind of intended parents they hoped for, many stated that they wanted a couple that "really needed a child," as one of the surrogates said, and that would "love, love, and love" this child, as another woman put it. They did not want to carry a child for a woman who simply feared losing her good looks. This was connected to the assumption that women who merely did not want to gestate themselves would not be good mothers. For surrogates, however, it was crucial to know that the children would end up in good hands, as they felt great responsibility for the future of these children. Yana also mentioned that children—more precisely, having one's "own," that is, genetically related, children—were a top priority in her life. The need for fertile women who "helped out" in situations of infertility was therefore logical to her—a thought that made it easier for her to take the decisive step.

Once women felt they were "prepared" to enter a surrogacy arrangement, those who were married needed to convince their husbands to agree to the program, since the law required their written consent (Federal Law No. 323, 2011). In almost all cases in my research, it was the women themselves who first had the idea of surrogacy. I did not encounter any cases of forced surrogacy by husbands or other family members (as reported, e.g., by Pande 2014), but I heard that such cases existed. Husbands were typically skeptical about surrogacy, anticipating that their wives might suffer emotionally. The women would then share their insights from the online forums and "educate" their husbands on what surrogacy was about and that they would not become genetic mothers (Jacobson 2016; Teman and Berend 2018; Ziff 2019). Some women were noticeably proud of the amount of time and effort they had invested in this process and often concluded their descriptions with such sentences as "and then he finally understood that this child is really *chuzhoj*."

The way surrogates described their alignment made clear that the right words and the right understanding are part of a linguistic repertoire "proposed, suggested, imposed" (Foucault 1997, 291) upon the surrogate worker through television, magazines, online forums, or conversations with other people working in the field of surrogacy—they help surrogates determine the "ethical substance" (Foucault 1990, 1997) of their conduct. Several researchers have argued that the surrogacy market provides particular understandings of surrogacy that surrogates are expected to lean on (Berend 2016; Jacobson 2016; Pande 2014; Vora 2009). These findings indicate that work on the self is crucially shaped by already existing "legitimate" understandings and feeling rules. At the same time, however, surrogates do not passively adopt these understandings but engage with them "in an active fashion" (Foucault 1997, 291), creating their own meanings.

It is important to contextualize the surrogates' technologies of alignment within the broader popularity and prevalence of "work on the self" in the post-Soviet space, where it is closely tied to ideas of neoliberal entrepreneurship and personhood and has given rise to a plethora of advice and self-help literature. Alexei Yurchak (2003) has argued that such discursive formats were particularly crucial in shaping the "neoliberal subject" in the post-Soviet countries, where individuals were forced to adapt to radical economic, political, and moral transformations in a short amount of time—as opposed to the more gradual process in the West. This adaptation has been facilitated through numerous magazines and books that, for instance, teach men how to become businessmen and "true careerists" (Yurchak 2003) or women how to invest in their personalities and bodies in order to become subjects of value (Salmenniemi and Adamson 2015). Work on the self has also become a crucial way of achieving moral personhood through emotional control and containment—for instance in relation to education, lifestyle, health, sexuality, and reproduction (Matza 2009, 2012; Rivkin-Fish 2005; Zigon 2011). This suggests that engaging in technologies of alignment was neither necessarily novel nor exceptional to the surrogates, as the importance of "work on the self" (*rabota nad soboj*) was frequently stressed in different spheres of social life.

Modes and Moods of Alignment

Seeking the right understanding, actors in the field of surrogacy selectively appropriated some cultural norms in order to undermine others. While the constant mantra that "this child is *not mine*, it's *chuzhoj*" reflected the primacy of genetic relatedness over gestation, the surrogacy-internal discourse drew on this primacy to stress that "natural" maternal bonding did not—and in fact *could not*—take place if there was no genetic bond. This logic worked as a basis for the surrogates' emotional labor while simultaneously helping them "naturalize" and "normalize" (Thompson 2005) what might otherwise be seen as unfeminine behavior. Speaking with Sara Ahmed (2010), surrogates used this repertoire to repudiate being perceived as "affect aliens"—women who do not experience the socially appropriate affects for the children they bear. This was particularly reflected in one surrogate's statement that she "cannot love somebody else's child." According to her, alignment was not so much concerned with *de*taching but rather with *not* attaching. This required no effort because there simply was no attachment. The Israeli surrogates in Teman's (2003) research reported similar dynamics when they used the "artificial" character of the pregnancy to explain the absence of maternal feelings: The hormonal medication had changed their bodies to an extent that these did not produce the emotional attachment to the fetus they had experienced during their own "natural" pregnancies. Through such statements, surrogates could thus naturalize and demoralize their lack of attachment. Another surrogate worker I spoke with even mentioned she was afraid that negative feelings toward the child might erupt, suggesting that because she was not the genetic mother, she might have less patience with or tolerance for the child's needs. Thus, the surrogates' emotional labor not only needed to entail keeping attachment at bay but could also require allowing a certain amount of bonding for the child's sake. Marina Nikitichna's words, for instance, show that her mode of alignment included a "responsible form of bonding" (Toledano and Zeiler 2017, 170) by caring but not loving, by being a nanny but not a mother. Surrogates thus used technologies of alignment to carefully balance responsibilities toward themselves, toward the children, and—ultimately—toward the waiting parents. This balancing also became apparent in the way surrogates described their relation to the child. Many showed a caring attitude, while simultaneously stressing the limits of their affection. Masha

Arkadyevna, for instance, a former two-time surrogate and now agency owner from Ukraine, stated:

> I can't say that it felt like I was carrying my child, but I felt some kind of love or tenderness for him. Like to any other child. I always wanted to stroke my belly and smile to the child. [. . .] But I wouldn't say that I loved him so much that I didn't want to give him away.

Olga Georgyevna, a woman from the Russian city of Belgorod, who at the time of our conversation was approaching the end of her surrogate pregnancy, also stated that she took good care of the child, being interested in whether she was comfortable and happy in her belly. "But nothing more. She's somebody else's . . . It must sound to you like we're all wild and uncivilized," she said and laughed. She was aware of the social discourse about maternal bonding and that in the eyes of many she was crossing a moral boundary by being a surrogate.

The balancing of responsibilities took place within the context of specific "moods." Drawing on Heidegger, Jonathan Flatley conceptualizes moods as "a kind of affective atmosphere" (2008, 19), "a state of readiness for some affects and not others" (17). Atmospheres support the feeling rules, as became clear to me during some of my visits to the surrogate flats of the Altra Vita IVF Clinic. At times, it felt like the surrogates were cultivating a certain "group attitude," one that foregrounded their monetary interests while also being ostensibly indifferent toward "their" intended parents. When, during one of my afternoons in the kitchen, I asked the group of women sitting with me whether they knew who their intended parents were, one of them cried out: "We're not interested." She laughed and said the most important thing was that they received the money. None of the other women objected. Indifference seemed to be a certain feeling rule, and the mood created by such statements supported these rules. Foregrounding their monetary interest and downplaying the importance of any other factors in the surrogacy arrangement could be read as a way of coming to terms with how agencies, clinics, and intended parents took control over the surrogates' bodies during pregnancy. Moreover, it could be read as a way of boosting detachment. Thus, in contrast to Indian surrogates, who were also in financially precarious positions but resisted the image of the contractual and commercial nature of their arrangements by underlining that they were selfless mothers (Pande 2010, 2014) and "morally superior gift givers of life" (Rudrappa 2016a, 157), most of the Russian and Ukrainian women I met embraced their image as self-interested workers. This image was an asset that gave the women power and agency and that was, in some way, culturally legitimized in post-Soviet Russia.

Redirecting, Sharing, and Containing Feelings

The surrogates tended to present alignment as a state that, once achieved, remained stable and continuous. Consequently, none of them reported additional alignment efforts during pregnancy. This is particularly interesting in comparison with, for instance, the Israeli surrogates Teman spoke with. Teman writes about certain body maps through which pregnant surrogates distinguished parts of their bodies that belonged to them and parts that belonged to the intended mother. Some of her research participants also mentioned that they would deliberately refrain from practices that might provoke attachment, such as touching their pregnant bellies (Teman 2010). The surrogates in my research never mentioned such strategies. They also did not worry about seeing the child on the screen during ultrasound—usually a very emotional moment for mothers (Sänger 2020). Rather, they stated that they were happy to see these images and often recounted in a tender tone what they saw on the screen and how the child was positioned in their womb. The "switch" and the "moods" thus seemed to do the necessary work of alignment once and for all.

A more careful reading of the surrogates' narratives, however, shows that emotional labor was a continuous process in the context of surrogacy, and the shape it took varied throughout the pregnancy. This was not surprising, for most women embarked on their surrogacies without knowing how the pregnancy would affect them. Like Marina Nikitichna and Yana Timurovna, most other women had "done the research" (Speier 2011), browsing the Internet and the online forums for information on the medical and organizational aspects of surrogacy, but, of course, questions remained, and clinics and agencies often did not provide the necessary ambiance to thoroughly discuss the different stages of the surrogacy program and the anxieties this may cause. Consequently, many women who entered a surrogacy program for the first time were nervous and worried about what to expect. On numerous occasions women on their first visit to the clinic, or who were about to take the crucial step of signing the contract, took out their phone and showed me pictures of their children posing in front of a giant birthday cake or of their families during the last summer vacation at the Black Sea. Not knowing what triggered the women to do so, I can only suggest that they felt the need to bring their children to mind for reassurance that subjecting themselves to all the uncertainties of a surrogate pregnancy was worthwhile. The photographs and memories seemed to give them the opportunity to redirect feelings of anxiety toward their children, thus turning negative feelings into positive ones. Doing surrogacy "for" their children also made it possible to construct themselves as good mothers (Pande 2010) rather than greedy women without morals, as parts of the public discourse implied.

The processual and thus changing character of alignment comes into view when contrasting the different stages of pregnancy with each other. For some women, the (nonexistent) relationship with the parents became an important issue as the pregnancy progressed—even for some of the "indifferent" women. Lena Mironovna, for instance, initially told me that she did not want to meet the intended parents. She knew that the mother's name was Alevtina and that she was thirty-six years old. However, she did not know her family name—"I tried not to remember. I don't need this; this is unnecessary (*lishnaya*) information for me," she said and laughed. When I asked her in a later conversation whether or not she would like to know more about the intended parents, Lena answered that, firstly, nobody would tell her more, and, secondly, she did not want to know. Then she added that "they don't want contact with us (i.e., her and her husband), not even via the Internet. What should we want? [. . .] If they wanted to, then I would agree. But they don't want to." Marina Nikitichna made a strikingly similar comment. When I asked her the same question, she said "No," but then immediately reconsidered: "Maybe. On the one hand, *I would like to know them*, but on the other hand, what for? If the agreement is such that *they don't want me to know them*, then that means I shouldn't (*nye nado*)." She added that according to the clinic it was better not to have contact and she trusted their experience with this issue. However, she also stressed that if somebody was carrying *her* child, she would want to know who this person was and she would want to "feel" the child. Both Lena's and Marina's ways of speaking about contact suggested a reluctance to articulate the wish to know the intended parents while simultaneously linking this reluctance to an awareness of their lack of power concerning this issue. The surrogates' words implied that there was no point in even thinking about what they wanted themselves, poignantly phrased by Lena when she said: "What should we want?" Hoping for something that seemed out of reach went against the approach of "pragmatic realism" many women adopted, as "practical realists focus on what seems feasible given limited options" (Utrata 2015, 108).

In an even later conversation with Lena, she told me that being in contact with the parents would actually help her emotionally, because then it would feel much clearer that the child was not hers; now, without the contact, it instead felt like a "regular" pregnancy, like she was carrying her own child. Once the pregnancy was well underway, many surrogates started wondering who the parents were, whose child they were carrying. Katya Yefimovna in particular said over and over again how much she wanted to meet them. She did not give up hope that the parents would eventually initiate contact with her and therefore mentioned at every one of our meetings, without me asking, that they had "not yet" done so. She seemed somehow offended by this lack of contact—it not only made her sad but also hurt her deep inside. She suffered from depression throughout the pregnancy, and it is quite probable that the lack of contact with the parents in some way contributed to her mental state. Katya thought she would be more "optimistic" if she knew who they were. "As it is, I am doing this just for the child," but if they had a relationship, then she would also be doing the surrogacy for the parents. She wanted to be in this together, she wanted it to be a "group activity" (*gruppovoe dyelaniye*), she added with a laugh. As I describe below, she finally met the parents after giving birth—just like Lena—only to find out that they themselves would have wanted contact during the pregnancy.

Experiencing surrogacy as a "group activity" would also have opened up the possibility to redirect feelings from the child to the parents, hence making it easier to *stay aligned* and realize that "it is not my child and there are people waiting for this child," as Lena said. As mentioned, other studies have shown that "sharing" and "shifting" the pregnancy between bodies are crucial elements of the emotional labor that both surrogates and intended mothers fulfill—they enable the former to disembody the pregnancy and the latter to embody it (Teman 2009, 2010; Toledano and Zeiler 2017). While I have not been able to observe these processes during my fieldwork, the narratives of intended mothers and surrogates who were in direct arrangements suggested that similar forms of sharing and shifting took place. And many surrogates who opted for direct arrangements did so because they explicitly wanted a relationship that enabled such intimate practices. This was the case for Raya Antonovna: "If I went through an agency, I think I would get some kind of depression," she told me. She had been in contact with agencies and once even had an appointment but then cancelled at the last minute, noticing that it did not feel right. "Agencies are for those who don't want personal contact," she told me, while for her, contact was essential. Raya went on to say that she really enjoyed giving presents and seeing the happiness in other people's faces. "If I give birth to the child and just give it to the doctor and then get taken to another room *without seeing* that this child was really a present for *these parents*, then it's really just a waste of time. That would be like giving birth to a child and then abandoning it." Her statement suggests that surrogacy without seeing the parents' joy was not worth it, while she could not responsibly give birth to the child and then let it go without knowing that it would have a safe new home. Raya had been in a direct arrangement with intended mother Rita Tikhonovna, but ultimately, their embryo transfer was unsuccessful. Within the short time between getting to know each other and the pregnancy test result, the two women had grown very close. Raya emphasized how sad she was that another surrogate was now carrying the intended mother's baby: "Of course I feel sorry that it is not me, because I would want that (i.e., being pregnant for Rita) *very much*. I would send her a picture of the belly every day, of the belly that is kicked and that bulges and grows." Since having met Rita, she had been looking for other intended parents with whom she would have a similar "connection," but so far without success.

Surrogate worker Masha Arkadyevna also stated that knowing the parents was an essential part of feeling well during the pregnancy, which was why she had opted for a direct arrangement. In fact, she and her intended mother had "really gestated together." She told me how one night she could not sleep because the child was moving so much that she thought it was going to "jump out" of her belly. Early in the morning, the mother called and asked worriedly whether everything was alright. She had dreamed about a huge room with a bed inside that her child was lying on, heavily turning from one side to the other. The mother ran to one side to catch the child, in case it fell, but then it quickly rolled over to the other side and the mother had to run there. "We both had to cry," Masha said laughing. "How is that possible?" She said that there were many such cases, and other intended mothers I interviewed experienced this connection to the child that made them "feel" when something was not going well. "Very strange things happen. This is all on a psychological level," she stated. "I very much approve of this kind of relationship. I support this, and it makes me happy to see a relationship like this between the mother and the *surr-mama*." She had been a surrogate twice and felt proud of what she had done. Being a surrogate had boosted her self-esteem. In 2007, she had decided to open her own small agency in her home country, Ukraine. She now carefully selected the intended parents and surrogates she worked with, as she was looking for people who appreciated a close relationship and would not treat surrogacy "like a business." Masha regarded the business approach as "inhumane," a perception that was shared by Lyuba Dmitriyevna. The latter said she would feel like a "commodity" (*tovar*) if she did not know who the intended parents were. The moment she met them and heard about their suffering, she immediately noticed that the "human" (*chelovyecheskii*) aspect suspended the monetary one. This was a dynamic that agencies sometimes made use of. While most recommend no contact, a few do suggest meeting once, so that the surrogate could understand the couple's history of suffering. This affectively bound them to the intended parents, making them more responsible workers.

Lyuba was very happy about her intended parents. When we met in the surrogates' flats, she had just had her embryo transfer but was in frequent contact with the couple. She said that she already saw her body as the mother's body, indicating that she had somehow transferred ownership. Lyuba added that the intended parents felt like parents to her, because of the caring way they looked after her. Many of the surrogates who wished for contact said they wanted to feel that they were cared for and that their pregnancies mattered to someone. They did not always see this as something unique to surrogacy but rather stated that this was important to pregnant women generally. However, when I asked her what the intended parents did for a living, she said that she did not know and was not interested in knowing. Then she reconsidered and stated that she *would* like to know but that she was afraid of becoming too close to the parents and then being disappointed later on. She assumed that they would keep the surrogacy secret and therefore might not want contact after the birth of the child—"At some beautiful moment I'll write them a text message and not receive one in return." Lyuba's account made clear how important but also how fragile these bonds were. Like Lena Mironovna and Marina Nikitichna, she also was unsure about what she wanted or what she *could* want. She knew that she was not in a position to insist on contact after delivery, that the two people who felt like parents now might vanish from her life once the child was born. Being aware of the fragility of their bond, the emotional labor she performed entailed drawing certain boundaries, such as not knowing too much about the intended parents and thus keeping them at a distance.

Filling the Void

The act of redirecting attachments became particularly evident in postbirth narratives, for example in my conversation with Katya Yefimovna the day after she was discharged from the maternity hospital. We were standing at the edge of a playground close to the surrogates' flats, watching her five-year-old daughter on the swings. Katya seemed melancholic, and as soon as the other young mothers in the playground were out of earshot, it became clear why: "I have a feeling of emptiness, of mental and inner emptiness. Someone should be here but they took him away," she said with a weary smile:

> Of course you understand in your head that the child is not yours; you have made an arrangement and the mission has been successfully accomplished—everything is good, everything is fine, everything is wonderful. You did a good deed, you received money for it, both sides are happy and satisfied. But inside it's difficult, we're all human. . . . Good that they gave me pills straightaway to stop lactation. If there had been milk, I don't know, it would have been horrible for my maternal feelings. Nature doesn't think of it that way—the child is meant to be *yours*. It's very difficult to trick nature; instinct remains instinct.

The doctor had been reluctant to show her the child after birth. "Of course she was afraid I would develop a maternal instinct and that I'd have a hard time." But she insisted and now described in great detail how "good" the baby was. Like many other surrogates, she stressed the importance of "seeing the result" in order to let go. There was a certain tension concerning the issue of seeing the child after delivery. Agencies usually stated that surrogates would not see the child once it was born, assuming that this moment might be emotionally too hard for the women. Most surrogates I spoke with before or at the beginning of their pregnancies found this aspect comforting. However, some of them later changed their mind, particularly during childbirth, as they realized that they might not have "closure" (Ragoné 1994) and be able to "let go" without seeing the result of their hard labor. Agent Alina Ruslanovna confirmed this importance by stating that most surrogates wanted to see the child at least once. "Maybe this sounds strange," she said, "but I think somehow they need to see that everything is OK with the child." She told me about one surrogate who had given birth by Caesarean and had been "really stressed out" because—having been under anesthesia during delivery—she did not see the twins for three days. Only after seeing them did she finally calm down. The surrogates' anxiety in this regard must also be understood in relation to their promised compensation, for if things were not "OK" with the child, there would certainly be an investigation into whether this was the surrogate's fault. If this were the case, she might be denied the entire compensation and made to pay a monetary sanction. And even if this were not the case, she might not receive the full compensation, because many contracts state that the full amount was only paid for the birth of a "healthy child." However, none of the surrogates explicitly mentioned concerns surrounding their contracts or the salaries when talking about their deliveries. Seeing the child seemed to be more of an emotional necessity.

For many surrogate workers also knowing that the child would be in good hands was crucial. Masha Arkadyevna recalled very positive memories of the delivery. Having chosen not to work through an agency but to look for intended parents herself, she had been in close contact with the "bio-mother" throughout the pregnancy. "When they first saw the child, this was a moment of indescribable happiness. I realized, oh my God! I made this happen! (laughs)." She liked experiencing the intended parents' joy. But when she came home,

> things became really difficult, psychologically. I was constantly worried about whether the child was OK and whether they were treating it well. And then late, late at night the mother called me and told me in great detail how they fed the child and how they washed her, that both grandmothers had come by and helped and showed them how to change the Pampers and how to heat the milk (laughs). And then my

soul was calm and I had no more worries. I understood that everything would be alright (with a smile).

She felt responsible for the child and thus worried about "whose arms it will fall into after I give birth to it." But the mother was great, Masha said; "she obviously sensed my concerns."

Katya Yefimovna had had similar worries. Having always wanted to meet the parents during the pregnancy, she was very happy—and also nervous—to finally get to know them and see that they were a loving couple and interacted with the child in an affectionate way. There was no reason for her to worry, for she could see that they had really wished for this child, both of them, and that they would provide a good and stable future for it. With a certain pride in her voice, she mentioned that they were very intelligent people, foreigners, from Poland. Because they could not make it in time, they were not present during the delivery, and Katya was glad about that. A few weeks earlier she had told me that she wanted the intended mother to be there, so she would witness what it meant to give birth and would thus value the surrogate's labor more. But she later reconsidered, because "giving birth ... you know, it's like oh la la," she said, probably hinting at the painful and intimate character of childbirth. She met the parents on the second day, when she had to sign off her maternal rights in the clinic. They sat together and drank tea. "I told them a little bit about myself and they told me about their lives. We had things to talk about." Then they gave her ₽5,000 for the taxi back to the clinic's flats, and when she said that it was too much, they responded that what she had done for them could not be measured in money: "They were very thankful. . . . I can't even put into words how happy, really happy, they were."

But the day after, still in the maternity clinic, Katya was not doing so well. She even had to take tranquilizers on the third day after delivery because she was "going crazy." It was difficult without having her own daughter around, and she only calmed down once she was released from the maternity clinic and could finally see her. Some agencies considered this in advance and let the surrogates' husbands and children visit them in the birth clinic, so they had their families' emotional support. One of the surrogates, who had been in a direct arrangement, even insisted on taking her son with her to Moscow before delivery, "so that I would see him and concentrate on him." This made it easier for her to keep in mind that the child in her womb was not hers. In most cases I am familiar with, however, this was not a common practice, not least because the surrogates' families usually lived too far away.

I asked Katya to describe what she meant when she referred to "maternal feelings." She struggled to find the right words: "How can I explain this? ... Well, it's like when there are newborn babies and you (laughs) want to hold them . . . it's how we're conditioned. Some develop a stronger instinct, others less." She paused for a few seconds, then added:

> The important thing is to align yourself; it is important to see the result (i.e., the child). Of course, there was the instinct but you have to align yourself and let go. You need to see things with your head. The more you cling, the worse it gets. So you have to let go of all this, with happiness, with God, with peace (laughs).

Taking her sadness as a natural given, she actively tried to counteract nature by "seeing things with the head"—thus with rationality—as opposed to with the affective body. Her words speak of the tension between what one should feel and how one really does feel. She also reminded herself—in one of the quotes above—that the surrogacy arrangement was an economic one and that she therefore had no reason to be sad. She experienced an excess of affect that she actively sought to attach to other objects. She was aware that she needed to redirect her feelings toward her daughter as well as the golden retriever she had decided to buy the day after our conversation. To fill the void, as she suggested.

Katya Yefimovna's account illustrates how she actively and consciously searched for an object of affection. Moreover, the quotes also exemplify another aspect concerning the difficult moment of birth—the uncontrollability of affects and the "naturalness" of instincts. She could explain and rationalize her feelings by referring to nature. I encountered several instances in which surrogates used these discourses in order to make sense of affects they did not "feel" or did not want to feel. Consciously or unconsciously, they strategically essentialized and naturalized their own bodies in order to legitimize their affective responses and explain why these were beyond their control—not only during or after delivery but also throughout the entire pregnancy, as becomes clear in Marina Nikitichna's statement:

> The pregnancy was like an emotional roller-coaster ride. Sometimes you want to cry; you feel really sorry for yourself. But at the same time, you know that these are just the hormones and you know that actually everything is OK. You understand that it is just temporary, so you can calm down and let yourself be a bit capricious for a while.

Referring to the power of hormones calmed her down, since she could hold on to the thought that there was a biological reason for her emotional turmoil, one that was only temporary. She therefore did not have to fight this feeling but could give in to it.

"My Emotions Just Ran Wild"

The influence of affects, instincts, and hormones was even more apparent in the postbirth account of Lena Mironovna, whom I spoke with four days after the delivery. I met her and her husband, Aleksej, at the corner store to buy drinks and snacks to celebrate the successful completion of the surrogacy process. They had spent the day at a huge market in the outskirts of Moscow, buying new clothes for themselves and presents for their son, whom they had not seen for five months. Both were in a great mood. Lena told me that she had given birth the day she had arrived at the maternity clinic. "It all went so fast. Everything was wonderful, honestly, wonderful. Everything was good. The clinic is really . . . " She made a facial expression that signaled how fancy it was, and she stressed how relieved she was that everything went well, because she had been "very nervous" about the delivery. But the doctors were great, they treated her in a respectful way, and she liked that they cheered her on during delivery. After giving birth, she was immediately taken to a room that she shared with another, very friendly woman. The woman asked her about how her delivery went and whether she had given birth to a boy or a girl, but their conversation did not go any deeper. She felt comfortable and not like "everyone had a child and it was only me who didn't." The room was nice, they had a TV, the food was brought on beautiful plates, and they were even provided with teabags. "Maybe this is normal," Lena said, "but I am not used to this treatment." Indeed, many of the surrogates were impressed by the equipment in the private infertility and maternity clinics and felt like they received a kind of medical treatment they had not had in public clinics when they were pregnant with their own children. The latter do not have a good reputation and are often compared to those in Soviet times, being perceived by some women and professionals as marked by overcrowded wards and a lack of care and comfort (Temkina and Zdravomyslova 2018). However, not all surrogates delivered in private maternity clinics, and either way, receiving good medical treatment did not always equal being treated well, as some women reported being looked down upon or insulted for being a surrogate.

Lena Mironovna's first narration of the time in the maternity hospital included no mention of the baby. Only when I specifically asked about it did she mention that she caught a glimpse of the child right after delivery. She described in great detail and with affection how tiny the baby's toes were and how much hair it already had. She did not have much opportunity to look at the newborn, because instantly there was a "huge crowd of people" around her: doctors, nurses, the mother. She mentioned, almost in passing, that the mother had been present during the birth. She had wanted the bio-mother to be present during the delivery so "I don't have to see or hear the child and it goes straight into her arms.

I know what kind of maternal instinct I would develop otherwise." In an amused tone Lena told me that she was not sure exactly when the mother had appeared, because she was not informed and thus only realized after she had given birth, when one of the doctors called out the intended mother's name. Everybody in the room was wearing protective clothing, so Lena could not tell staff from visitors anyway. She only saw the mother's eyes—the rest of her body was covered. At some point they called in the father, and then the couple and the child left the room.

The two parties only met properly on the second day, as in Katya's case, when they signed the documents. I asked Lena whether they had the chance to talk to each other:

> Yes. Well, "talk"? You really can't call it a "talk." We just exchanged a few sentences. We sat like this (gestures), on a corner bench: they sat on one side, I sat on the other . . . There was no "thank you," they didn't thank me. . . . Well, they were just like normal parents. . . . I can't say anything, nothing good and nothing bad. I didn't . . . Well, how long did I talk to them!?

She did not dwell on this point but went on to say that she was happy to hear that the child was calm and slept well, because it had been very lively in her belly. The parents had not taken the baby to the meeting with Lena, so I asked her whether she saw it again after the delivery. "No!" she exclaimed. "That would already have been dangerous. You know, these children . . . The female organism can react in very different ways." And after a brief pause she laughed and commented again on the moment of giving birth: "Tears were running down my cheeks. It just happened. I was looking at her—she was so *small*. The mother was standing there taking photos and I was just like boo-hoo (simulating crying)." Lena said, still laughing at herself, "My emotions just ran wild. I was holding and holding back for such a long time. And you know, shit, giving birth is hard. It just got me. I don't know, whether I was crying for joy or was I . . ." She did not finish her sentence but instead spoke of her concurrent feelings of self-pity, pride, and happiness. "You know, there has to be some kind of outlet for all these emotions. And these were good emotions; I saw these toes, it was above all the toes—I saw them and that was it . . . These *small toes*." Lena thus suggested that it had been the child's toes in particular that made her cry, that made feelings come to the fore that she had held back for so long. But it remains unclear what kind of affects these were and why she felt that she had needed to hold them back. She said they were "good emotions," and she was happy that the whole process of surrogacy and delivery was finally over. At the same time Lena clearly stated that the affects she experienced were triggered by the child and that ultimately these affects were dangerous, suggesting that they could cause harm and pain. She thus seemed to imply that she was feeling happy, while simultaneously being aware that her body—her hormones—could easily corrupt this feeling by imposing a physical response beyond her control. Picking up what Katya Yefimovna had said, I asked whether she experienced any feeling of emptiness. "We immediately filled this emptiness with tequila," her husband joked. He was sitting next to us with a two-liter bottle of beer, refilling my plastic cup over and over again. Lena laughed but then said in a more serious tone that there was no emptiness to be filled. She did not understand where such a feeling would come from but suggested that it might be linked to "other problems," problems not connected to the surrogacy. In fact, none of the other surrogates I spoke with reported any similar feeling of emptiness or any great emotional difficulties after giving birth. "I did my work. I'm calm. The child is healthy," Lena said. And her husband added: "Now we await the money."

"I Shouldn't Have Done This"

The story could have ended here, and in fact it nearly did. It was only in the course of writing a first version of this chapter in 2017 that I decided to contact Lena Mironovna again, because her words had left too many question marks in my head. There were too many things that indicated tension, contradiction, rupture: Her laughing while telling me that she had cried. Or her telling me that she had "held back for so long" and was really happy about the surrogacy being over, while not acknowledging that relief implied having gone through negative or wearing experiences.

I wrote to Lena via Vkontakte, a social media platform similar to Facebook. We had maintained contact over the years, and she immediately replied to my message and agreed to read over the parts of the interview transcript that had caused the question marks. In her brief answer she merely repeated what she told me that very day but then, out of the blue, she mentioned that she regretted the surrogacy: "This money didn't bring me anything good; I shouldn't have done this, now I regret my decision. [. . .] It was a mistake!" She added a smiley emoji with a tear in one eye. I was taken aback by this message, and when I asked her what had prompted this change of heart and why the money "didn't bring her anything good," Lena answered that "it's not about the money, it's about the soul (*dusha*) and the conscience (*sovyest'*)." And it was not so much a change of heart; rather she had already felt this way when she was in Moscow. She did not know why she had this feeling or how to describe it. "Life is such a turbulent (*stryemityel'no*) thing! You want to live in a happy and unconstrained way and without sin! But that doesn't work out. [...] Time goes by, they say that time heals all wounds." Overwhelmed by these words and struggling to find an appropriate reaction, I responded that I was sorry for bringing up this issue. "It's alright!!! Everything is OK!!!" she replied, clearly rejecting what she seemed to read as pity on my part. As only Aleksej and I knew about the surrogacy, I thought that maybe she wanted to talk to someone about the way she felt, but this was not the case. "Actually, I had completely forgotten about it. I try to forget it. There are so many new problems, I don't think about what's already in the past." Her son had had a serious accident a few months before, and this was what troubled Lena now, not what had happened in Moscow two and a half years ago.

I was thrown off balance by the fact that Lena had been experiencing regret during the pregnancy while always presenting herself as a happy and carefree woman toward me. In fact, I had often wondered about the surrogates' reluctance to talk about the emotional side of surrogacy and was never sure how to interpret their silence. However, I was also trying to critically challenge my own assumptions about there *having* to be emotional challenges in surrogacy; in addition, aside from the practical obstacles to discussing these issues (e.g., lack of privacy in the communal flats and lack of shared time due to the fact that many surrogates only came to Moscow for brief checkups), I wanted to respect the surrogates' boundaries by not pressing them about these issues.

Retrospectively, I could not help but wonder whether or not it was a coincidence that exactly those two women I accompanied over such a long and intense time voiced "emptiness" and "regret," and whether more surrogates would have voiced such feelings had we developed a closer relationship or had there been more spaces for exchange—a question that will remain unanswered. However, while Katya Yefimovna's and Lena Mironovna's experiences were certainly not "representative," I suggest that they were not exceptional. Instead, what was exceptional was that they *articulated* these experiences—which could be explained by coming back to the metaphor of the switch, which, as mentioned above, implies that emotional labor is a one-time act with a stable effect. In a context where surrogacy is understood as an economic relationship largely free of emotions and affects, I can assume that there was little space for surrogates to articulate their feelings during and after the pregnancy, especially when the arrangement was mediated by an agency. Agencies reproduced the notion of the switch, however, in an ambivalent way. On the one hand they propagated the idea that surrogates had to be controlled throughout the pregnancy, for one never knew what might come into their heads in these states of hormonal turmoil. On the other hand, they suggested that emotional problems could be avoided from the beginning by "picking the right surrogates." This was clearly expressed by agency representative Konstantin Pavlovich, who argued: "We don't take girls who might get too attached to the child. Well, there are some who just have this kind of disposition or character. The separation from the child would be an emotional trauma for them. We *don't take* such girls." Or agent Sergej Petrovich, who answered my question about whether some surrogates experienced emotional difficulties upon relinquishing the child with the simple statement: "We don't take women for whom this might be difficult." From the perspective of agencies, emotional well-being was thus merely a matter of "disposition" and "character," and not connected to possible difficulties during the process. Their psychological examinations were thus treated as a panacea to avoid any further problems. A good worker should know from the start that she would not encounter emotional challenges during the process. This emphasis puts responsibility for the surrogate's well-being entirely in her own hands. Such assumptions can be seen as one of the reasons why psychological counseling for surrogates was not widely offered. Some clinics and agencies did offer psychological support, but none of the surrogates I knew opted for support, and I am not sure how aware they were of this provision. Moreover, psychological counseling seemed to be conceptualized not as a matter of prevention and accompanying support but rather as troubleshooting. Upon one of my visits to the surrogate flats, the women there told me about an incident in which a surrogate who had just given birth did not want to relinquish the child, assuming that it was biologically her own. In this case, the psychologist was called to the maternity ward to explain the IVF procedure to her again and convince her to sign off her maternal rights. This was one of the few times I heard that an interaction between the psychologist and the surrogates after the initial tests had taken place.

From such a perspective, affects and emotions that cannot be rationalized away by referring to instincts or hormones became signs of individual alignment failure. This, of course, did not invite an open exchange about or an "outlet," as Lena Mironovna termed it, for the emotional challenges surrogacy can entail. Sayani Mitra and Silke Schicktanz (2016) have made a similar point, showing how Indian surrogates' grief over failed conceptions is disenfranchised by clinic staff, who read grief as inappropriate attachment to the embryo. Not wanting to be dismissed from the clinic, surrogates thus officially silence their feelings of loss—that they were not evoked by the embryo itself but rather by the lost opportunity for upward mobility. Different as they are, the two cases reflect a conflation of two very distinct aspects: experiencing challenging or negative emotions during a surrogacy program was automatically seen as a sign of attachment to the child. In Russia and Ukraine, the fear that surrogates might develop a bond and might not want to relinquish the child seemed to be so dominant that any emotional articulation turned into a potential threat. Experiencing emotions for the child was thus equated with not wanting to give the child away. This conflation sometimes made it impossible even to just speak about this issue. The examples of Konstantin Pavlovich and Sergej Petrovich show that doctors and agents often did not directly answer my questions about the relationship between surrogate and child, but rather explained to me how their selection process and their control mechanisms prevented surrogates from wanting to keep the child.

What attracted my attention in this regard was a certain difference between the accounts of women who had worked through agencies and those who had made direct arrangements. While the former frequently approached surrogacy as a business transaction free of affects and emotions, the latter more readily addressed such issues. In addition, those few surrogates who articulated that surrogacy was a rewarding process were all women who had been in direct exchange with the intended parents. While money was certainly the primary motivation of surrogates, many also longed for a feeling of recognition, for a word of gratitude. In her ethnography on surrogacy in Israel, Teman has shown how surrogates (who likewise participated in surrogacy for financial reasons) initially perceive their relationship to the intended parents as contractual but gradually develop the sense that the relationship is rather based on a gift. From the perspective of the surrogates, then, what they expected in return was more than money: the "payment does not eclipse the gift" that they made by turning a woman into a mother (2010, 211). While surrogacy relationships in Israel are not directly comparable to those in Russia and Ukraine, since they often entail profound emotional bonds between surrogates and intended mothers, I believe that there is an important parallel: that surrogacy is not a type of work like any other. To the Russian and Ukrainian surrogates, it was without doubt work, and yet, it was significantly more intimate and more embodied than their usual occupations, making them hope and expect that this would also be recognized—not in the form of gifts but rather in the form of mere acknowledgment. Listening to the stories of the surrogate workers, it seemed like clinics and agencies continuously failed in transmitting this recognition. Furthermore, they hindered contact between intended parents and surrogates by constructing this contact as dangerous, thereby acting against what some intended parents and surrogates actually wanted. For instance, when Katya Yefimovna finally met the parents after giving birth, she found out that they had wanted to get in touch with her during the pregnancy but had been discouraged by the clinic. Had they been in touch earlier, she could have received the recognition she was longing for already during the pregnancy.

Another aspect that caught my attention—and that my written conversation with Lena Mironovna clearly illustrates—was that emotional labor not only extended beyond flicking the switch but also beyond giving birth. Her ongoing attempts to forget can thus be read as the continuation of *alignment*. This was similarly manifested in Masha Arkadyevna's response to my question about whether she still had contact with her first intended mother—with whom she was not as close as with the second one:

> No, never. Sometimes I look her up on social media, but I never write to her, I never call her, I don't get in touch. They have their own life; I guess they have long forgotten that their child was born through a surrogate.... If they wanted to, they would have contacted me.

Her words expressed that the intended parents were still on her mind, that she kept asking herself about how their lives had developed. Masha would have liked to maintain contact, but she sensed that she did not have the right to know anything about their life. As mentioned above, this was what many other women suggested when I asked them about the issue of contact with the intended parents during but also after delivery. Even though she opted for a direct arrangement, she was aware that "this was really not her story," as the Ukrainian agent Anastasia Anatolyevna had phrased it.

Individualizing Surrogate Labor

The way the surrogates in my research engaged in technologies of alignment stands in stark contrast to research from other contexts, where surrogates are invoked as altruistic helpers or caring mothers rather than workers. Nevertheless, as this chapter shows, there are related aspects of emotional labor across these different contexts, and such similarities are not surprising for cultural settings in which affective bonding between gestating woman and child is considered natural as well as a sign of proper motherly/feminine behavior. In dialogue with their cultural context, surrogates perform emotional labor in order to align themselves with the predominant feeling rules. They engage in technologies of alignment, on the one hand, through internalizing a clinic/agency discourse that stresses the importance of *understanding* and *being prepared*. By making these technologies sound like they are merely a matter of operating the "switch" (Zhenya Pavlovna) or "finding the right words" (Marina Nikitichna), they become concrete and controllable. Alignment implies aligning oneself with a specific mood, making the self receptive to some but not other feelings. On the other hand, surrogates selectively appropriate social and medical discourses when it comes to explaining "hormones" or "instinct," which they perceive as beyond their control. Their physical responses are explained by "strategically naturalizing" (Thompson 2005) the female body. Reference to their "natural" bodies allowed Lena Mironovna to rationally explain her tears and Katya Yefimovna to make sense of her feeling of emptiness. Moreover, the surrogates also tried to tackle unwanted affects by redirecting them toward others (e.g., in latter's case, to her child and the dog) or by trying to avoid them (e.g., in the former's case, not wanting to see the child). Through these distinct technologies of alignment surrogates make sense of their emotions and aim at "dis-emotionalizing" their pregnancies. This enables them to remain effective workers while preserving their ethical integrity as good women and mothers.

However, this attempt at "dis-emotionalizing" reveals cracks, as the tension between the economic and the affective/emotional cannot be entirely dissolved. While these two spheres are supposed to be held apart, because the affective/emotional threatens to pollute the economic (Zelizer 2013), Katya Yefimovna's and Lena Mironovna's stories show that the intimate aspect sometimes finds its way back into the equation. While affects can be more easily tamed during pregnancy, the moment of delivery is one of great physical and emotional force that can cause the neat divide between the economic and the intimate to collapse. It is also this moment that entails the most potential to experience surrogacy as rewarding, as sometimes the surrogates can apprehend the profound happiness they bring to "their" intended parents, making this their "trophy moment" (Teman 2010; see also Jacobson 2016). This was the case for Katya, who seemed profoundly relieved that the pregnancy had taken a positive turn, that she could finally meet the parents, and that they expressed their gratitude multiple times. It was through this happiness and gratitude that surrogates like Raya Antonovna and Katya Yefimovna felt that their exceptional labor was adequately recognized, as opposed to the ways in which they were treated by agencies and clinics as "only one element in the cure for infertility."

The historian and psychologist Lisa Malich (2017) has shown how historically dominant gender norms and social/medical body imaginaries shape ideas about the "natural" feelings of pregnant women. She argues that the affects/emotions pregnant women experience have often been psychologized, locating them "inside" of women, thus concealing the social, political, and economic factors that influence how we feel. It is also this concealment that Tomas Matza (2009) refers to in his analysis of the rising popularity of narratives of self government on Russian talk shows. Drawing on James Ferguson's (1994) notion of the antipolitics machine, Matza argues that turning the self into a site of government results in the "emergence of a feeling subject, left to negotiate a denuded landscape of pure affect" (2009, 513). Along similar lines, Michele Rivkin-Fish (2005) shows how the neoliberal transformation of the Russian healthcare sector has resulted in blaming individuals for failing to care for themselves in appropriate ways. The concealment of structural inequalities, as both authors conclude, thus significantly limits the ways in which individuals can conceptualize, tackle, or organize against such inequalities (see also Salmenniemi and Adamson 2015).

Translating these thoughts to the field of surrogacy, it becomes obvious that "hormone-talk" was precisely what allowed agents such as Larissa Osipovna to dismiss the surrogates' discontent as hormonal mood swings that had no legitimate trigger but were rather interpreted as a sign that surrogates needed to be strictly controlled. In such a setting, then, experiencing emotional challenges becomes a sign of alignment failure. Those who fail in the post-Soviet economy are simply "not trying hard enough" (Utrata 2015, 104; see also Attwood, Schimpfössl, and Yusupova 2018). As Matza (2009) and Rivkin-Fish (2005) have argued, it becomes difficult to share and conceptualize feelings of "failure" when they are individualized. Few of the surrogates in my research seemed to have opportunities for exchange, as they experienced their pregnancies largely in isolation. Exchange among the surrogates was limited, and those who spent several months or their entire pregnancies in the flats of clinics and agencies did not experience the sense of community and support that some Indian surrogates report (Pande 2014). Moreover, those who worked through agencies had no or only restricted contact with the intended parents and could therefore not turn their pregnancy into a "group activity," as Katya Yefimovna would have wanted. Finally, due to the secrecy surrounding the endeavor and the general lack of involvement of many husbands and partners, surrogates could also not make the pregnancy into a "family project," as many U.S.-American and Israeli surrogates did (Jacobson 2016; Teman and Berend 2021). To be sure, not all women in my research would have wanted or needed more exchange but were happy to participate in anonymous business transactions. However, when engaged in a practice that is socially condemned as immoral, it might be more difficult to keep such reproaches at bay as an individual. It is thus no surprise that after the completion of a surrogacy program, some surrogates might be left with the sense of having committed a "sin," as Lena Mironovna implied.

Part III

6

LABORING WITH HAPPINESS

When I zoomed out from the Russian and Ukrainian context in order to get a better understanding of the global surrogacy market, I could not help noticing that this sphere was shaped by very different moral concerns, discourses, and practices. Being intrigued by these differences, in part 3 of this book I examine the shifts in moral economy that occur when surrogacy involves intended parents from western Europe (notably Spain, Germany, and Austria), Russian and Ukrainian agencies that mainly cater to these foreign parents, and Spanish agencies that facilitate surrogacy arrangements through direct collaborations with clinics in these two countries. The following two chapters thus focus on these groups of actors, who formulate and circulate truths not in relation to the dominant moral concerns in the post-Soviet surrogacy market but rather in relation to those that structure Western debates around commercial surrogacy. These debates mainly revolve around the issue of the surrogates' potential exploitation, an issue that was raised and contested by almost all foreign market actors I interviewed, especially the intended parents, without my asking. The fact that this is not unique to my research but that other surrogacy researchers have reported similar experiences (e.g., Arvidsson, Johnsdotter, and Essén 2015; Rudrappa and Collins 2015) reflects that many individuals involved in transnational surrogacy arrangements, especially in countries with high levels of poverty, feel troubled by the danger of exploitation and by the reproach that they might contribute to this. Many explicitly distanced themselves from the businesslike character of surrogacy in Russia and Ukraine and said they wanted to prevent or work against such an approach in their own surrogacies. Since they are under enormous pressure to legitimize their decision to pursue surrogacy, it is not surprising that some of my research participants actively brought this up. Being aware that financial issues were central for Russian and Ukrainian surrogates, they needed to find arguments and practices that nevertheless refuted the allure of exploitation.

These factors crucially affected the way foreign intended parents imagined, desired, and experienced their surrogacy programs and, consequently, also the forms of ethical labor they engaged in. Two forms were particularly relevant in the context of my research. Both cast the surrogate as a "choosing subject" and thus made her a "biodesirable" surrogate to work with (Gunnarsson Payne 2015). On the one hand, some research participants emphasized that (their) surrogates acted not *only* on financial grounds or that they hoped this would not be so in their case. They "accepted" the surrogates' economic motives and highlighted the normality and ubiquity of money. Nevertheless, most viewed this aspect as undesirable, as carrying the aura of exploitation and polluting the potentially beautiful experience of surrogacy. Commercial aspects were therefore downplayed, and actors engaged in practices and rhetoric that affectively saturated the relationship between intended parents and surrogates. In other words, their ethical labor was one of "affective de-commodification" (Smietana 2017b), which aimed to create narratives and experiences of "happiness." On the other hand, some of my research participants readily embraced economic motivations for surrogacy but legitimized these by stressing the surrogate's free choice. The perceived "freedom" of the surrogate thus enables them to accept her financial motives but nevertheless allows for stressing the win-win situation. However, in these cases, too, most intended parents did not view surrogacy merely as a business transaction. Rather, they imbued the process with affective meaning by foregrounding the surrogate's "thankfulness" or the benefits of the surrogacy for her. The first aspect thus evoked notions of "gendered altruism," while the latter referred to surrogacy as a form of "gendered empowerment" (Markens 2012). Existing research has shown that the former is more prevalent in the United States, while the latter is more prevalent in low-income countries (Jacobson 2016; Markens 2012; Pande 2014; Rudrappa and Collins 2015). As I show in part 3, the conceptualization of Russia and Ukraine as "middle ground" allows for the presence of both moral framings.

In the following chapters, I will explore these two aspects in greater detail. My approach here is somewhat different from that in the prior parts of the book, in which I have focused on delineating the organization of surrogacy, unfolding my research participants' experiences and backgrounds, and contextualizing these within the post-Soviet setting. In part 3 I concentrate on the specific notions of happiness and free choice, explicitly scrutinizing the moral power they carry. I chose this approach not least because—as mentioned above—my interviews with foreign market actors as well as with those catering to foreign intended parents often reflected a degree of anticipatory justification (through which I was "presented" with the notions of happiness and free choice) that I did not encounter in other interviews. Their ethical labor was more palpable, particularly since part of it seemed to be directed toward me as researcher, as if wanting to eagerly convince me of their perspective. This dynamic compelled me to investigate why, when, and how these notions were evoked and shaped, and what was, consequently, concealed or de-emphasized.

The current chapter will deal with the question of how happiness becomes incorporated into the ethical labor some of my research participants engaged in. Following Sara Ahmed (2004a, 2004b), I ask what it is that such affective dimensions "do." For this purpose, I not only draw on my interviews, but also include agency websites, forum discussions, and other forms of text produced with the clear—yet sometimes concealed—aim of promoting surrogacy in general, and surrogacy in Russia and Ukraine in particular. The focus lies on two aspects of happiness and how they contribute to shaping the ethics of commercial surrogacy. The first emerged from an unease about the commercial aspects of surrogacy. As mentioned, many foreign intended parents wanted surrogates who were happy to help and not financially coerced into an arrangement. Moreover, intended parents and agents actively engaged in—or wanted to actively engage in—practices that reduced or "humanized" the commercial aspects. The second aspect I scrutinize is the way happiness was instrumentalized on a rhetorical level. Some of my research participants cast happiness as a human right that should be free from state regulation, so that all actors could decide freely what happiness means and how they would pursue it. Overall, the affective labor detailed in this chapter reflects how happiness becomes what I call an "ultimate argument."

The Promise of Happiness

Happiness is a notion that carries considerable affective potential because it is often presented as the universal and ultimate goal in life (Ahmed 2010). Happiness is also an affect that "sticks" to the object of the child, in the sense that it is seen as causing and spreading happiness—an image re/produced by numerous agency websites: "A baby is sunshine and moonbeams and more brightening your world as never before," writes one surrogacy agency.[1] Or: "When your child looks into your eyes and you know it's yours, you know what it means to be alive."[2] Such claims evoke the baby as necessary for a good life and, as such, the desire for a child as universal fact (see also Riggs and Due 2017). Furthermore, such claims can be understood as a form of marketing, for they nourish desire and hope, and make it difficult to resist what assisted conception can offer (Franklin 1997)—after all, who would want to miss out on an opportunity to brighten up their world? And who would not want to feel "alive"? As Ahmed argues, "happiness describes not only what we *are* inclined toward (to achieve happiness is to acquire our form or potential) but also what we *should* be inclined toward (as a principle that guides moral decisions about how to live well)" (2010, 199). Seeking these kinds of feelings, the "promise of happiness thus directs life in some ways rather than others" (41). It is through this promise that the child becomes a "happiness means" (34) and people are affectively directed toward surrogacy. Agencies and surrogates are thus dream-makers in a double sense—their existence makes dreams come true, but at the same time they contribute significantly to creating these dreams.

When investigating what happiness "does" (Ahmed 2004a, 2004b), it is helpful to work with the concept of "affective labor," which can be situated within the broader framework of "economies of affect"—a notion used by Analiese Richard and Daromir Rudnyckyj (2009) to analyze how affect enables economic transformations and produces economic subjects.[3] What I call "affective labor" has been termed "emotional labor" by Arlie Hochschild. In the previous chapter, I used this latter term to describe the "technologies of the self" (Foucault 1990, 1997) that surrogates engage in to get and stay aligned with the "feeling rules" (Hochschild 2003) of surrogacy. I was thus interested in the way actors conceptualize what they feel and what they do not feel. According to Hochschild, emotional labor—as work that is performed on and with the emotions in a commercial setting—has a second dimension: that of producing a certain feeling in others. In her analysis of flight attendants, it makes sense to subsume these two aspects—working on one's own emotions as well as working on creating emotions in others—under one term, for flight attendants are compelled to engage in what Erving Goffman (1959, cit. in Hochschild 2003, 35) calls "deep acting." They must not only *put on* a smile, but they must actually *feel* the smile in order to convincingly transmit a sensation of comfort and ease to their passengers. For my endeavor it is more productive to analyze these two elements separately and maintain a conceptual distinction between inward-oriented (toward ourselves) and outward-oriented (toward others) ethical labor. Therefore, I draw on Michael Hardt's (1999) notion of "affective labor," which partly overlaps with Hochschild's concept of "emotional labor." As the example of the flight attendants illustrates, affective labor is "corporeal," even though it produces something "intangible" (Hardt 1999), by aiming at inciting or inhibiting a certain feeling in another person. Both authors argue that affective labor has increasingly become part of the labor market with the rise of the service sector since the 1970s. Affect can be a commercial end in itself if it becomes a *good* to be sold. At the same time, it can be a *means* through which other goods or services can be sold. In the sphere of surrogacy, both of these purposes can be observed.

In order to explore the affective labor of happiness, I first want to provide some context as to how Russia and Ukraine are discussed among intermediaries and intended parents as a "moral middle ground" between different surrogacy destinations. The intermediary position of Russia and Ukraine allows actors to draw on a diverse repertoire of arguments that differently locate and explain happiness.

A Moral Middle Ground

According to Spanish intended father Juan Romero, the field of surrogacy is a highly differentiated terrain, in which "there is white, there is black, and there are several tonalities of gray." For Juan Romero, as well as for many other foreign intended parents I spoke with, the United States constituted the best option. The country represented the color white, because its legal and medical conditions offered a great deal of security.[4] Even though this was never explicitly mentioned by my research participants, I would contend that the United States as a surrogacy destination also offered them some kind of "ethical certainty," because intended parents and surrogates were believed to meet on a more equal footing there (see also Smietana 2017a). Traveling to the United States for surrogacy did not have the neocolonialist aura that traveling to India or Mexico did (Nebeling Petersen, Kroløkke, and Myong 2017). The color white, evoked by Juan Romero, has an ambiguous meaning in this context: not only is it the color of innocence, but it also symbolizes the mostly white bodies of U.S.-American surrogates, as opposed to the brown bodies of their Indian or Mexican counterparts. U.S.-American surrogates are often seen as free and altruistic actors, who are therefore also imagined as happier surrogates than those who turn to surrogacy for financial reasons. This framing dominates the U.S.-American understanding of surrogacy but also serves as a point of reference on a transnational scale, not least because the United States remains the "epicenter" of surrogacy (Jacobson 2016, 17).

Some of my interview partners implicitly or explicitly criticized the "ethical hierarchy of destinations." Alberto Cabello was one of these critics. At the *inviTRA* International Fertility Fair in Barcelona in 2015 he introduced himself to me as the representative of a Spanish association for parents who were going through or had gone through surrogacy.[5] He expressed unease about another association that was present at the fair and that was campaigning for the legalization of surrogacy in Spain, by promoting the way surrogacy in the United States was based on "the urge to help [...] other people to be happier and live a better life," as Anahi Molina, one of the association's members, had told me. Many of the members had themselves gone through surrogacy arrangements in the United States. In the eyes of Alberto Cabello, promoting the U.S. model in such a way equaled the disqualification of arrangements in other countries, which he found problematic:

> The United States as panacea? *Definitely yes.* The country that works best [in regard to surrogacy] in the world? *Definitely yes.* I wouldn't say "no." Are there problems with the U.S.? *Yes.* Is it really expensive? Yes. [. . .] And then, of course, there are other destinations like Ukraine, Mexico, um, Greece, Russia, which are a bit . . . *a lot* (laughs) cheaper and maybe there is a group of people [. . .] who *can't afford* the U.S. So we should give these people an opportunity.

Alberto Cabello made a plea for taking the concerns of *all* intended parents seriously, regardless of which country they traveled to, because "the need to have children can be found across all social classes." Consequently, while he deemed the United States the best option for surrogacy, he seemed to imply that it is a matter of reproductive justice to offer "opportunities" to those who are economically less fortunate but nevertheless "in need" of children.

The issue of ethical hierarchy had also troubled the German intended mother Teresa Wagner. She would have liked to travel to the United States for surrogacy but the US$100,000 or more would have exceeded her budget. Like many other intended parents she and her husband had to make this decision "according to our wallets," making them opt for Ukraine. Teresa Wagner considered it unfair that surrogacy destinations other than the United States are portrayed as morally opaque and wrong. She told me about the heated discussions in online forums, where people who could afford the United States judged those who chose to go to other countries. "When you say that you are considering going to Ukraine, some people get really angry. They say this is exploitation and ask how you can do such a thing."

Many foreign intended parents and agents eagerly argued against this perception, often re/locating exploitation to the other side of the planet, to India, Thailand, or Mexico, where there are "surrogate farms" and "women are treated like cows" (intended mother Sara Blanco) or like "ovens at your disposal" (intended father Juan Romero). Within these imaginaries, the United States is located on the bright side of the ethical spectrum, and countries such as India, Thailand, and Mexico on the dark side. Russia and Ukraine are positioned in between. According to Sara Blanco, Ukraine, the country she was currently considering for a surrogacy program, constituted a good intermediate option (*término medio*). It was not comparable to the United States—particularly in regard to the situation of the surrogates and the warm relationships between intended parents and surrogates that can develop—but also "not that bad," she said laughing. Both countries, I contend, could be seen as a "moral middle ground" in comparison to the available surrogacy destinations worldwide: While Russia has a reputation for good educational, medical, and technological standards, Ukraine has the advantage of being seen as more "European." Neither is viewed as a "third world country," as Spanish intermediary Pedro Monte confirmed, but as "totally occidentalized" and as enabling women to "freely" choose to become surrogates, while remaining affordable destinations for a broad range of incomes.

Choosing between Result and Service

Agencies and clinics in Russia and Ukraine actively work toward establishing their image of operating on a "middle ground" within the competitive global surrogacy market. One way of doing so is by arguing that intended parents have to sacrifice happiness *during* surrogacy in order to achieve happiness (in form of a baby) *after* the process. This rhetoric goes hand in hand with an affective labor based on fear and hope to direct the promise of happiness toward Russia and Ukraine.

The primary location for this form of affective labor is the anonymous and vast space the Internet offers for expressing one's opinion and experience in forums, in commentary sections, and in blogs. The difficulty of discerning authorship in this space becomes an important asset for affective labor: as I show below, the ubiquity and similarity of the narratives as well as the missionary and appealing language of these posts are striking, and strongly suggest that their authors—often posting as intended parents—are employed by surrogacy agencies and clinics. Based on the assumption that these posts are a marketing strategy, I wondered what kinds of images the narratives convey and the ends to which they are employed.

Ukraine's biggest "center for human reproduction"—as BioTexCom calls itself—in particular has turned to an aggressive and invasive form of advertising.[6] Its website assembles a collection of articles about the center from all over the world. It is clearly secondary whether the articles give praise or are unfavorable, as the center states that "criticism is the key to success and it does not matter what people are talking about; it is important that they are already talking!" Furthermore, it is claimed that "journalistic investigations are the most truthful and interesting"[7]—a statement that, unfortunately, did not translate into giving me an interview during my stays in Kyiv. The fascinating aspect about BioTexCom's maneuvering is a strategic play with negative and positive attributes of Ukraine in general, or the center in particular. The lines quoted above about criticism being "key to success" refer to an article that is an illuminating example of this strategy. The title "Ukraine Has the Worst Roads and the Best Reproductive Medicine in the World" (Chak 2013) reflects the content: throughout, the author claims to balance the disadvantages and advantages of Ukraine as a surrogacy destination. The text is accompanied by a picture of a pregnant woman dressed in white, standing in a wheat field and stretching her arms and upper body toward the sky. A critical reading of this image could interpret it as representing two of Ukraine's national resources—wheat (Ukraine used to be the Soviet Union's granary) and wombs. Both these resources are natural and nurturing: wheat fields and wombs signify fertility in two complementary ways. The image can be seen as illustrating the claim of one of my interlocutors that Ukrainian women are "very healthy," and even "much healthier" than surrogates in the United States.

The author of the article takes into account potential stereotypes intended parents might have about Ukraine. In online forums on surrogacy, intended parents often mentioned that they had never been to eastern European countries, that they thought of them as culturally very different, and therefore found the idea of doing surrogacy there somewhat "scary." The author claims to be a freelance journalist, who herself went through surrogacy with another woman's eggs. Such statements as "conditions and service were not at the appropriate level" and that "it gets worse and worse as it goes on" crisscross the article. The author complains about long waiting hours in the clinic and huge lines of people from all over the world, hoping for appointments and examinations. Simultaneously, she refers to other intended parents who underline that "BioTexCom really work wonders in the field of reproductive medicine." At the end of the article, she concludes:

> Let us suppose Ukraine is considered to be a third world country that lags behind other European countries in development by all indicators and has roads as ploughed land but it does not prevent Ukrainian doctors give happiness to people all over the world and help them in such an important issue of a global importance as continuation of human genus.

The article is followed by a long list of comments that—almost without exception—praise the miraculous workings of the agency. One user even goes beyond that and describes how much she was taken aback by Ukraine as a country and Ukrainians as people:

> People are so kind, they are so happy, they laugh and smile, have a rest in parks. After such horrible events that took place in [Kyiv] and have

been taking place still in eastern Ukraine citizens of this country can smile and be kind to another people. They are so patriotic! [...] I have liked this city so much! Sometimes people write not so good things and comments concerning Ukraine, [Kyiv], level of service there and so on. But I can say for sure! It's very beautiful and strong nation, country. And I hope in the nearest future it will be better. I pray for Ukraine and these fantastic people! They deserve happiness and good comfortable life. (MarryJ, comment poster, December 22, 2016)

Written a few years after the upsurge of violence in Kyiv's Maydan Square (2013/14) and the subsequent military conflict between Russia and Ukraine, this post can be read as restoring Ukraine's image as a safe, proud, and happy country. The other comments below the article are very similar in tone to both the article as well as numerous other commentaries I have found online. Within recent years, the name "BioTexCom" has appeared in many online discussions about transnational surrogacy destinations. Often, there are numerous users posting in these sections in poor English and discussing Ukraine and BioTexCom with each other, taking different—even contrary—positions. These users make little effort to disguise their agendas. I found a particularly provocative example of such a discussion in one of the forums on BioTexCom.[8] Calling the thread "Other side of Biotexcom" (September 11, 2014), a user named Sarah12 describes her experiences of traveling to Kyiv. While her remarks are surprisingly similar to those of the freelance journalist mentioned above, her conclusions are different. Sarah12 and her husband decided to leave the clinic because they were unhappy about the long waiting hours and the way they were treated. In a later post, she states that she is "very disappointed and scared" and that "all that attitude to business in that clinic made me frustrated. [...] I know that I want to have a child. But the same time I want to be happy making my baby." The posts by other users unanimously and vehemently attack Sarah12 for having the wrong "priorities":

> I think you should decide your priorities. It is you decision whether you opt for result [or] whether you opt for service. [...] For me it was the most important to have a healthy child. Biotexcom helped me with this. Perfectionism is not always good. [...] Biotexcom has a very high success rate. [...] I also find surrogate mothers and egg donors very beautiful in Ukraine. [...] Surrogate mothers live in rather good conditions here. Maybe it is because Ukraine is a European country. Surrogate mothers have an appropriate medical examination and psychological and social control. They have enough rights. They sign a contract that is clear and precise. [...] I am sure that you will change your opinion. (Amapola, forum user, September 16, 2014)

Amapola goes on to state that she had started a surrogacy program in Georgia and that while the service was better than in Ukraine, the three IVF attempts "failed," just as with many other couples she had met there. The description of such a "route" is common in online discussions. Users claim to have been to numerous other countries—for instance to "luxurious" clinics in the United States—and to have lost a lot of money and hope along the way. Once broke and desperate, they overcame their fears and traveled to Ukraine, where their dreams finally came true. One user in the same discussion also goes to great lengths to explain that Georgian clinics implant the embryo too early, while several users on other sites refer to an article—posted on the same platform as the abovementioned article—that "unveils" that Spanish clinics work with frozen egg cells, leading to low results, while Ukraine works with fresh egg cells. Mexico is also attacked for having surrogates that "are infected with the most terrible diseases." Furthermore, India and Mexico are said to not have "proper medical control" over their surrogates.

Often, women's complaints about long queues at BioTexCom and loud crying children in the accommodation that the clinic offers are interpreted as "evidence" of success. Patricia75, for instance, does not understand how these small inconveniences mentioned by Sarah12 can be "more important for you then having a baby [sic]." She continues that maybe Sarah12 is too young or still too inexperienced in the world of infertility and has thus not yet gone "through hell of infertility": "I don't know the reason of your attitude. But you made a mistake. [...] try to be serious and think better. If you have a chance to come back in clinic, do it" (Patricia75, September 25, 2014).

The posts and discussions reveal the logics and argumentation underlying Ukraine's success as a surrogacy destination. Prospective parents are told to overlook the disadvantages of traveling to this country and to focus on the "results" rather than the means. Considering the many faults clinics in other countries are said to have, the reader is made to believe that it is only a matter of time until all other prospective parents come to realize that they need to tolerate queues, crying babies, and unfriendliness if they really want a child. When Sarah12 writes that the "attitude to business" in the clinic frustrated her and she wanted to "be happy making my baby," she is educated by others that she should get her "priorities" right and that one cannot have it all ("Perfectionism is not always good"). The most important and enduring form of happiness is that which comes after the surrogacy process, when parents can hold a baby in their arms.

The atmosphere these words create underlines the affective labor performed by forum users and comment posters, who play on the hopes, fears, and despair of prospective parents. The comments are accompanied by statements about Ukraine's orientation toward Europe and that as opposed to in other countries, surrogates are healthy, live in good conditions, and have "enough" (but not too many?) rights. Through strategically swinging between acknowledging the negative aspects encountered in Ukraine and stressing the positive aspects, these users and authors construct Ukraine as a "middle ground" for surrogacy. BioTexCom must have been particularly successful with this strategy: When talking to an employee of the German consulate in Kyiv in 2015, I was told that almost all German couples who came to Ukraine for surrogacy were working with this center.[9]

However, not all intended parents are willing to postpone happiness to after the child's birth. Considering the intimate character of the wish for a child as well as the fact that parents would have to account for their decisions to others—including to their own children—many were inclined to create happiness along the way and therefore turned to other agencies.

She "Obviously Has Some Kind of Calling"

David and Christoph Hauser were one of the couples for whom a happy experience of surrogacy was central. I interviewed the two men via Skype (mainly the former, as the latter was cooking dinner and taking care of their eighteen-month-old son at the time and, thus, only sporadically participated in the interview), when I was in Moscow and they in their apartment in an Austrian city. I want to present their story in greater detail, because the interview was highly interesting, in that they were not simply telling me their story but also conducting a certain affective and ethical labor on me. They were eager to present a specific impression of surrogacy, as if wanting to dispel any reservations I could possibly have.

The gay couple had been thinking about having children together for a long time, weighing different options. They eventually made an arrangement with an Indian surrogate and a Ukrainian egg donor, but when India made headlines about a possible ban on surrogacy for foreign couples, they pulled out and in 2010 decided on Russia. Russian legislation only explicitly allows surrogacy for heterosexual couples and single women (Federal Law No. 323, 2011) but at the time—before the Gay Propaganda Law was implemented in 2013—gay couples could pass as "single men," which was accepted by many clinics. This meant that officially David Hauser was doing the surrogacy alone: his partner accompanied him to the clinic in Moscow but could not participate in the consultations because the clinic did not want anyone to suspect they were a couple. They had opted for a program "with guarantees," which proved to be a good choice, since it was only after the thirteenth embryo transfer—involving different surrogates and egg donors—that one surrogate, Venera Igorevna, finally became pregnant. In the sixth month of pregnancy David Hauser flew to Moscow to visit her. "It is difficult to experience a pregnancy online," he said. Being there helped him realize that it was all true and happening: "It was very *nice*. I went to see her in the clinic and I *felt* her belly and I saw that she was doing well and she seemed very cheerful." In the last month of pregnancy, Venera flew to Prague. The agency collaborated with a Czech clinic and could, upon request, arrange for delivery to take place within the EU, a convenient option for many European intended parents.

David and Christoph Hauser were the first gay couple in their community to have a child through surrogacy. Their endeavor was met with a mixture of support, interest, envy, and sometimes hostility. Hostility particularly came from one "bull dyke," as David called her, who argued that women only become surrogates because they "had to." He vehemently countered this critique:

> I'm of a different opinion. Because Venera, for instance, said that she is of course doing this for financial reasons, because she wants to support her family by buying a flat, but, also, because she *can* help, she said. She is very Christian and you really notice she is a warm-hearted, generous person who obviously has some kind of calling for this.

He underlined his point by arguing that now—one and a half years after the birth—they were still in contact with Venera and that she regularly demanded (*verlangen*) photos of the child. The couple had hoped for a surrogate who would serve as a mother-figure in the life of their son, and Venera had agreed to this idea. David and Christoph were thus trying to establish a relationship between their son and Venera, for instance by referring to her as "mama" or by giving the child a photograph of Venera to hang up in kindergarten. And when they decided to decorate their son's room with pictures from Russian fairy tales—for "this is already part of his identity," as David Hauser said—Venera enthusiastically gave them a book as a present. He also started learning some Russian, and they regularly Skyped with the former surrogate, with the help of Google Translate.

David felt lucky that things worked out so well with Venera, for they had known little about her before the program started. When I asked him whether the woman's motive mattered to them when choosing a surrogate, he answered that they had, "of course," delegated the selection to the agency, assuming they would not pick women who were merely greedy for money. David and Christoph made the final decision based on a selection of portfolios, containing a photo and information such as birth date, citizenship, place of residence, number of children, job, and education. They only got to know the surrogate during a Skype meeting once the third month of pregnancy had been reached. According to the agency, it would have been too much pressure for the surrogate to commence contact while the pregnancy was still in the critical early stage.

When recently Venera had agreed to carry another pregnancy for the couple, David said he had to cry, because this was the ultimate proof that their relationship was "much more human than a mere financial transaction." Initially, the clinic did not want to take her on a second time, because she had delivered the couple's child via C-section and for most clinics this was a reason for exclusion from further programs. "Venera really fought for it, because she really wanted to work with us," David said with a slight tone of pride in his voice. Ultimately, the clinic gave in, and at the time of our interview Venera had just started the hormonal preparation. However, the legal situation in Russia had changed, and this time David could not take part as a "single man." He and Venera had to sign a document stating that they were a couple going for egg donation. "It's a don't ask, don't tell policy," he told me. "As long as you keep up appearances, people don't care, it just works."

David Hauser's narrative is compelling, for he put considerable effort into demonstrating the affective dimension of his relationship with Venera Igorevna, foregrounding the "exceptionality" of his surrogacy experience (Førde 2017). He acknowledged that money was an important motive for Russian surrogates but that Venera was somehow special, because she had a "calling"—a term that is somewhat reminiscent of the way women's reproductive labor is often idealized as inherently altruistic (Almeling 2007). He also emphasized that Venera often acted in ways that went beyond what was written in her contract, like keeping the couple updated on examination results, which was actually the agency's job. In her research on gay fathers' paths to surrogacy in the United States, Julia Teschlade (2019) argued that the emphasis on such small "rebellious" practices contributes to affirming the intimate relationship between intended fathers and surrogates—an important element in reducing the commercial character of the arrangement. Moreover, David repeatedly emphasized how "normal" Venera was and how she managed to continue her life in a "normal" way, despite the surrogate pregnancy—statements that could be read as normalizing and naturalizing the procedure of surrogacy per se (Thompson 2005).

David distanced himself from the United States as an ideal destination and criticized the overly commercial programs there, while in Russia, according to him, surrogacy took a more natural form. He was shocked about the "catalogues" for egg donors and surrogates in the United States, saying that they were much more superficial and commercial. "In America, you pay five thousand for a housewife and sixteen thousand for a doctoral student. I think this is really bad." While criticizing this, he nevertheless stressed that they had chosen a woman with an academic qualification, "so that we could be sure this person has at least a minimal intelligence quotient"—implying that it was not the choice per se that is problematic but that you have to pay an extra fee. David was also disturbed that

U.S.-American catalogues listed women who had been surrogates seven times already, giving him the impression that many surrogates "only do it for money" and have no other possibilities in life. As if to suggest that financially motivated women were not taken as surrogates in Russia, he referred to his conversation with his Russian agent, who had assured him that only 10 percent of the surrogacy candidates passed the elaborate physical and psychological examinations. However, these examinations followed a whole different logic, and agents usually *encouraged* financial motives.

Knowing the agency the couple had worked with and having briefly met Venera in Moscow, I have reason to assume that things might not have been as bright as presented by David. Venera told me that she earned around ₽15,000 (roughly US$310) a month in her job as cook in a school canteen. The amount of work was out of proportion to her salary. In her hometown, over a thousand kilometers from Moscow, this was barely sufficient to cover basic expenses, and being a single mother, there was no additional income to support her child. David was certainly not wrong in stating that Venera was a "normal middle-class woman," but what does this mean in a country in which many who might belong to this middle class struggle to make ends meet? And what did it mean if the couple stressed their frequent communication and that Venera "demanded" photographs, while she told me that she enjoyed the contact but only ever reacted to messages rather than initiating them? I do not wish to imply that David deliberately presented his surrogacy journey as something it was not. And my aim is certainly not to "dismantle" his story and delegitimize the efforts he made to humanize the (at least initially) commercial relationship to Venera. Rather, I present and challenge his narrative here in detail, because it is illustrative of the ethical labor invested when turning surrogacy into a story of shared happiness. The ethical labor finds its expression in a neat account of a surrogacy experience that seems picture-perfect. On a manifest level, there are no insecurities, no frictions, no problems. This was also echoed in David's way of talking. His narrative was clearly meant to prove to me—and consequently to the readers of this book—that surrogacy was a morally viable option for family-making. The strong justificatory element in his narrative can also be read as a reaction to the contested status of gay parenthood. As opposed to heterosexual couples, David and Christoph needed not only to normalize surrogacy but also to normalize same-sex fatherhood in order to claim a place in contemporary society (Lustenberger 2016; Rudrappa 2014; Smietana 2017a; Teschlade 2019). Being exposed to "reproductive vulnerability" (Riggs and Due 2013) and increased "bioprecarity" (Leibetseder 2020) and, hence, confronted with many ideological and legal obstacles to becoming fathers, it would make sense for the two men to be careful how they presented their story, for their sake but also for the sake of their children.

Making It "More Intimate and More Beautiful"

The way David Hauser described his relationship with Venera Igorevna corresponded to Spanish intended mother Sara Blanco's wishes for the surrogacy process. Sara, a teacher living in northern Spain, had recently had her ovaries removed due to a cyst that had formed as a result of her endometriosis. Consequently, she needed to finally bury her hopes for birthing a child, but she and her male partner immediately signed up for adoption. At the time in Spain the waiting list was at least six years, she said, so they looked into international adoption from China or Vietnam. But the process was long and tedious, and everything seemed to be morally "obscure." Sara participated in all the preparation courses intended parents have to go through, but it was a frustrating process throughout. She felt like she was constantly under suspicion of not being a good mother and not worthy of a child. After doing some research into the option of surrogacy, she realized that with considerable effort, she and her partner could scrape together the €40,000 (at the time roughly US$43,000) for a program in Ukraine. They decided to remain in the adoption process but at the same time go for surrogacy in combination with egg donation. This seemed like a safe and fast alternative that, moreover, restored her sense of autonomy (see also Becker 2000; Speier 2016). The sphere of surrogacy was also an "underworld" and "a space of deception and trickery," she said, but in the end they found a Spanish agency that they felt comfortable with. The founders were parents through surrogacy themselves, and the relationship with them was "very personal and close." At the time of our interview, Sara was still at the beginning of the process; in a few months she and her partner would travel to Kyiv to sign the contract, choose a surrogate and egg donor, and leave a sperm sample.[10]

Sara was profoundly distressed by the commercial character of surrogacy in Ukraine. She hoped to find a surrogate whose motives would not only be monetary, for she wanted to establish a relationship with this woman. She spoke longingly about how surrogacy in the United States was considered a very normal procedure, during which intended parents and surrogates grew close and after which the latter often became an important person in the child's life (Dempsey 2015; Jacobson 2016; Smietana 2017b). "This would be what I want, for sure," she said. "A relationship of care, of gratitude, not only commercial." But even though she could not afford what she regarded as the best option (the United States), she did not feel like she was compromising her moral standards. She was upset that the media always portrayed intended parents as so desperate that they would do whatever necessary to obtain a child:

> It hurts to hear these sensationalist programs, where they say that "people are so desperate that look what they end up doing," right? They even

contract an agency, they do all these obscure and illegal things, without caring about the surrogate's conditions, because their despair is so great.

Sara stated that these moral issues mattered a lot to her and that she would do what she considered right. Surrogacy might be an "extreme measure," but she did not feel desperate and she would not put her wish for a child above everything else. Similar to some of the Russian intended mothers, she perceived herself as a person who was merely looking for a solution to a problem. She also stressed her own agency in shaping the surrogacy experience by doing "fair play in a dirty field" (Førde 2017). Stating that "even at the supermarket I can buy a kilogram of sugar that was made by exploiting people in South America, or I can buy fair trade, right?" Sara hoped to be able to "overcome the commercial barriers and make it a bit more intimate and more beautiful" by "removing the obscure bits and putting in a bit of color," as she said with a laugh. The language barrier might make things more complicated, but "there is also the universal language of looks and smiles and hugs." She did not want the surrogate to feel like she was just a "uterus": "Regardless of how well I get to know her, for me this person will be someone I will feel thankful toward for my entire life."

Even though the intended mother recognized that "no money in the world could pay for this," she emphasized that surrogacy had always existed and that capitalism had turned it into a business, just as everything else is made a business nowadays:

> The problem is that we live in a capitalist world and capitalism changes everything a little bit, right? It commercializes and changes all things that could be beautiful even if there needs to be an *exchange*; well there needs to be an exchange. I can't ask for everything for nothing, right? I am asking for something very important; I'm asking for the most important thing in my life that I have not asked of anybody else. I understand that there needs to be an exchange and the economic aspect nowadays is important to all of us, right?

Sara's words illustrate an argument that was made by many other research participants: that surrogacy could not be moved completely out of the commercial sphere, because payment was not only legitimate but also fair. Consequently, it was altruistic surrogacy that was considered unfair, because "everyone earns money apart from the surrogate," as intended father Diego Torres argued. He and his wife had gone through surrogacy in the United States and were now three-time parents, living in a suburb of Barcelona. Diego's line of reasoning was very similar to Sara Blanco's when he said that it would be great if one could "pay" for surrogacy by "giving 1,000 thank-yous (*mil gracias*)" but that there needed to be monetary compensation because "she is doing us the *favor of our lives.*" In Diego's eyes, this monetary compensation was thus a sign of respect. "If an independent, free woman decides to do this (i.e., surrogacy) [...] it is one more insult if they can't receive money for this. It's like 'oh those poor people, they're exploiting them,'" he said, emphasizing that it would be exploitation not to pay the surrogate, while everyone else was paid. Such statements point to a certain need to normalize payments in the intimate context of childbirth. Coupled with his comment on a woman's "free decision," Diego seems to suggest that receiving money for childbirth is not only fair but even emancipatory (see also Shalev 1989). Despite embracing this logic, the wording some of my interview partners chose seemed to reflect a certain unease about the topic. While in Russian, the term "salary" (*gonorar*) is mostly used to describe the surrogate's final payment, the foreign surrogacy participants I interviewed mostly spoke of "compensation."[11] For instance, when angrily telling me about feminists and "the left," who accused parents through surrogacy of "trading" human beings or eggs, Spanish intended father Juan Romero said:

> And I'm like: *No.* I'm giving her, I'm giving the carrier, compensation because she will suffer physical, um, inconvenience. She will have to, um, if she's working, she will have to be absent from work, at least three months. [...] She will have to buy clothes. She will have to do this; she will have to do that. And I'm compensating her.

By speaking of "compensation," Juan implied that surrogacy is not a service or a job, but rather a favor that comes with certain inconveniences and necessities that need to be compensated. Like the claim that capitalism pervades all spheres of life and that it would be unfair to pay everyone but the surrogate, these statements are attempts to normalize and humanize a process that takes place in the market sphere. The term "compensation" attributed a new "social meaning" to the money, moving it from the market sphere to the sphere of favors (Førde 2017; Zelizer 2013). Moreover, it allowed intended parents to emphasize that they were not paying for the baby and that the child was, therefore, not commodified (König 2018; Stuvøy 2018).

Intended parents such as Juan wanted the public but also the surrogate to see them not as paying clients but as caring individuals with a personality and a history of suffering. The thirty-six-year-old Spaniard wanted the surrogate to "think that she's contributing to a family, to making their life happy." She should be interested in him and his male partner, and she should be looking for "good intended parents" who would take care of the child. He had been researching the different options available for several months and had been in contact with over fifty agencies around the world: "I have seen all the tonalities of gray and even black during the surrogacy process, the legal process, the medical process; I could see everything and I dislike this world a lot." Concluding that agencies "convert something lovely and beautiful into something ugly" by "exploiting surrogates and intended parents," Juan decided to go "freestyle" and search for a surrogate himself. He was highly suspicious of agencies, as they were the ones who made big money and set the rules. In contrast to Sara Blanco, who did not want to be seen as a victim, many other intended parents, including Juan Romero, regarded themselves as deprived of agency, equally vulnerable as surrogates, and therefore exposed to the power of agencies.

Producing Happy Surrogates

While many Russian and Ukrainian agencies and clinics failed in transmitting the warm feelings intended parents such as David Hauser, Sara Blanco, and Juan Romero were longing for, some were nevertheless "attuned" to narratives of altruism. As the prior sections have illustrated, the position of the surrogate plays an important role in contributing to making surrogacy a happy process, not least because her happiness can fundamentally undermine critical positions on surrogacy. If the surrogate is "happy to help," then who can criticize surrogacy for being morally wrong or exploitative? Some agencies have therefore learned to wrap their services in a language that appeals to foreign couples. But many attempts at producing "happy surrogates" seem half-hearted and reveal cracks and contradictions.

Particularly striking in this regard was a Skype meeting I participated in as translator between the German intended parents Teresa and Stefan Wagner, surrogate Alyona Timofeyevna, and surrogacy agent Marina Romanovna. The Wagners had been excited about this opportunity: it would be the first time they saw and talked to the Ukrainian woman carrying their twins. The agency had advised the couple against personal contact before the critical phase of twelve weeks was over and the pregnancy was well under way. And even then, they required all conversation to be mediated by them, to avoid unreasonable demands from the surrogate. The couple did not have total confidence in the agency and preferred to have me translate from Russian into German for them, rather than relying on the agency's translations. Having five people in three different places speak to each other through a bad Internet connection proved to be a challenging undertaking. After overcoming initial technical problems, the agent initiated the conversation: "Alyona is shy," Marina Romanovna said with a smile. "She does her work in order to help other people," she added, without any question having prompted such a statement. "Her motivations are altruistic. She does this with love." Stefan and Teresa Wagner gave me incredulous looks—via the screen—when I translated these sentences. They realized that the entire setting told a different story: Alyona Timofeyevna did not appear shy but rather intimidated and nervous. She was positioned right in front of the computer and stared into the camera. Next to her, yet much closer to the screen, stood the agent, who kept answering questions on her behalf. Marina Romanovna's attempts at conveying the surrogate's altruistic motives were in stark contrast to Alyona's distant conduct. The situation was somewhat comical and tragic at the same time, because the agent's efforts seemed too calculated. Marina Romanovna did not engage in "deep acting" but in "surface acting" (Goffman 1959, cit. in Hochschild 2003), and so her affective labor failed to produce and transmit the desired affect. But her words nevertheless showed that she was aware of her role as cultural translator, of mediating between what she assumed to be different approaches and expectations toward surrogacy. The agent mirrored the wishes of foreign intended parents for "the human feeling," as one of my interview partners had phrased it, even though Teresa and Stefan were not among those for whom this was of central importance.

Another revealing experience in this regard was my encounter with the psychologist of a fertility clinic. When we first met, in her small consultation room, Aleksandra Denisovna told me about her years working in Italy, where she had realized that people thought of Russia as a poor and underdeveloped country, which clearly offended her. She wanted to set the record straight and explained to me that Russia had so many egg providers not because of poverty but because of a specific historical mindset: "This goes back to the Soviet Union. It is just our Eastern mentality, to think not only about yourself," she stated. That was why, according to her, people in Russia more readily risked their health in order to help others, in contrast to "Europeans," who only thought about their own lives. Wanting to learn more about the psychologist's view on this "Eastern mentality," I returned to Aleksandra Denisovna a few weeks later. When I brought up this issue, she gave me a confused and irritated look: "A successful person would never participate in such a program. They all do it for the money . . . I mean, would you donate a kidney just like that?" While I do not know for sure what prompted these contradictory claims, I assume that they were connected to the way she perceived me—at first as an outsider who knew little about surrogacy in Russia and then rather as an insider who was aware that financial motives were central for Russian surrogates. There were numerous incidents during my fieldwork in which I had the impression that agents who knew I had been doing long-term fieldwork were more direct in this regard, while others were keen to stress the altruistic nature of surrogates.

Some agencies and clinics—particularly in Ukraine—have learned to integrate "altruism-talk" into their self-representations, to create the "human feeling," a feeling that transforms the otherwise cold and distant commercial exchange into a happy and warm encounter. The Ukrainian agency Vittoria Vita, for instance, includes testimonials by former surrogates on its website. Five women from cities all over Ukraine express their gratitude toward the agency for "this marvelous opportunity" (Tetiana) or for enabling them to realize their "potential as a surrogate mother" (Anastasia).[12] All former surrogates stress the support and help they received during their pregnancy and the way they always felt well cared for. The agency has also learned to incorporate the critique of exploitation into their discourse and portray surrogacy as a matter of free and informed choice. Tetiana, for example, states that "we have discussed all questions in great detail, considering the opinions and wishes of both sides." This resonates with the account of intended father Juan Romero, who said that the agency he had been in contact with had told him that in Russia and Ukraine intended parents and surrogates choose one another:

> You have to write a report and say, this is who I *am*, this is my *partner*, this is what we *want*, this is how I *live*, and then the surrogate mother can *opt* for you. She can say, "well, I would like to, um, do the process for him, for her, for them" and, um, in turn they offer you the chance to choose between the different surrogate mothers that have *opted* for you and so there must be a connection; you get to know the surrogate mother [...] more or less the same process as in, as in, um, as *in* the U.S.

Whether Tetiana's and Anastasia's statements reflect the reality of surrogates who worked through this particular agency, and whether the information given to Juan Romero is accurate for the agency he had spoken to, is, of course, impossible to evaluate. However, I can almost certainly say that none of the thirty-nine surrogates I met during my research would have phrased their experiences in this way, especially not if working through agencies. Considering that surrogates often have high levels of financial stress, they are seldom in the position to lay out and fight for their opinions and wishes. As one of the surrogates I spoke with said: "It's a market, a business; there's nothing you can do about that. Either you swim with the flow or you drown." I have also never heard about "mutual selection" in any of my interviews in Russia and Ukraine. I suggest that such narratives are produced and circulated by agencies in order to silence moral concerns. Testimonials in particular can be powerful in such a context, as they are personal and immediate—inevitably presenting some sort of truth. The testimonials quoted also reflect the importance of "happiness" in countering moral concerns, as Tetiana and Anastasia are portrayed as happy to have been able to help. As Maria Kirpichenko (2020) has argued based on the analysis of Russian surrogacy websites, such images and messages facilitate "reproductive consumption."

The Spanish agencies seemed more experienced in conveying "the human feeling." I was intrigued by their enthusiasm and their means of conveying this feeling. A particularly memorable instance in this regard was my visit to Ricardo Delmonte's office in Barcelona. He was the founder and director of an agency that facilitated surrogacy arrangements in Ukraine. During our interview, Ricardo Delmonte continually underlined his statements by showing me photographs and short videos of the surrogacy process. "Look at these pictures," he said blissfully, and turned the screen of his laptop in my direction:

> This is the couple. And this is the surrogate. She was so charming, really. She was a really calm woman and with a *super positive attitude*. I was there when they met the first time and, honestly, I nearly had to cry, because . . . it's just such a beautiful thing. This situation between two women. [. . .] They (i.e., the intended parents) sent me a photo. They said: "Look, this is Fernando" (showing me a picture of a newborn). And I was like "how great." They were all really happy. The thing is, this is really an experience, it should be like this, a positive experience and beautiful.

Then the agent opened another couple's file and showed me pictures of the woman who had carried their children. He told me that the intended mother and the surrogate were both crying when they met each other, because "it was a lovely moment." The parents expressed their gratitude by giving the surrogate more money than stipulated in the contract. Ricardo Delmonte repeated: "It was lovely, the truth is, it was really . . . Look at their happy faces." He seemed so passionate about the encounters of intended parents and surrogates that he again and again interrupted his answers to my questions by showing me yet another batch of photographs. Also Álvaro Fuentes, director of another Spanish agency working in Russia and Ukraine, got excited about the moment intended parents and surrogates meet for the first time: "It's a magical moment, really," Álvaro Fuentes said. "I wish you could experience it one day. And it's so emotional, because the surrogates, they are usually very open and then they all kiss each other and hug. They are very affectionate."

The quotes by these two agents show that "the human feeling" requires making use of affects and emotions, which produce a general feeling of happiness for all involved. This affective labor of happiness also creates bonds. It makes the relationship between the intended parents and the surrogate appear to be one of mutual support, of being in this together (see also Teschlade 2019). All of the Spanish agents stressed how important it was that intended parents and surrogates know each other. Moreover, this was referred to as "normal," "natural," and "healthy," while not knowing each other was considered "cold" and "a bit strange." Most argued for this stance by mentioning the intimate character of surrogacy and stating that one could not negate the "human aspect." One of the agents I spoke with, Pedro Monte, became particularly upset about my question regarding whether the two sides should or should not be in contact:

> Well, personally, I have to say that someone who doesn't want to know who'll give life to their child, this is neither *polite* (*fino*) nor *ethical*. Because at the end of the day, this woman is doing you a great favor; it's not a question of money. This is not a supermarket. You are not going to buy a bottle of Coca-Cola. No. You are asking this person, a human being, a favor.

Parents who did not want to know the woman who was going to carry their child should go to one of the "commercial agencies," because he would certainly not work with them. Pedro Monte's "agency" was among those that do not want to be labeled as such, as the term has strong connotations of profit-making.[13] Rather, as he told me, they see themselves as "consultancies" or "associations" that act as facilitators and companions during the surrogacy process, because their involvement in surrogacy is not a matter of profit but of personal commitment. These "facilitators" are deeply emotionally involved with their clients, not least because many founders of the Spanish agencies are parents through surrogacy themselves. As Amy Speier (2016) has argued in relation to reproductive tourism in the Czech Republic, personal experience gives intermediaries special credibility in the reproductive market. They are part of the community they construct, for example by actively updating their clients and fans on Facebook with news and photos about the latest trips, the latest births, and the latest positive pregnancy results. In this way, affective labor creates social networks, communities, and collective subjectivities (Hardt 1999), specifically a collective body of intended parents, united by "shared histories of suffering" (Schurr and Militz 2018, 1636). At the same time, such online spaces can be understood as "echo chambers" (Whittaker 2019, 121), where particular understandings of surrogacy were shared and affirmed.

Through researching surrogacy, I sometimes became part of these collective online spaces: My visit to Álvaro Fuentes's agency, for instance, resulted in a Facebook post, accompanied by photographs I felt obliged to consent to. Like the surrogates' testimonials on the Ukrainian agency's website, the use of photographs can be seen as a form of evidence: in this case as evidence of my visit to the agency but more generally also as evidence of the intermediaries' intimate involvement as well as of the happiness surrogacy brings. Photographs add an affective quality to words. I, as a researcher, would not have to believe his words, for I could surely see with my own eyes that these people were truly happy. When I asked Ricardo Delmonte whether his clients might object to his showing me the entire photographic record of their time in Kyiv, he looked at me indignantly and reminded me that his agency was not a commercial one and that these parents should help "the project" if they wanted to work with him. They should not hide but be proud of their mutual effort. The "project" he had in mind was one aimed at normalizing surrogacy within society and in building what Sharmila Rudrappa (2014) has called "caring communities"—meaning safe and accepting future surroundings for the children born through such forms of assisted reproduction. Ricardo Delmonte and Álvaro Fuentes were thus keen to create affective communities between intended parents and surrogates and between intended parents themselves, for they believed that surrogacy should be a positive and beautiful experience. At the same time, they were engaged in ethical labor to further social acceptance for surrogacy by distributing displays of happiness through social media or by sharing them with researchers like me. Their approach was thus fundamentally different from that of my Russian and Ukrainian research participants, who felt compelled to choose silence over disclosure. Nevertheless, they were united by the wish to create safe spaces for themselves and their children in the future.

Happiness as Human Right

Another aspect that united the different participants in my research was a specific way of "laboring with happiness" through which happiness was rhetorically presented as an end in itself, embedded in a discourse of discrimination and rights. As Sara Ahmed observed, happiness per se can be used as moral argument:

> To refer to happiness might suspend obligation to refer to anything else in making good an argument. Happiness becomes our defense; you can defend anything by saying it is necessary for happiness, whether that happiness is the happiness of a certain one, or the happiness of many. You can attack anything by saying that it is the cause of unhappiness. Happiness adds weight to arguments. To be on the side of happiness or to be for happiness (as a way of "being for being for") means you are on the side of the good. (2010, 204–5)

Happiness is thus not only *one* of many arguments for or against something but can be seen as the *ultimate* argument that overrides all other ones. In the context of surrogacy, the moral power happiness entails in refuting any possible moral concerns is well illustrated on a Ukrainian agency's website. It starts with the following lines:

> There is no doubt, being a mother is a real happiness. It's a pity but some women can only wish to hold a tiny hand and hear merry laugh of her such a "desired little happiness." Others dream about the wealthy life for their children but don't have an opportunity to provide it.[14]

The text goes on to state that surrogates are motivated by love toward children, the desire to offer a helping hand, the joyful feeling of creating a new family, or the financial compensation. After listing these possible motives, the agency concludes that in the end these aspects are not decisive. Either way, surrogacy is an "honorable thing to do" and "one of the greatest gifts one can give to another person." The agency reminds readers that there are many women who would be willing to become surrogates for free, even though—not very surprisingly—they only offer arrangements with women who take this "noble step" in return for "some gratuity." These statements reveal two interesting aspects. On a more explicit level, the agency employs the notion of happiness as an argument for surrogacy. The quotes underline the manifold ways in which positive affect "sticks" to the figure of the baby, making it a "happiness means" (Ahmed 2010, 34). This means is not questioned; rather there is "no doubt" that "being a mother is a real happiness." A similar logic was reflected in my own interviews. One of the Russian doctors, for instance, stated: "Of course, surrogacy is somehow against nature but seeing all these happy parents you understand that it cannot be such a bad thing." And another stressed that surrogacy enabled people to experience "the joys of motherhood and fatherhood" and therefore "this is all very good and human and ethical." Such assertions show how the evaluation of something as ethical and good is shifted from the conditions and means of surrogacy to its end—happy children and happy parents—just as forum user Amapola (quoted above) had reminded others that it was the "result" that counted when choosing surrogacy.

On a more implicit level, the agency in question suggests that happiness is something everyone deserves. Constructing happiness as the ultimate argument thus transforms the issue of happiness into a matter of individual rights. Many surrogacy participants and advocates argue that individuals should be given the right to define for themselves what it is they need. In this logic both intended parents and surrogates are satisfying each other's needs via the market, and—from this utilitarian approach to morality and justice—it is the mutual satisfaction that makes the exchange good and ethical (Sandel 2009). Most Russian and Ukrainian professionals were thus satisfied with the minimalistic legal regulation of surrogacy in their countries. They preferred little state regulation, arguing that laws—as well as any other "norms"—were inhibiting "possibilities" for happiness, as doctor Valeriy Ivanovich contends:

> Religious and legal norms practically inhibit possibilities for those people who see in this (i.e., surrogacy) a solution to their problem. So why should this be forbidden if it is not something that damages people, no one is killed, and in the end a healthy and happy baby is born that is loved and needed. This is what is most important.

That "no one is killed" and that quite the opposite happens, because a happy baby comes into being, was a recurring phrase in interviews. The surrogacy market "produces a good that is inherently *good*" (Spar 2006, 196) and, according to many, essentially "necessary" in life. Even though infertility is not a fatal illness, as Valeriy Ivanovich contended, it leads to unhappiness. It is therefore crucial to "provide maximum possibilities," so that individuals can choose for themselves what they need—"this would be ideal," the doctor said, "because then there will be a higher number of happy people."

While Valeriy Ivanovich claimed that infertility is not an illness one dies from, the Moscow-based family lawyer Konstantin Svitnev seems more pessimistic when he writes that "infertility, childlessness, lack of somebody to care about leads to moral suffering, lower social status and even premature death" (2012, n.p.). Svitnev is well known in the reproductive market, as he is the founder and director of Russia's central law firm that deals with surrogacy and attracts many foreign clients. He is active in promoting Russian surrogacy and has published extensively in English, mainly on his firm's website but also in several handbooks on surrogacy. The lawyer presents himself as a tireless advocate for those affected by medical and social infertility, often drawing on a language of compassion and pathos. Framing access to assisted reproduction as a human right, he states that "refusing to allow people with limited reproductive possibilities to become parents [. . .] means discrimination. [. . .] washing out their unique genes from the gene pool of humanity" (2012, n.p.). In another article, he even extends his discrimination argument to "those to be born" (Svitnev 2016). Furthermore, he claims that "any unrealized human life which could have been realized is a missed chance to change the world to the better and make people happier" (Svitnev 2006, n.p.).

Konstantin Svitnev's statements reveal several inconsistencies. His strong argument for maximum individual rights can only lead to a conflict of interests. For instance, he states that abortion is murder—not only of the individual child but also of the children this child could have given birth to—while in the same article making a plea for legal sex selection (Svitnev 2006). He underlines his argument by referring to the case of an Indian woman who had "died of grief" after realizing that she had given birth to a girl. Anticipating that Russian couples might feel the same, Svitnev argues for the legalization of sex selection even in the absence of a medical indication. In his texts, the lawyer also makes a number of other legal recommendations that mainly entail removing those few regulations that currently exist. He himself summarizes his stance in the following two polemic sentences: "Everything which helps a new person to come to this world is ethical and acceptable. Everything which impedes it is immoral and unacceptable" (Svitnev 2007). His words unarguably reflect a utilitarian approach to issues of justice. Again, the assessment of surrogacy is shifted from the conditions and means to the result of enabling a maximum number of "unique genes" to continue in a new person—a person that is expected not only to make her or his parents happy but also to "change the world to the better." Imbuing children with this positive affective power, the opposition to surrogacy becomes unfair or even irrational. This was most evident in a bizarre comparison made by the Spanish surrogacy advocate Alberto Cabello:

> I think that if someone is against someone else being happy, I don't know, this is like if I wake up tomorrow in the morning and say: "Ah well, clowns, I *really don't like clowns*. I'll make a law that forbids clowns." But there are people who like clowns. What's going on, just because I woke up that morning and went out and, um, I'll take away other people's happiness? This is horrible.

From this perspective, then, banning surrogacy is a random act of cruelty, primarily motivated by the wish to make other people's lives less happy. The quotes from both Alberto Cabello and Konstantin Svitnev thus demonstrate how the "language of happiness converts swiftly into missionary language" (Ahmed 2010b, 204) when seeking legitimation for a contested practice. Conceiving of intended parents as vulnerable individuals deprived of the right and the opportunities to reproduce, these intermediaries become ethical actors because they help make desperate people happy. Their stances imply that it would be unethical to "abandon such people and leave them without any hopes," as one agency states in an online contribution titled "Is Surrogacy Ethical?"[15] Constructing themselves as altruistic actors, intermediaries and advocates not only reduce the contested nature of surrogacy but also mask their profits—by means of which, in turn, profits can be increased, for surrogacy becomes more morally acceptable (Jacobson 2016, 43). Illustrative of this argument was one of my interviews with a Russian lawyer who argued that he would like to dedicate more time to research than to facilitating surrogacy but that he needed to keep up with the many requests from intended parents, who were forced to travel to "cold Russia, with all the bears in fur hats on bicycles drinking vodka" in order to "fulfil their dreams." Considering that this man is head of a large firm mediating surrogacy arrangements, his complaint about having to "help" so many infertile couples can only be read with cynicism.

Finding Happiness in the Marketplace

This chapter has traced the affective labor of happiness, investigating how happiness operates and circulates in the moral economy of surrogacy. I have illustrated how intermediaries and doctors evoke the baby as a "happy object" (Ahmed 2010) and thus become dream-makers in a double sense: they make dreams come true, but they also play a significant part in producing and upholding these dreams by actively engaging in affective labor. This type of labor not only works through the notion of happiness but also draws on hope and fear. These affective practices are directed toward promoting an image of Russia and Ukraine as a "middle ground" between the ethically superior United States and countries such as India, Thailand, and Mexico, which are associated with exploitation and scandals.

Moreover, the affective labor some of the foreign surrogacy actors engaged in aimed at an "affective de-commodification" (Smietana 2017b) to "humanize" otherwise commercial relationships. This wish for humanization stemmed, on the one hand, from a shared cultural assumption that the child and the family are not supposed to belong to the sphere of commerce and money but that the latter would corrupt the former (Zelizer 2013). On the other hand, the way in which transnational surrogacy is criticized for exploiting women crucially shapes these discourses and practices, as surrogates who are "happy to help" are regarded as women who are not forced into surrogacy. As such, happiness has the affective potential to undermine the two most prominent critiques—the so-called "coercion critique" and "corruption critique" (Sandel 2013)—in Western discourses regarding surrogacy.

Agencies and other intermediary actors, as I have shown, actively respond to wishes and desires for de-commodification. While some join humanization efforts and want to create happiness as part of the surrogacy process, others advertise their services by stressing that they are cheap and successful and that trying to achieve happiness along the way might result in never achieving happiness as an end, through becoming a parent. Yet others employ happiness to make an argument for individual human rights. In such a libertarian view of society, the market is seen as providing everyone with what they need. Norms and morals are regarded as negative and impeding, and surrogacy opponents are constructed as irrational beings that take away other people's happiness. Opponents, critics, and skeptics—or in fact all those who question the libertarian notion of rights—are thus cast as "killjoys" (Ahmed 2010). They "disturb the very fantasy that happiness can be found in certain places," by pointing out what some might want to cover up, and by investigating "how happiness is used to justify social norms as social goods" and what power relations underlie these dynamics (Ahmed 2010).

In contrast to the impeding character of morality, the free market is imagined as a "neutral" arena that "affords possibilities," as the Russian doctor Valeriy Ivanovich phrased it. His argument is in line with legal scholar Martha Ertman's views on the "upside of baby markets." Such a market, according to Ertman, allows minorities, such as those who are LGBTQI+, to form families in ways that might not be welcomed by a majoritarian morality and are thus prohibited by law: "Market mechanisms present a different moral vision, which gives priority to liberty and innovation, rather than tradition and divine or biological mandates" (2010, 23). Affording possibilities, a free market is also imagined as bringing political freedom, because the market is thought to support human rights. In such a logic, however, "consumer sovereignty" and "getting people what they want" become disguised as a democratic project (Fourcade and Healy 2007, 289).

7

AMBIVALENCES OF FREEDOM

Many surrogacy advocates suspect a moral double standard among feminists criticizing surrogacy for potentially exploiting poor women who have to sell their reproductive capacities to secure a living. As Spanish intended father Juan Romero put it: if feminists campaign for the right to abortion with the slogan "my body belongs to me," what right do they have to deny other women, who would like to sell their reproductive cells or services, this kind of agency? Taking this tension as a starting point, this chapter addresses how actors in the field of surrogacy negotiate moral concerns in relation to the notion of free choice. In the previous chapter, I indicated that this notion is at the heart of many discussions around surrogacy in Western countries, and I detailed how choice can find its expression in the altruistic motives of the economically stable surrogate who wants to *help* an infertile couple. This narrative, however, often cannot be applied when surrogacy is conducted in regions with high levels of poverty (Pande 2011). Russia and Ukraine are such countries; however, they also constitute a certain "moral middle ground" between countries such as the United States and India. This means that the framing of the altruistic surrogate can coexist next to another framing: one that locates the surrogate's "freedom" in a neoliberal rhetoric that casts her as a choice-making market actor in a win-win transaction (Gunnarsson Payne 2015). This rhetoric has become incorporated into neoliberal (development) discourses since the 1970s, which have added an "entrepreneurial spirit" to the libertarian notion of the autonomous individual, positioning poor women as self-improving and "enterprising subjects with limitless capacity to 'cope'" (Wilson 2013, 87). Moreover, since structural constraints on people's lives are downplayed, choice is conceptualized as being equally available to everyone, resulting in a logic of individual self-responsibility (Hemmings and Treacher Kabesh 2013, 34).

From this perspective, surrogacy emerges as a form of gendered empowerment in a field where self-responsibility plays out in very particular ways. While surrogates are presented as autonomous women who happily and voluntarily sell their reproductive capacities in the marketplace, intended parents often stress their lack of freedom and choice in pursuing the path of surrogacy. In this chapter, I am interested in these "contradictory logics of reproductive choice" (Gunnarsson Payne 2015) and in teasing out how and when surrogacy actors accepted, rejected, redirected, or negotiated notions of choice. My focus here lies on the perspective of foreign intended parents, and I will dedicate much ethnographic detail to one particular surrogacy arrangement that I was able to follow closely and for a long period. While neo/liberal rhetoric—and its repercussions on issues of self-/responsibility—was also reflected in my interviews with local actors in Russia and Ukraine, the notion of free choice was much more present in the interviews with foreign market actors. Confronted with the reproach of exploiting poor women, references to "free choice" offered them a moral tool to grapple with the inherent power inequalities surrogacy entails and justify this contested social and medical practice. This tool is all the more effective because "ideas of freedom," as Nikolas Rose argues, "have come to define the ground of our ethical systems, our practice of politics and our habits of criticism" (2004, 10).

As I will show in this chapter, the notion of freedom or free choice is also particularly powerful, as it can be flexibly filled with meaning and, hence, adapted to changing situations, which alleviates the need for actors to take responsibility for one another. Freedom and choice thus constitute central elements in the moral economy of surrogacy and can be seen as moral values that are made profitable in the reproductive market.

Embodied Subjects or Fragmented Objects?

Feminists have for a long time fiercely argued about whether women are "embodied subjects" or "fragmented objects" of the new reproductive technologies (Gupta and Richters 2008). In the United States, early debates about women's agency culminated with the famous Baby M case in the 1980s, when a "traditional" surrogate—meaning, a surrogate who was also genetically related to the child she carried—refused to relinquish this child upon birth. The case went to court and while in the end the intended father won custody, not all of the judges involved were comfortable with this decision. One of them pronounced the surrogacy contract invalid, arguing that "any decision prior to the baby's birth is [...] uninformed and [...] any decision after that, compelled by a pre-existing contractual commitment, the threat of a lawsuit, and the inducement of a $10,000 payment is less than totally voluntary" (cit. in Phillips 2013, 149). Some feminists reacted to the statement with rage, for it suggested that women's decision-making was tainted by the influence of hormones and financial promises. Arguing against this claim, Carmel Shalev (1989), a human rights lawyer and active supporter of surrogacy in Israel, even stated that a surrogate's freedom was greatest when she demanded pay for her reproductive services.

Since the internationalization of the infertility business in the 2000s, these debates have become even more heated, and international surrogacy has often been discussed in terms of trafficking in women and baby farming in the "Third World" (Spar 2010, 187). These tropes have been taken up by contemporary initiatives such as Stop Surrogacy Now, who depict surrogates and donors as exploited women deprived of agency and forced into this kind of labor and therefore in need saving. Such discourses are highly reminiscent of the way other forms of intimate economies—such as sex work (Agustín 2008; Kempadoo and Doezema 1998) or marriage markets (Constable 2006)—have been publicly discussed. They tie into the construction of the category of "Third World Women," who, as Chandra Mohanty has famously argued, are cast as "a homogenous 'powerless' group often located as implicit *victims* of particular socio-economic systems" (1984, 338). Numerous surrogacy scholars (e.g., Lewis 2019) have criticized these stances for their normative and paternalistic assumptions about what women want and what "free choice" means. These assumptions are often linked to the explicit or implicit statement that women who do not see their own oppression suffer from a "false consciousness."

This tension was also noted by several intended parents, who stressed that women are not "forced" into surrogacy and that they are capable of making their own decisions. "The thing is, I'm not harming anyone. I'm paying, yes, but this girl is an adult; she knows what she's doing," Marta Pérez—an intended mother who had recently started a surrogacy program in Ukraine—said. And Diego Torres, a three-time father through surrogacy in the United States, argued that surrogates were "true feminists," because they were self-confident enough to say: "As a woman I can give this, I can offer this. Who are you to judge me?" His quote suggests that "judging" others would not be "true feminism," thereby disqualifying all those who might critically comment on questions of choice and coercion in the context of surrogacy. Diego's reference to feminism was probably not incidental: from the perspective of many surrogacy advocates, feminists embody key adversaries and were thus often commented on in my interviews, especially in the one I conducted with Juan Romero, the above-mentioned intended father from Spain:

> It's easy to let feminists see that they fall into contradictions. They're like: "Oh I must be able to say what I want to do with my own body, when it comes to abortion. I must be able to terminate my pregnancy. Nobody can tell me what to do with my body." OK. But they're telling you not to have a pregnancy for *me*. If *you* want to have a pregnancy for *me*, the law doesn't allow you to do it. So are you free to do what you want with your body or *not*? If you defend a woman's right to be free to do what she wants with her body, shouldn't you *allow* surrogacy? I'm not asking *you* to do it for me; I'm asking you to understand that somebody else wants to do it for me. *Freely* and *voluntarily*.

Such statements reflect how tricky feminists' engagements with notions of choice are, as they have to navigate a certain dilemma due to the double goal they pursue: on the one hand, pointing out power structures and showing how these affect the different possibilities individuals encounter in their lives; on the other, opposing victimization, making agency visible, and accepting that different people pursue different projects in their lives. But while the points mentioned by Juan Romero constitute a significant challenge for feminist engagements with surrogacy, it is also important to put his comment in perspective: while he emphasized that many of his female friends would be willing to carry a child for him, such a statement cannot be equated with committing to becoming a surrogate, with all the medical interventions, risks, and uncertainties it involves. It is therefore not surprising that those countries that only allow altruistic surrogacy or egg donation usually have a shortage of women who "*freely* and *voluntarily*" offer such services, while commercial arrangements are booming in low-income countries.

We Are "Getting One Family out of Poverty"

Unlike Juan Romero, most foreign intended parents I spoke with readily accepted that surrogates in Russia and Ukraine acted on financial motives. Their comments about the surrogates' "free choice" often came with an emphasis on the win-win nature of surrogacy that enabled a simple transaction of a "life for life" (Cohen 1999; Vora 2013)—one life was created in the course of the pregnancy, the other significantly improved, or even saved, by money. This was particularly reflected in intended father Diego Torres's hypothetical example of a woman who could avoid being thrown out of her house by becoming a commercial surrogate:

> It's difficult because this woman is acting with full liberty and she wants to do it because otherwise they will chuck her out of her house, right?

Who am I to say "what you are doing is bad"? No, "it is bad if I am left on the streets with my children." So it's complicated. [...] "I am helping someone and at the same time I am saving my own life. We're all winning here." There is no way of saying "No." Because really everyone is a winner. Who am I to say that your decision seems bad to me?

Diego acknowledges the difficulty of evaluating other people's lives, priorities, or necessities and insists that all parties emerge from surrogacy as winners. Despite the fairly radical conditions under which the woman in question would become a surrogate, he circumvents any reference to issues of coercion by emphasizing that the woman is nevertheless "acting in full liberty" when wanting to "help." The example illustrates how the framing of win-win obscures the material inequalities that underlie such exchanges, as Lawrence Cohen (1999) has argued in his work on organ selling and Kalindi Vora (2013) in her work on surrogacy in India.

Some intended parents even connected the win-win argument with highlighting their agentic role in "getting one family out of poverty." Intended mother Marta Pérez, for instance, said the following in relation to her surrogate's motives and living conditions:

> They wanted to buy a house [...] and she told us "well, thank you for choosing me, because I can solve a lot of things with this money," right? She wanted to start studying; because she had only studied a bit, she didn't have the opportunities ... well, with this money her and her family's quality of life would improve a lot, right?

For Marta, it was precisely the monetary exchange aspect and hence economic benefit that countered the reproach of exploitation: "We're not using (i.e., exploiting) her, because she will receive money for this." More so, as her quote implies, she was doing a good deed that was greeted with thankfulness by the surrogate (rather than the other way around).

As studies have shown, such arguments are particularly prevalent when cross-border family-making involves surrogacy or egg selling in poorer countries. In a paper with the subtitle "Gifts for Global Sisters?" anthropologist Amrita Pande (2011) juxtaposes the gift-metaphors encountered in the context of U.S.-American and Indian surrogacy arrangements, concluding that wealth disparities between Indian surrogates and foreign intended parents are too great to foreground the "giving" nature of the former, as is the case in the United States. In the Indian context, intended parents and the clinic become the altruistic "givers," as they enable women to improve their lives—a finding echoed in much research on surrogacy in India (Førde 2017; Rudrappa 2016a; Rudrappa and Collins 2015; Vora 2013) or Mexico (Schurr 2019). Moreover, some surrogacy firms officially register as nonprofit or social work organizations, to conceal their economic interests (Rudrappa 2016a, 148). Through such framings and practices, money is converted into "ethical value" (Førde 2017). The most obvious example of such "charity" is inarguably the Indian infertility doctor Nayna Patel. Sophie Lewis (2019) elaborately unpacks the rhetoric of the world's most famous surrogacy specialist. After coining the phrase "women helping women" on TV on the U.S.-American *Oprah Winfrey Show* in 2006, her words have entered the canon of the global justification discourse, stressing the altruistic and selfless orientation of such clinics as Patel's. In a show for Russia TV, Patel states: "To my critics I say: *can YOU give this poor couple a child? Can YOU give this poor woman's family a better life?* When you do, I will STOP doing SURROGACY!" (cit. in Lewis 2019, 5). In numerous articles, interviews, TV appearances, and other contributions, Patel has negated her economic motivations, while emphasizing her commitment to empowering surrogates, who, according to her, suffer not only from financial constraints but also at the hands of their abusive husbands. In her clinic, they learn to take care of money and have to attend English courses. Patel has also created a charitable trust that aims to assist former surrogates with medical problems or provide help with schoolbags and books for their children. Even though her "philanthrocapitalism" rather appears as a marketing strategy in disguise, her efforts allow intended parents who have worked with Patel to now claim their choices as moral ones—as having chosen a morally safe clinic as opposed to other clinics in India (Lewis 2019). Through such framings, surrogacy is presented as a "solution to, rather than a symptom of profound social and economic injustice" (Fixmer-Oraiz 2013, 127). Consequently, some intended parents report deliberately choosing low-income countries, so that they could make what they thought of as a life-transforming contribution (Schurr 2019). While surrogates certainly share these hopes, Sharmila Rudrappa and Caitlyn Collins (2015) argue that—for a number of reasons—this hope did not often materialize in the case of Indian surrogates.[1]

Balancing the Double Bind

Despite surrogacy payments not being life-transforming in most cases, Rudrappa (2016a) shows that while many of the Indian surrogates in her research endured pain and suffering during the process, they experienced their surrogacies as more empowering and fulfilling than other employment opportunities available to them—mostly work in garment factories.[2] Indian surrogates were thus active protesters against the proposed ban on commercial surrogacy in 2015, arguing that surrogacy was a unique opportunity to support their families.[3] This example shows that in the capitalist and highly unequal system we live in, allowing as well as banning surrogacy can have harmful effects—a dilemma legal scholar Margaret Radin (1987, 2005) has referred to as "double bind."

On an individual level—rather than on a legal or structural level—the issue of the "double bind" was also troubling to some of the intended fathers and Spanish intermediaries I spoke with. A particularly telling encounter in this respect was my meeting with Álvaro Fuentes, the founder of an agency that operated in Ukraine as well as in Russia. I took a seat in his office in Spain and waited while Álvaro Fuentes sorted out a few things with one of his employees, and hence allowed me to get a glimpse of his daily work at the agency. "So you will fly from Barcelona to Kyiv on the fifteenth of August, right?" a blond woman with a slight Slavic-sounding accent asked him. He nodded and gave her instructions to organize a taxi that would take him from the airport to the hotel. "And then we also need an appointment at the clinic, maybe around midday, then Arnau and Lucía can still have a shower before." "How many couples are going with you?" the woman asked. "I think, three . . . I still have to arrange the meeting between Arnau and Lucía and their surrogate. We already have one for them, but we still need to find one for Paloma and Eduardo." The woman was already through the door when Álvaro Fuentes called after her to please book an apartment for several months close to Thessaloniki—obviously another city the agency operated in. Then he turned toward me with a big smile and asked me to tell him more about my research interest.

A doctor and father through surrogacy himself, Álvaro Fuentes managed the entire surrogacy program and accompanied all of the intended parents during the process. He regularly traveled with his clients to Russia and Ukraine, and personally screened all the surrogates the local clinic proposed. This usually took four to five hours of conversation, in which—among other things—the agent looked for the woman's "freedom" (*buscar la libertad*): "I need to know about your *entire* life in order to know whether you can gestate a *child* and whether you *freely* enter this process," he said. The conversation often began in an informal way, with coffee and small talk, so that the surrogacy candidates could get to know and trust the agent, before coming to the more formal part of the procedure.

Álvaro Fuentes told me about his trip to Ukraine two weeks before, where for the first time he had to turn a surrogacy candidate away, because she did not seem to be acting freely: "This woman wasn't doing it voluntarily, she was doing it out of necessity, for purely economic reasons. She was very poor," he said. "A woman who has no money isn't free to decide. [. . .] So we couldn't allow this, because we would be abusing the poverty of one person to fulfill the desire of another." He acknowledged that there was always an economic motive, but according to him, this should not be the only motive and the woman should certainly not be "starving to death." He was annoyed about the Ukrainian clinic, which was mainly concerned about the woman's uterus and did not understand his point about the "freedom" of the surrogate. Álvaro Fuentes saw his role as "blocking" these kinds of things from happening. However, he was glad this had up to now been the first and only time he had had to turn away a candidate:

> It was the first time I had to say "no" and it was really traumatic for me. Professionally, I felt really bad because I was denying this woman the opportunity to (clicks his tongue) have more money. But we figured that she was not free and I couldn't, ethically I couldn't say "yes."

He felt very sorry for the woman but again emphasized: "Ethically, we can't accept such a case. Right? Just because you are poor, this doesn't necessarily mean that you have to sell your body to have a child." It was interesting how his prior discourse on the joys of surrogacy and the altruism of the surrogates suddenly changed into talking about surrogacy as body trade. While "free" surrogates seemed to be able to give the gift of life, poor surrogates were merely "selling their bodies"—a rhetoric that can also be found in the context of other forms of reproductive labor. Charlotte Kroløkke (2014), for instance, showed how in Denmark Spanish egg providers were commonly imagined as having agency and as "donating," while eastern European women were seen as selling their eggs for financial reasons, in a shady market dominated by untrustworthy clinics. The "freedom" of eastern European women thus emerged as something questioned from the beginning, as something that needed to be searched for (as implied by Álvaro Fuentes's expression *buscar la libertad*), as if it was well hidden and could be retrieved merely after hours of digging around in their biographies—resulting in a stark form of exposure for the potential surrogates. Álvaro Fuentes did not clearly define what he meant by "freedom," but I would suppose the circumstances of many of the surrogates I met during fieldwork would not have met his standards, and I was surprised that to date he had only turned down one woman. But as became clear from his further comments on this particular woman, his concerns about a woman's poverty were not only linked to issues of exploitation:

> If you are a person who has always lived with a lot of poverty, then there is no culture of care. And as much as I will pay you compensation so that you can eat well, you won't be eating well. Because there is *no* culture of good nutrition. [...] Because this is something you learn from an early stage. [...] *This part* I want to control. [...] You will buy (laughs) another pretty bag but you'll keep eating bread, because this is what you consider normal. [...] So there are things that can't be changed *in me*, *in you*, and in *any other* person.

Invoking Pierre Bourdieu's (2007) notion of "habitus," Álvaro Fuentes suggested that a woman who had always lived under financial constraints would not be able to take proper care of herself during the pregnancy. He seemed to imply that the surrogate's inadequate behavior might damage the child. His concern about the surrogate's freedom thus served a double purpose: It undoubtedly reflected an ethical concern regarding the surrogate, but it also reflected a medical one regarding the fetus and the paying clients. This is why his screenings took so long and involved taking into account the state of the woman's teeth, her hair, facial color, etc. and evaluating what he termed her "roots," "education," "culture," and "habits of life."

"Women Making Big Money"

While many of the foreign intended parents in my research stressed the win-win situation of surrogacy by foregrounding their own "giving" nature, some regarded the surrogates as mere "service providers" who earned a big amount of money for what they were doing. This understanding was particularly evident in my conversation with Stefan Wagner, on a cold but sunny day in L'viv, Ukraine. We were sitting in a restaurant in the Old Town, enjoying our "day off." The next day, I would be accompanying him to the clinic where he would sign the contract and leave his sperm sample, which would then be used to fertilize the provided eggs. Five days later, two of the embryos would be implanted into the womb of a surrogate carrier. Her name was Alyona Timofeyevna, a twenty-eight-year-old single mother to a one-and-a-half-year-old son. That was all the German couple knew about the woman who would make them parents by the end of the year.

Over lunch, Stefan Wagner told me about a friend who had turned out to be a clear opponent of surrogacy, arguing that surrogacy arrangements exploited poor women. "Of course she is right," he exclaimed. "But exploitation is everywhere. When you buy a T-shirt for five euros you can be sure that it was produced by exploited women and children in India or Bangladesh." He shrugged his shoulders. "But at the end of the day, women like Alyona decide for themselves to become surrogates. It's not like forced prostitution; it's a business model. Women do this because they can earn a lot of money." When I told him that his words surprised me because many of my interlocutors spoke only reluctantly about the commercial side of surrogacy and stressed altruistic motives, he laughed:

> I don't believe in these altruistic motives. If as intended parents you have misgivings that the women might be exploited, or if you feel sorry for them, then you can't get involved in this business. You have to regard these women as service providers, who earn good money for what they do.

"So you would say that surrogates are being exploited?" I asked cautiously. "They're not exploited. I'm simply saying that they themselves offer to do this." He continued: "You can see this as exploitation or you can see it as women making big money within just a year. Financially, this is a great deal for her."

According to Stefan, it was necessary to see the surrogates as enterprising "repropreneurs" (Kroløkke and Pant 2012), who actively shaped their future through the calculating choice of a "great deal" that *allowed* them to make "big money." The circumstances under which this choice was made did not matter, as long as these women were not physically coerced into surrogacy. He seemed to have internalized a specific neoliberal logic that stripped the notion of free choice of its structural aspects. From this perspective, questions of choice were sidelined by reference to the "adequate" financial compensation. The story of the Wagners offers a good opportunity to explore these logics further. In the following pages, I would therefore like to zoom in on this story in greater ethnographic detail.

Having read about my research upon Googling "surrogacy" and "Ukraine," the couple had contacted me in 2015, and what began as a distant exchange of information soon developed into an intense relationship. Teresa Wagner was born with a heart condition, and when she and her husband thought more seriously about having children, her doctor told her clearly that a pregnancy would be too much for her body. Struggling to live with this verdict, Teresa went to see numerous specialists but finally came to accept that pregnancy would be "like suicide" for her. She then turned to adoption, but the employee at the government office for youth welfare said that her chances were slim. The waiting list was long, and by the time they might have been able to adopt a child, the couple would have already exceeded the age limit. Teresa's illness would also pose severe difficulties in being considered as adoptive parents. The employee suggested signing up for foster care, with the possibility of later adopting the child. Teresa immediately felt that foster care entailed too many emotional risks, as she could already anticipate the painful separation in the event that the child was taken from her. It was her gynecologist who finally raised the idea that the two of them might be the "perfect couple for surrogacy" and that she had already accompanied three other couples in their surrogacy process. These other couples had traveled to the United States, but the Wagners could not afford this option. They did not have a "high income," as they had once told me. Of all the foreign intended parents I had spoken with during fieldwork, they were the only ones who both had no university degree and worked in less prestigious jobs—as opposed to other intended parents who, for instance, worked as schoolteachers, university lecturers, or in human resources. Teresa and Stefan owned a house in a small town in Germany, which they shared with the latter's parents. Happy to have already repaid the mortgage on their house, they seemed to live a fairly modest life, not going out much for dinner and usually not spending their holidays abroad, as they told me.

It took the couple two years to finally end up in Ukraine. First, they went to see a clinic in the Czech Republic that had worked with German couples before, but in the end this option proved too complicated and too risky. The clinic would have only taken care of the medical part of the process, leaving the Wagners to find a surrogate themselves. In addition, surrogacy is not regulated in the Czech Republic and they felt unsure about this legal gray zone. They nevertheless started to look for surrogates online and were in contact with a German and a Czech woman, but the first turned out to be taking psychiatric medication and the other was severely overweight—both not ideal preconditions for surrogacy, according to the doctors. After a number of other attempts at finding private surrogacy arrangements, the couple decided to consider Ukraine. This was approximately the time they contacted me. Not being able to find an agency or clinic that would take on their complicated case—considering the illegality of surrogacy in Germany and the heart disease—Teresa was eager to get advice from me. Though I was reluctant to offer "advice" and felt uneasy about being put in such a position, she seemed comforted by the fact that she could share her experiences, hopes, and anxieties. A few months later, she asked me to join her husband on his trip to L'viv, to sign the contract and leave the sperm sample. Not speaking English, Russian, or Ukrainian and not being used to traveling much abroad, Stefan welcomed my company as translator, organizer, mediator, and tour guide. His wife stayed in Germany. Her health condition had deteriorated, and so she preferred to avoid the strenuous trip. From a medical and legal point of view, her presence was not necessary, as the embryos were created with the eggs of a Ukrainian provider.

The trip to L'viv must have also been strenuous for Alyona Timofeyevna, who lived in Kharkiv, a city on the other side of Ukraine, almost nine hundred kilometers and a thirteen-hour train ride from L'viv. The Kharkiv-based agency offered foreign clients the possibility of conducting the embryo transfer in L'viv, because the city was geographically closer to such countries as Germany and was also regarded as more European. Where the egg provider was originally from, we did not know. She must have been at the clinic the same day as us, but to preserve anonymity, we were not allowed to meet her. We also did not meet Alyona, who arrived only five days later, when the embryos were ready to be transferred to her uterus.

The first embryo transfer proved successful. Teresa and I maintained close contact over the course of "their" pregnancy, and eight months later the couple asked me to travel with them to Ukraine to pick up their newly born twins and get to know Alyona. Because she had given birth a month early, the delivery took place in Kharkiv and not, as planned, in L'viv. The intended parents and the surrogate had only seen each other twice via Skype before—illustrating that digital technologies play a crucial role in transnational surrogacy, forming a kind of "digital umbilical cord linking the intended parents to the pregnancy" (Whittaker 2019, 123). This cord, however, was not direct: the two Skype talks were "mediated" by the agency, which had restricted the contact—as most agencies in Ukraine and Russia do. Considering the effort to keep both parties apart, it surprised me that only the official translator and no one from the agency was present when the Wagners and I went to the birth clinic to visit Alyona and the newborns. This provided an exceptional opportunity for me to get to know two perspectives on a shared story, and thus learn about how the agency had controlled and manipulated information. Under circumstances in which intended parents and surrogate do not share a common language and cultural background, agencies are in a powerful position to shape their relationship, as much surrogacy research has shown (Deomampo 2016; Lustenberger 2016; Pande 2014; Rudrappa 2016a).

"We Had Just Hoped . . . Our Souls Would Be at Ease"

"So? Are you satisfied?" Masha Radionovna asked with a mischievous smile. Hands on hips, she stood next to the cot with the two babies that her stepdaughter Alyona had given birth to. Only later would I realize the anxiety and skepticism this sentence entailed. For the moment, though, it was her self-confidence and her piercing look that struck me, the way her words marked her own involvement in the pregnancy. Alyona had carried the twins, but Masha had, in a way, managed their lives "around" the pregnancy and seemed to have become her stepdaughter's spokesperson. The surrogacy was a joint project, and with her question Masha made obvious the contractual nature of this deal. She was inviting, if not demanding, the clients to evaluate the fruits of their labor, as one could fittingly say. Stefan and Teresa laughed. They seemed to find this directness unpleasant but were happy to finally see and hold their children. "It all still feels so unrealistic and so far off," they had told me just an hour ago, before we left for the birth clinic to visit the surrogate and the twins for the first time.

Alyona was still lying in bed, in a pink dressing gown adorned with small sparkly rhinestones. She looked tired. I sat down on her bed, and Masha came over to me, letting the new parents take pictures. "Why did they only come now? The birth was five days ago!" she hissed at me in a low voice, pointing with her chin at the German couple. "We were really worried they would leave us with the children!" Her words were not meant for immediate translation—she was hoping that I could offer an answer to a question she might have deemed too rude to ask directly of the parents. But before I could answer, one of the babies started crying. Alyona glanced at the sheet of paper next to her. "It's time to feed the children. They are still weak; they need to be fed every three hours." Her face was twisted with pain as she carefully moved herself out of bed. She was still suffering from the Caesarean section that had left a fifteen-centimeter scar on her lower belly. Unable to stand up straight, she looked frail as she walked past me to get the milk powder and show Teresa how to feed the children. Masha turned toward me again: "It was not part of the contract that Alyona has to take care of the kids! It shouldn't be this way. What kind of deal is this!?" she said, widening her eyes with indignation. The contract had stated that the surrogate would not even see the children in the event of a Caesarean. But the clinic staff just put the children in her room, and she had to look after them day and night, "like her own." Alyona sat down next to me. She showed us pictures of her son on her phone. A few weeks ago, he had turned two but she could not celebrate with him. When her cervix shortened in the twenty-eighth week of pregnancy, the doctors sounded the alarm and sent her straight to the birth clinic. She had been there for nearly two months, unable to leave the building.

The German couple was filled with dismay that Alyona had had to take care of the children. "This is really cruel," Teresa said, explaining that she had not known any of this. Within seconds a lively debate developed, with me and the translator mediating between the two parties, while more and more details about their collaboration emerged. The weeks in hospital had been traumatic for Alyona in several respects. Despite the fact that the intended parents had chosen the "premium package" in order to secure maximum safety and comfort for the woman carrying their children, she was assigned a three-person room she had to share not only with a succession of other women but also with several cockroaches. "They had to sleep with the lights on because they were so afraid of all the pests," Masha told me. The hospital did not even provide patients with food, so in addition to taking care of her stepdaughter's son, Masha had to make daily visits to bring food. Alyona felt neglected and not well cared for, assuming that this was because she was "only" a surrogate and as such not worthy of good treatment. Her perception was corroborated by the way in which the clinic explained why she received no information about her and the babies' health after tests or ultrasound: she was simply told, "You don't need to know this. We will let your agency know the results." However, Teresa complained about not having received any ultrasound pictures. She had written to the agency every second day to ask how the surrogate was doing and was told that the agency was in frequent contact with her and that everything was fine. Alyona, however, said that the woman from the agency only called in on her once a week and usually did not bother conveying any of the intended mother's greetings and wishes. While the agency's website stated that they are happy to enable contact between intended parents and surrogates, they were actively hindering what would have been of vital importance to both women. Alyona was dependent on the agency, because she herself had no computer or Internet access. "If I had a computer, I would have written to them every day and every hour," she stated. Marina Romanovna, the agent, however, did not find this important and kept telling her: "What do you need this contact for? We write to them every day. They ask about you and we write that everything is OK." Before the first mediated Skype conversation between all parties the agent had told Alyona to refrain from complaining to the intended parents. I asked her what it felt like being held back during the conversation, while there were so many things she wanted to know from the Wagners:

> Marina was looking over my shoulder. I couldn't say a word; she was breathing down my neck. I wanted to ask something, but I kept quiet. I had *a lot* questions, *so many* questions for Teresa: where she works, what her husband does, many questions. But when there is a person breathing down my neck, I lose this desire. I was afraid that afterward Marina would shout at me and ask why I was asking these questions.

She went on to tell me that the agent once came by the maternity clinic to take a picture of her for the intended parents. Alyona had been told to stand up and smile, even though she had not felt like smiling at all. I remember the picture, which Teresa Wagner had forwarded to me via e-mail. The photograph depicted the surrogate standing in front of a few plants in the clinic corridor, her big belly showing beneath the pink dressing gown. She smiled, but there was no happiness in her smile.

Not having direct contact was particularly troubling for Alyona, since she feared the intended parents might have been shocked about the twin pregnancy and did not want to have two children. In a later conversation with her, she told me that she did not even know that two embryos were implanted and only found out during the first ultrasound. Alyona also criticized the lack of information when it came to the decision about performing a Caesarean section. While the intended parents knew a week in advance that there would be a Caesarean (although they did not know when, which was one of the reasons why they came to Ukraine so late), the surrogate was only told minutes before the operation was performed. She was devastated. She said, although C-sections were apparently fashionable, she believed a birth should happen naturally. Such a scar was "shameful," and Alyona feared she would no longer be able to go to the beach. She complained about the scar from when her appendix was removed that still hurt when the weather changed. In addition, she was planning to become a surrogate again, but hardly any agencies take on women who have had a Caesarean. With a scar as a reminder, she might also possibly have anticipated not being able to "forget" the surrogacy (Teman 2010). It was never explained to her why this procedure was medically necessary, but she nevertheless had to sign a document consenting to it. She clearly did not see this document as reflecting her *agreement*, since she emphasized that the C-section was performed "by fraudulent means, without my consent." The agent later told her that there had been a legal change, which from then on required surrogate children to be delivered by Caesarean—a claim for which no evidence could be found on the website of the Ukrainian parliament.[4]

The lack of information Alyona had received became even more evident when Stefan asked her whether she would be able—despite the Caesarean—to travel to Kyiv in the following week to sign the necessary documents at the German consulate. She answered that she did not know she had to travel to the capital. "This is awful," her stepmother intervened; "it gets worse and worse."

"What about L'viv?" Stefan asked. "Did you know the delivery was supposed to be in L'viv?"

Alyona shook her head. "We were not told a single word about that."

The translator intervened and tried to calm everyone down: "The agency can't give every piece of information at the beginning. It would just be too much," he said.

"But that's unfair," Teresa exclaimed; "then Alyona can't make a real choice."

"Well, probably if they said everything at the beginning, they wouldn't be able to find any surrogates," the translator suggested with a shrug.

The intended mother looked frustrated.

"That's just the way it is," her husband replied in a pragmatic tone, as if to put an end to the discussion: "The agency wants to make money, and the less information they share, the more money they make. This is business. Why don't you get it?"

And then, in a more empathic tone to me: "It must be interesting to see how both sides are played off against each other. It's shocking how little information Alyona has received." It was indeed interesting and shocking, and the reason agencies usually did not want me to receive information from both sides—intended parents and surrogates—was surely in order to conceal this playing off. It was also interesting how Stefan did not seem to be at all shaken by the turn this day took, almost as if he had not expected things to be otherwise in this world of business.

When we arrived at the clinic two days later, Alyona and Masha were extremely nervous. It was the day that Alyona and the kids were to be discharged. The babies would then come to the Wagner's hotel with us, and Alyona would return home to her son. She and her stepmother knew we had just been to the agency to pay the final invoice, and now it would be their turn to go there to collect the money they were still owed. But they were worried about being tricked by the agency into signing all the documents without having received the entire amount. In the clinic corridor, I took out the piece of paper on which the agent had noted all outstanding payments. Of the €7,000 (at the time roughly US$7,400) final compensation, Alyona had so far only received 10 percent, plus €250 as a monthly payment during the pregnancy. Today, she would receive the rest of her salary, plus €1,000 as a bonus for "good behavior," an additional €1,000 for the second child, and €15 for every day she spent in the hospital. I ran Masha through the list. Then I added that the agent had proposed holding back half of the bonus until Alyona had made the trip to Kyiv. "I see," she nodded and gave me a look above the frames of her reading spectacles. "They are afraid we will run off with the children . . . And we are afraid they will run off with the money." I asked her whether she wanted to take the piece of paper with her, and Masha laughed. "My dear, I know these numbers by heart," she said. As she opened the door to return to the hospital room, Alyona rushed past her to the toilet, tears running down her cheeks. "Alyonoshka, what's wrong? . . . It's only a job!" she called after her. The Wagners and the translator had stopped packing the babies' things together and looked worriedly at her. "She has got used to the children . . . We had just hoped that everything would be fine, that the birth would take place as planned, that the parents would come on time, that our souls would be at ease. Well . . . it didn't turn out that way. [. . .] But when we meet in Kyiv, we will talk and we will kiss each other and everything will be OK." Masha tried to look hopeful.

Imaginaries of Disempowerment

While Teresa and Stefan did not touch on any of the above-mentioned issues when we met the agent, they did bring up the question of the insurance, as they had been unable to answer Masha's query about what kind of insurance they had for Alyona. The English contract between the "provider" and the "customer" stated that the latter needed to take out insurance for such cases as "festering and inflammatory processes, post-surgical treatment, infectional processes and fatal outcome, which pertain to the delivery and postnatal procedures" and present the documents to the agency. Teresa and Stefan had interpreted the contract to mean that the agency would take care of the insurance. The agency, however, did not do that and also did not insist on seeing any papers from the intended parents. The topic was thus not discussed until we gathered at the agency a week after the babies were born. However, the agent did not seem troubled about this. She claimed that in any case it was currently not possible to take out such an insurance policy, neither for cases of surrogacy nor for one's "own" pregnancy, because a few months previously legislation had changed—another supposed legal change that could not be found on the website of the Ukrainian parliament.⁵ "So if there are any damaging consequences for Alyona's health that would just be her bad luck?" Teresa asked, astonished. "Yes. But she took this decision consciously and she knows what she's doing," the agent answered, and after a brief pause she added: "Everything worked out fine, so no need to worry about that." She smiled and took out a stack of bills. She wanted to talk about payments, not about insurance.

The agent's statement reflects all too well the trope of "the rational individual exercising free will" (Wilson 2008, 83) and points to the elements of risk that choice always entails, as critical scholars of neoliberalism have argued (Gershon 2011). Enterprising subjects have to calculate and manage risks before taking a decision. In surrogacy, both parties, when agreeing to collaborate, take a great risk, as they hope and bargain that things will "work out fine." As becomes clear in the example of Alyona, she alone needed to carry full responsibility for this decision. This kind of neoliberal freedom can be seen as "inevitably unstable, especially since, in capitalism, calculating to one's advantage is all too frequently also calculating to someone else's disadvantage" (Gershon 2011, 540). This was underlined by Stefan, who, in one of our conversations, quoted the well-known German proverb: "One person's sorrow is another person's blessing." He stated that the contract was "rock-hard" and that this must have been tough on Alyona, but for the parents, on the other hand, a strict contract was reassuring.

With the expression "she took this decision consciously and she knows what she's doing," the agent indirectly pointed to what in medicine and bioethics has been termed "informed consent." According to the Council for International Organizations of Medical Sciences and the World Health Organization (2002), this notion refers to giving consent "without being subjected to coercion, undue influence or inducement, or intimidation" and after having received and understood all relevant information. Tracing the history of this concept, health researchers Klaus Hoeyer and Linda F. Hogle argue that the atrocities of World War II provided the "moral urgency and legitimacy" to reframe fears of legal liability as concerns over individual autonomy and self-determination—"packaged as a universally valid protection of the human subject, informed consent could then travel to new domains" and became part of a global moral economy of biomedicine (2014, 350). Many criticize the notion of informed consent as an "ethical panacea" for all sorts of problems, as an expression of an "empty ethics" (Corrigan 2003)—a universal standard principle of an autonomous individual with no regard to economic, cultural, and social aspects and to the structural conditions under which consent takes place. Critics, however, argue that consent does not take place outside the realm of power but is shaped by dominant discourses and norms that constitute the field of freedom and choice (770–71). According to Hoeyer and Hogle, informed consent in medical practice and research constitutes "a way of circumventing the problem of defining common goods" and "silences an open discussion of the actual ethics of recruitment" (2014, 350): "Just as it obscures the ways in which consent protects researchers [or in my case, agents] against liability, it can obscure exploitation of desperate patients seeking treatment through research" (352).

In the context of surrogacy in Russia and Ukraine, as I have shown throughout this book, there are not many requirements guiding an "ethics of recruitment" concerning the surrogate workers. Besides the minimal relevant legislation, clinics and agencies usually only consider issues of mental and physical health in the recruitment of surrogates. While giving detailed and clear information about the surrogacy process is vital to "informed consent," my data indicate that in Alyona's case the agent did not go to great lengths to explain the process to her. And as the translator quoted above implied, giving out such information might negatively impact the steady flow of available and willing surrogates. Several studies have shown that surrogates often experience a lack of transparency and information and have little negotiating power throughout the surrogacy process, often fearing that they would be discharged from the clinic if they were too demanding (Deomampo 2013a, 175; Rudrappa 2016a).

However, what sounded like a prime example of exploitation and the opposite of an informed and free decision got a twist in a different direction in my later talks with Alyona and her stepmother, after the former was released from the maternity hospital. When I met the two of them in Masha's small apartment on the outskirts of Kharkiv, Alyona mentioned that in fact food *was* given out in the hospital, but in terms of quality it was not close to anything she would consider edible. Her stepmother agreed: "They came with a big bucket made of enamel, like in the old days. The name of the department was written on it in red letters. This is really something from my time (i.e., from the Soviet era). They came with this bucket and gave out porridge (*kasha*)." But they did not just bring *kasha*, Alyona added with a laugh: "There was also macaroni with condensed milk and cold water poured into the macaroni. And buckwheat and potatoes that were not well cooked. Or oats with cheese." Both laughed and shook their heads. "I bet they get better food in prison," she joked.

Later on in our conversation, she also corrected her earlier statement about the place of birth and said that the agency *did* tell her that she would have to give birth in L'viv, but she had merely forgotten. I checked the contract both parties had signed, and it clearly mentioned L'viv as the location and also that two embryos would be implanted. One could easily assume that the two women had simply lied in order to gain pity and perhaps consequently more money, and that they therefore personified the "dangerous" women that agencies constantly brought to mind. But I sincerely doubt that this was the case. There was genuine outrage in their voices, and when they "corrected" their statement in retrospect, there was no apparent need for them to do so at that specific moment. I suggest that their words were not lies but rather imaginaries that resulted from the extreme power imbalance at stake. Not being treated well and not trusting the agency as well as not receiving adequate information during pregnancy opened up a space of precariousness and vulnerability that gave way to a conflation of what *might* have happened and what *really* happened. If not necessarily a reflection of reality in a strict sense, the two women's accounts can be seen as reflections of their sensation of disempowerment in light of the way they were treated by the agency. Living in a country where legal regulations have limited validity due to unprosecuted infringements of the law as well as the high level of corruption, Alyona knew that she would not be able to make legal claims against the agency or intended parents were something to go wrong.

"Why Should We Feel Bad?"

While intended parents and agents often cast surrogates as free women making informed choices, many of the intended parents constructed themselves as lacking choice and thus being coerced into "reproductive exile" (Inhorn and Patrizio 2012). With many countries introducing more restrictive laws on commercial surrogacy in recent years or banning the practice altogether, the number of prospective destinations had decreased for most of my research participants, due to financial constraints and/or the legal requirements. According to intended father Juan Romero, particularly gay men like him had "limited options." Already suffering from discrimination due to his sexual orientation, he regarded it as an additional layer of discrimination that he could not have children due to the legal situation in his home country, Spain. With adoption being a fairly hopeless alternative for gay couples, and surrogacy contracts being legally void (Orejudo Prieto de los Mozos 2013), Juan felt that he was "denied the right to be a father." Furthermore, while he had to pursue his wish for a child outside Spain by paying a great deal of money, other men could "be a father for free" and "if you have a uterus, you can do whatever you want." Juan was the most articulate of my interview partners in framing his lack of choice and his right to parenthood. This even triggered a conflict between us, when he read the abstract of an article I had written. In the short text I had stated that "surrogacy has often been discussed as the ultimate form of commodification processes that position surrogate mothers as the weakest links in global reproduction chains" (Siegl 2015)—a statement that

Juan perceived as "simply insulting" and "very unfair." In his eyes, my "interpretation of the facts was very very very biased and [did] not correspond to reality." In his reaction via a Skype chat, he wrote:

> Do you know who feels like the weakest link? [...] I feel like trash. I feel like nobody fucking cares about us. [...] I have searched and saw nothing about the discrimination we are suffering because we are denied access to public health. [...] We are constantly subject to discrimination. And that is the only way for us to become parents. If it is regulated, the abuse finishes.

The forcefulness of his words reveals the sheer scale of discrimination he perceived, while also illustrating a clear link between choice—or the lack thereof—and responsibility, when he set the conditions for "finishing abuse." In my preceding interview with him, he had phrased it thus:

> If surrogacy is not regulated in the European Union [...] we have to go abroad. And then a lot of people here told me: [...] "well, but they take advantage of Indian *women*, blah-blah-*blah*, they pay them too *little*." You're like "OK, then let's regulate it *here!*" [...] then people tell me, "You go to other countries, to poor countries, to take advantage of those poor ladies." No. I don't go there *because* of that; I go there because I don't have a legal framework here.

Juan claimed that intended parents like him did not go to other countries *because* they wanted to take advantage of poor women but seemed to imply that they did so *despite* the fact that there might be exploitation in these countries. "We go there because that's the only possibility to do it (i.e., surrogacy). Because we can't afford the U.S. End of story." Emphasizing that many intended parents had no alternative could also be read as a way of evading a discussion about the ethics of pursuing surrogacy (Riggs 2016). From this perspective, exploitation is thus just an "undesired by-product" of surrogacy (Førde 2017), which Juan hoped to circumvent by finding a surrogate himself rather than working with one of the agencies. From his perspective, the risk of exploitation was an issue that society or politics at large had to deal with, because the unfavorable legislation in Spain forced him to travel to eastern Europe, while his own financial situation did not allow him to start a surrogacy process in the United States, which would have been his first choice.

In contrast to Juan Romero, intended father Diego Torres *could* afford to start a surrogacy program in the United States. He said he felt lucky because of this, indirectly suggesting that he had no bad conscience to deal with when he described himself as having chosen the "ethical" path. What would he have done if their income had not have been sufficient? Diego was unsure. He would have liked to say that India—a popular destination at the time—would *not* have been an option, but he could not guarantee this. Indicating that the wish for a child was so fundamental that people would pursue this desire despite legal obstacles, he argued for legalizing and regulating surrogacy in Spain:

> The only thing that helps is good regulation. Because people will go. They will go to countries where the legal guarantees are minimal, where the conditions for the surrogates are bad. I'm not saying that they are bad people. But the wish . . . The thing is that a possibility for you to *become a parent* opens up. [This wish] is so strong, you won't [stop anyone] with prohibitions [. . .]. It's like a snowball that gets bigger and bigger. [. . .] I'm telling you, the culpable ones in the end are those who don't implement laws (i.e., laws legalizing and regulating surrogacy in Spain). If they don't want to give you laws, what are you to do?

Juan and Diego both shifted responsibility from the intended parents as participants in the global surrogacy market onto national governments that provided no "options" to fulfill a wish that they considered not only understandable and natural but also a human right, as I have shown in the previous chapter. From this perspective, intended parents had no choice but to travel abroad and become "patient-consumers" in the neoliberal marketplace (Gunnarsson Payne 2015; Kroløkke and Pant 2012; Nebeling Petersen, Kroløkke, and Myong 2017; Speier 2016)—with all the risks this implied.

Returning to the story of Teresa and Stefan Wagner and Alyona Timofeyevna for the remainder of this chapter, I would like to illustrate how a similar shift of responsibility took place in the argumentation of the former, this time toward the agency. The evening before the Wagners and the twins traveled back to Germany, we gathered in their cramped hotel room in Kyiv. I asked them to look back at the past three weeks in Ukraine and how the things that had "gone wrong" affected them. They repeated that they felt sorry for Alyona, but having received information that everything was going well, they could not have known that this was not true: "We can feel sorry, but there is nothing we could have done. We had very little to no influence at all on the surrogacy process," Teresa stated. She had complained about the lack of information and transparency throughout the entire process, and I had often wondered why the couple had made so few complaints and claims to the agency. "They have the upper hand; we can't risk blowing it with them. They can always put obstacles in our way," she said. Feeling vulnerable themselves, they did not dare challenge the agency. For the same reason, they also did not feel responsible for what had gone wrong:

> I don't have a bad conscience or lack scruples. I regard this merely as a service provided by this woman and we pay for the service. [. . .] When I look at the amount the agency asks for and how much of this the

surrogate receives [in this case, roughly one third], then this is really a dirty business. But if you compare it to what people here earn annually, then this is big money. So why should we feel bad?

Emphasizing that surrogacy was merely a service and comparing the surrogates' salary to the average income, Stefan could reject "feeling bad." Moreover, in light of this comparison, the couple could not understand why some people regarded surrogacy in the United States as ethically superior and Ukrainian surrogates as exploited. When I connected the issue of exploitation to the question of "choice" in a later conversation, they replied that "of course" surrogates acted on financial grounds. Nevertheless, "at the end of the day, I do think that she (i.e., Alyona) has a choice," Teresa said. "She *does* have a choice," her husband interjected but then added that there was obviously no other way of earning so much money in such a short amount of time.

> Considering all the things we know through you about Alyona—that her father never cared about her, that her mother died in a car accident, that she had a child but the father of the child doesn't support her, that she doesn't have a good education or a large income. Well, if I put two and two together ...

Stefan's quote implies that—considering her life circumstances—he did not think Alyona had much of a choice. But instead of finishing his last sentence, he repeated that probably all agencies in Ukraine operated in the same way. It was thus not their fault or general bad luck that things "went wrong," he said. He thus recognized the structural roots of "what went wrong" but nevertheless did not problematize these roots and did not see himself as part of this structure. Stefan also did not condemn the specific agency they had worked with, for—at the end of the day—the surrogate had received all the money she had been promised. Taken together, the couple's statements reveal that embracing the economic aspects of surrogacy makes it possible to reduce the question of exploitation to a matter of payment and of informed consent. If you pay enough, then surely it cannot be exploitative. And if you have put your signature on a contract, you have consented to a relationship. Stefan emphasized that the surrogate had received all the contracts. She had known how much money she would get when she signed them: "If she consented to all the conditions in the contracts, then there is no reason for her to feel exploited," he added. Their statements further show that while the Wagners acknowledged that Alyona turned to surrogacy out of financial necessity, they regarded her choice as "free" as long as she was not physically coerced into it. Such a conception "silences" other ethical concerns, because if a person has consented to a specific agreement, "then the action *must* be ethical" (Widdows 2013, 158).

The Flexible Ethics of Free Choice

Investigating "free choice" in an empirical context is methodologically challenging. What do we direct our attention to? Do we rely on what people say or on the background information we have? How far is "free choice" a neo/liberal concept, rooted in a specific historical and geographical context? I never dared to ask the surrogates directly whether they would speak about their decisions in terms of free choice. I feared that such a question might have sounded cynical, inappropriate, or simply would not have made sense. This was the case with Alyona, when I tried to bring up the issue in our conversation but repeatedly failed. When I asked her whether she had "freely" or "independently" decided to become a surrogate, she did not answer this question directly. She merely stated that she needed money to feed her son and provide him with adequate housing. Alyona wanted to buy a flat, but the money would only be enough to get a room in a shared apartment. The kind of "choice" I was implying did not translate into her life context. In my previous conversations with her, she had stated that she did not want to become a surrogate but decided to "risk it," due to her difficult circumstances. Like many other surrogates in my research, Alyona seemed to approach life as a "practical realist" (Utrata 2015) who made pragmatic choices among the options available to her. It was thus clearly her economic situation that made her body "bioavailable" (Cohen 2005) for the surrogacy market. And yet, as many reproduction researchers have argued, terms such as "agency" and "choice" and such dichotomies as active/passive are too simplistic to capture the complex realities of those involved (Banerjee 2010; Deomampo 2013b; Nahman 2008; Parry 2015).

Trying to steer away from simplified dichotomies, this chapter has explored the *work* that notions of "free choice" do in cross-border reproductive markets—more specifically, how surrogacy actors integrate these notions into their ethical labor, when negotiating concerns around issues of coercion and exploitation. This kind of ethical labor could be said to build on a flexible ethics of free choice. This form of ethics relies on a neoliberal and libertarian discourse that casts individuals as autonomous and self-responsible actors. In this logic, intended parents and intermediaries acknowledge the power relations and economic inequality involved but emphasize the win-win situation that surrogates voluntarily entered by putting their signature on a contract. But as Alyona Timofeyevna's case clearly illustrates, informed consent is much more than a simple signature. It is not a moment but a process that goes well beyond the signature and extends to the end of the pregnancy. This process includes transparency and the possibility to shape contracts and conditions. In addition, informed consent is more than a formal procedure: it is also about issues such as respect, trust, and care. Such attitudes create atmospheres in which questions can be asked and insecurities articulated. To be more than an expression of an "empty ethics" (Corrigan 2003) informed consent should rely not on the "logic of choice" but on the "logic of care" (Mol 2008). Alyona's different versions of truth arose due to the lack of exactly these qualities in the way she was treated. They arose from the precarity and vulnerability of her situation within the surrogacy program. It is precisely this context that facilitated the emergence of certain *truths*—not just in Alyona's case but also in that of Teresa and Stefan. The couple were aware of the fragile nature of their claims, and yet they seemed to have internalized the neoliberal discourse of free choice that offered them a powerful tool to repudiate accusations and responsibility, and to make sense of their situation. I was surprised that their experiences in Ukraine did not lead them to question surrogacy (as practiced by their agency) or their own involvement in such a practice. But feeling powerless themselves, there was only so much critique they could accommodate. Surrogacy was their only and last option to realize their desire for offspring. Many of the intended parents' narratives reflected such a feeling of vulnerability and powerlessness, for instance Juan Romero's and Diego Torres's statements that shifted responsibility for exploitative surrogacy arrangements to the state, while simultaneously legitimizing such arrangements by emphasizing the unique financial opportunity they posed for women.

The story of the Wagners and Alyona Timofeyevna illustrates the striking persistence with which intended parents and intermediaries hold on to this discourse, against all the odds. The case shows that the flexible ethics of free choice can be used as a moral tool, in order to reduce ethics to a matter of choice, free of context. Such a free-floating notion of "choice" becomes so meaningless that it can be flexibly filled with content, depending on the relevant circumstances. It mutates into a vessel that can be filled by different *truths*. Similarly to the discourse of mutual happiness, the flexible reference to "free choice" constitutes an ultimate argument for this contested medical practice. This allows intended parents and intermediaries to reject all responsibility for things that "go wrong" in this market exchange.

On the above-mentioned last evening in Kyiv, I asked the German couple why they had participated in a business they had numerous times described as a "dirty business." "Well ...," Teresa began her sentence, paused a few seconds and then continued, "I guess the wish to have a child is just too great." "And now, holding the twins in our arms, I can only say that the whole struggle was worth it. They really bring tears to my eyes," Stefan said, and wiped his wet eyes with the back of his hand.

Conclusion

Exploring the moral economy of commercial surrogacy exposes the struggles over what it is that makes the economic moral. It also draws attention to the fact that this moral meaning is made and sustained by the circulation of cultural norms and affective forces. Intimate markets in particular call for a constant negotiation of morality. In this book I have traced such efforts of "ethical labor" by analyzing forms of rhetorical justification and persuasion, strategies of protective care toward others and oneself, and practices of affective labor on others as well as bodily and emotional work on the self. I scrutinized how actors within and at the fringes of the surrogacy market in Russia and Ukraine—surrogate workers, intended parents, doctors, infertility psychologists, intermediaries, advocates, and opponents—ethically labored in order to find, internalize, create, and circulate specific truths about surrogacy.

Listening to the way many of my research participants presented their truths—and sometimes defended them against all odds—I was often reminded of the chorus in Leonard Cohen's song "Anthem," cited in this book's epigraph: "Forget your perfect offering," it goes, followed by the lines: "There's a crack in everything. That's how the light gets in." Cohen's observation seems fitting when recalling the narratives I collected and the observations I made in the course of my fieldwork. Interpreting the chorus in regard to my research, I would say that the neat and impermeable accounts left little space for the insecurities and ambiguities that are inevitably part of our lives, adding texture and complexity to our experiences. "Perfect offerings" also did not allow much critique or reflection—as if a trace of uncertainty would question the entire narration or the speaker's position and experience. Thinking in such dichotomous terms as true and false obscures the "everyday ambivalences which underlie our ways of making sense of the world and acting upon it" (Kierans and Bell 2017, 25). Following Ciara Kierans and Kirsten Bell (36), I regarded such offerings as "an invitation" to challenge them and ask when, how, and why they came into being.

Fragile Truths

Many of the truths I encountered seemed to be inherently *fragile* truths, revealing tensions, inconsistencies, and contradictions. Sometimes the "cracks" were obvious, but in other instances they were less evident and revealed themselves only in exceptional cases, as in two I presented in this book—those of surrogate Lena Mironovna (chapter 5) or of intended father David Hauser (chapter 6). Both their accounts outlined a "perfect" surrogacy experience. In very different ways, they presented their respective programs as carefree and unproblematic. Lena stressed the convenience and simplicity of a business relationship with an unknown Russian couple; David, in contrast, recounted a picture-perfect love story between him, his male partner, and the Russian surrogate. Only once a bond of trust had developed between Lena and me did she admit, two and a half years after her surrogacy program, that her alignment with the market's "feeling rules" (Hochschild 2012) had failed and that she regretted becoming a surrogate. And only upon interviewing the woman who had carried David's son could I see the inconsistencies between their accounts—such as the fact that he had spoken of her as a middle-class woman working in a school (which led me to assume she was a teacher), while she told me that she was employed in the school's canteen and could barely make ends meet with her salary.

These stories are exemplary of the way the moral economy of surrogacy builds on what economic sociologist Viviana Zelizer (2013) has called the "separate-spheres and hostile-worlds doctrine"—a doctrine that rests on the misconception that emotions and economic activity are separate spheres and that their intersection might lead to mutual contamination. The need for this separation was grounded not only in the unease many surrogacy participants experienced about this intersection but also in the recognition that the economic and the intimate *could not* be separated in the case of intimate labors such as surrogacy. Maintaining a neat work relationship became important *because* intended parents, professionals, and surrogates imagined it difficult for the latter to stay aligned; for other intended parents and professionals, emphasizing altruism and happiness was essential precisely *because* they were aware of and troubled by the surrogates' economic motives. But the stakes for those involved were too high to engage with these issues. They ethically labored to cover up the unsettling "cracks" they did not want to turn their or my attention to.

The fragile truths presented by intended parents and surrogates emerged from shared yet completely different forms of precarity and vulnerability between both parties that intimately tie them together in a bond of mutual dependency. The dependency is marked by great biopolitical and economic pressure, by medical uncertainty, and by a lack of trust—not only toward each other but also toward all kinds of intermediaries, who are feared as taking advantage of the vulnerable position of intended parents and surrogates alike. This creates a setting of high tension, in which actors have to consider their desires and how far they are prepared to go to satisfy them. Desperately needing what the "other" can offer, for them truths become flexible and situational, shift and mold around the given possibilities and constraints. This flexibility reverberated most explicitly in the accounts of the surrogates, who grappled with the negative connotations of being a surrogate as well as with the culturally dominant imaginary of maternal bonding. Their narratives highlighted that moral boundaries could be subject to economic factors and that it was the need or desire for money that gave them "a certain push," as one of the surrogates phrased it, to step beyond these initial boundaries.

Considering the contested nature of surrogacy, long-term fieldwork was crucial to see beyond the "perfect offerings." At the same time, fieldwork in such a contentious setting was highly challenging, because relationships with research participants had to be carefully navigated. I needed to constantly seek a balance between trying to see beyond my interlocutors' "perfect offerings," while trying not to cross what I often perceived as their protective boundaries. When surrogates like Lena Mironovna stressed their lack of emotional involvement and told me that they could not care less about the intended parents, I deemed it insensitive to keep asking along these lines. And when intended parents like David Hauser shared their stories of suffering, it was difficult to probe their narratives and respond with critical questions (see also Robben 2012). Likewise, they seldom addressed me as a source of information or discussion but rather as a listener. While many of my interviews with foreign intended parents revolved around the issue of the surrogates' exploitation, few used the opportunity to ask me about my fieldwork insights from Russia and Ukraine. They were interested in telling me their truths but not in hearing what could potentially challenge these. Their blind spots were thus not necessarily unintentional states of not-knowing but sometimes an active refusal to know, learn, or reflect (Mair, Kelly, and High 2016; Vitebsky 1993). The separation between the intimate and the economic needed to stay intact so as to avoid losing balance and questioning the very foundation of their intimate choices.

For the professionals involved, "perfect offerings" were not so much an intimate concern but rather served to facilitate their work and enhance the comfort of the intended parents. This was particularly evident in the way agency staff could flexibly oscillate between the spheres of the economic and the intimate, as if to get the best out of both. Money was never the only motivation for surrogates, one Russian lawyer stated, only to go on to say that surrogacy was "just a job" and that many surrogates were therefore not interested in meeting the parents. Another professional, a Spanish agent, initially went to great lengths to describe how "magical" the first encounter between surrogates and intended mothers is, and then contrasted this with the moment of delivery, after which going their separate ways and breaking off contact are legitimate on the grounds that surrogacy is based on a contract with a clear end. This oscillation works toward alleviating the intended parents' feeling that women might be financially coerced into surrogacy, while also freeing them from certain responsibilities after the end of the program. Many of the intended parents gratefully adopted the truths that agencies offered. As such, while most of the foreign couples in my research criticized the commercial character of surrogacy in Russia and Ukraine, they inevitably profited from the way the market prioritized them as paying clients. It was *their* needs and desires that counted and were—in many though surely not in all cases—represented and facilitated by the agencies, the market's masterminds.

Constructing the intimate and economic as oppositional spheres (which, nevertheless, allowed for oscillation) thus clearly covered up and reinforced the power relations at stake. And while many intended parents stated that they wanted surrogacy to be legalized in their home countries, they also emphasized the benefits of an arrangement with an "intimate stranger," so with geographical, cultural, and emotional distance: they would not have to include the surrogate in their lives or fear meeting her unexpectedly in the street, and if she suffered a permanent injury from the pregnancy, they could feel less responsible. This was also true in regard to the Russian intended parents, who held the surrogates at bay by maintaining a business relationship or by entering anonymous programs. The distance meant that the couples could leave behind the surrogates and concentrate on their new lives and new identities as parents. As such, national and transnational surrogacy arrangements rely on specific local moral economies—be it in Russia or Ukraine, where surrogates are said to understand what they do as work; in India, where surrogates are constructed as poor but noble mothers (Pande 2014; Rudrappa 2016a); in Thailand, where surrogates are presented as motivated by the Buddhist notion of merit-making (Whittaker 2019); or in the United States, where surrogates are seen as self-determined and proud women (Berend 2016; Jacobson 2016). Agencies knew how to make use of these local moralities in ways that brought them profit.

However, their attempts at legitimizing surrogacy often seemed somewhat staged, exaggerated, or out of place: just as in the Skype conversation between surrogate Alyona Timofeyevna and intended parents Teresa and Stefan Wagner, when the Ukrainian agent clumsily emphasized the surrogate's happiness and altruistic motives, while the latter sat quietly in the background, with an intimidated look on her face; or when one of the Spanish agents argued that the prohibition of surrogacy was equivalent to the prohibition of clowns or—according to lawyer Konstantin Svitnev (2016)—even the discrimination against "those [yet] to be born." While such comparisons and analogies were employed to point out the absurdity of making claims *against* surrogacy, they seemed to work in the opposite direction, revealing a certain argumentative desperation and thus, again, pointing to the fragility of their claims.

Regimes of Truth

Throughout this book, I have paid attention to how specific words, metaphors, practices, affects, arguments, and logics traveled within the reproductive market, and thereby became part of a trans/national ethical repertoire of truth claims. This repertoire provided a diverse and powerful toolbox for circulating intellectual, emotional, and corporeal "understandings" that surrogacy participants could draw on. The "right understanding" was something that intended parents and surrogates could discover or achieve. It was through engagement with surrogacy that they came to understand what it was *really* about and could, hence, resolve the tension between the intimate and the economic.

The notion of the "right understanding" speaks of a particular "regime of truth" (Foucault 1987, 72–73) that upholds the moral economy of surrogacy. This regime establishes which individuals are "truth bearers," who thus have the power and legitimacy to speak truth, and sets the rules for distinguishing between true and false discourses. In the context of my research, the regime of truth was best captured in a statement I encountered over and over during fieldwork, with only slight variations: Any "normal" person, who had the right understanding of what surrogacy was about, would—without doubt—accept this practice. Reflecting on the "effects of power attached to the true" (74), it becomes obvious that framing the acceptance of surrogacy as a matter of understanding served to legitimize one's own position while delegitimizing other positions by claiming that they were based on a *wrong* understanding, a *not*-understanding or a *mis*understanding.

My research participants often explained such other positions by referring to positionality, backwardness, or ideology. Many, for instance, claimed that lack of understanding was rooted in the fact that most people had not experienced infertility themselves and were thus not in a position to make judgments in this field. Larissa Osipovna, the agent I introduced at the book's outset, underlined this argument by comparing infertility with bad eyesight: "I don't have anything to say about problems with eyes, because I have perfect sight. I can't feel the same as my husband, who has lived all his life with lenses. [...] Okay I understand him [...] but I will never *feel* the same way." Her words emphasize the importance of experience and of what one could call an "affective understanding" in order to gain the "right understanding" and, hence, the legitimacy to participate in discussions on surrogacy. The effect is to exclude a significant number of potential discussants from the beginning by delegitimizing their speaking position and by claiming that only those directly affected could be regarded as bearers of truth.

Other ways of delegitimizing critical voices included classifying them as backward and/or ideologically tainted. Such endeavors were often directed toward the diverse group of conservatives, left-wing supporters, and feminists, whose truths were presented as strongly biased and therefore invalid. This kind of delegitimization, for instance, manifested itself in the way one of my research participants, a man living in a same-sex relationship, labelled those who criticized surrogacy as "candle suckers" (a self-created term ridiculing religious authorities) or—referring to a lesbian acquaintance—as a "bull dyke" (*Kampflesbe*) and "man hater." Such derogatory terms clearly imply that the stances of these individuals could not be taken seriously, because they were strongly biased.

Apart from these forms of "wrong understanding" or "not-understanding," surrogacy participants also spoke of specific "*mis*understandings." Critics were presented as falsely assuming conditions in Russia and Ukraine to be as bad as in India, Thailand, or Mexico, while this was not the case (see chapter 6); as thinking that surrogates inevitably bonded with the children they carried, while affective bonding without a genetic link could not take place (see chapter 5); or as assuming that intended mothers were exclusively rich women who did not want to spoil their figures, while they were women who suffered an illness and "really needed" a child (see chapter 1).

Such statements illustrated the assumption that being in favor of surrogacy is a matter of having information, understanding this information, and being "objective" enough (i.e., not ideologically tainted) to translate this information into a surrogacy-friendly attitude. One intended father I interviewed had dedicated a significant amount of his time to disseminating the truths of surrogacy. He had taken up an active position in fighting for the legalization of surrogacy in his home country, Spain, and saw his role as educator: "There is a lot of pedagogy to be done still; I need to lecture a lot of people. [...] They don't understand what surrogacy is. Still today."

Likewise, many other people I spoke with in the course of my fieldwork believed that the normalization of surrogacy was merely a matter of time. One of the Spanish intended mothers stated that society was not yet ready for surrogacy, but that people would gradually "open their minds a bit." And two agents referred to surrogacy as a "twenty-first-century profession," claiming that in around ten years surrogacy would be a job comparable to that of a lawyer, an economist, or an accountant. Considering that commercial surrogacy mostly rests on significant economic inequalities between "consumers" and "providers," this is a somewhat cynical comment. However, the analogy is clearly meant to portray surrogacy as progressive and future-oriented. Framing the acceptance of surrogacy as a question of information and understanding cast it as a natural and self-evident social development, while making it possible to dismiss critique without properly engaging with it. Such a regime facilitates holding on to certain truths that—on the surface—appear to be intact and without cracks.

Casting an eye over the recent past and considering events in the field of surrogacy, it is highly unlikely that surrogacy will become a profession like any other, as some of my research participants suggested. As indicated in the introduction, many countries (such as India, Thailand, Nepal, or Mexico) have banned or severely restricted surrogacy since 2012, leaving Russia and Ukraine as two of the few countries in which commercial surrogacy remains legal and regulated. Debates around the scandals and legal changes in 2012 and the following years have also led to the formation of numerous citizens' initiatives in Europe (e.g., Stop Surrogacy Now), and both the European Parliament and the European Council have signaled their disapproval of this reproductive procedure. By now, however, the global outcry seems to have faded, and in recent years several European states—such as Germany or Switzerland—have witnessed the emergence of new movements that call for legalizing surrogacy (and egg provision) in the name of social progress and equal reproductive rights. These movements also argue that legalizing such procedures would reduce the potential harm caused by reproductive travels to countries with more lenient regulation (see also chapter 6). But, as we know from other contexts, the forms of altruistic surrogacy and egg provision they envision will not decrease reproductive travel: limited "supply" and high costs in these countries will continue to keep transnational reproductive mobility alive and thriving (Siegl et al. 2022). The global routes, however, might be about to change once again, as the latest developments in Russia and Ukraine indicate that surrogacy laws in these countries might be significantly curtailed soon.

In the remainder of this final chapter, I would like to zoom in on these developments, which ultimately reflect a renegotiation of the "regime of truth." It is probably no coincidence that these renegotiations emerged in early 2020—at a time when the COVID-19 pandemic had spread to most parts of the world and the subsequent travel bans and border closures had severely "disrupted" global surrogacy (König, Majumdar, and Jacobson 2020; Vlasenko 2020). These disruptions, which attracted significant political and media attention, shed new light on the dimensions and dynamics of international surrogacy.

Babies for the World?

In April 2020, the Ukrainian infertility center BioTexCom released a curious YouTube video in seven languages.[1] The video begins by taking the viewer into a large hotel room in Kyiv, filled with the ear-splitting cries of forty-six babies. From above, the camera pans over the three rows of newborns lying in plastic cots, one next to the other. We are told that with every week the number of babies in the hotel rises. They were born to Ukrainian surrogates after the country shut its borders in March, due to the global outbreak of COVID-19. In the meantime, they are being taken care of by a dozen nannies, who hover around them in pastel-colored outfits, protective masks, and gloves. The women have been living in the hotel in quarantine with the children. As the crying in the video is gradually replaced by soothing piano and violin music, one of the nannies, holding a newborn in her arms, explains through her mask that the intended parents come from the United States, Italy, Spain, Britain, China, France, Germany, Bulgaria, Romania, Austria, Mexico, and Portugal. "It's difficult for us but we handle it well. We show babies to their parents online, and our managers arrange video calls. It's necessary for us to inform parents how much their babies eat, how they sleep, and what their weight is," she says. "It's heartbreaking to see how parents miss their little ones. We wish they were allowed to pick up their children soon."

The video clearly intends to prove to parents that their children are in good hands. The infertility center presents itself as a reliable savior in difficult times, illustrated by a close-up of a "Thank you very much!!!!" card that displays six babies propped up on a brown leather sofa. Toward the end of the video, the clinic's lawyer appears—a young man with a MacBook—and appeals to consulates and governments to take a stand for their citizens to enter Ukraine to collect their long-awaited newborns.[2]

It is impossible to watch these four minutes without associating the babies with commodities produced on an assembly line that now cannot be delivered to the customers. The video is a carefully staged ensemble of images and statements, so this is no coincidence or by-product. Rather, I assume that BioTexCom is deliberately playing with the image of the global baby factory that can cater to anyone who has the necessary money. "Look here," the video seems to say, "we have an excess of babies! We will also have one for you!" This image fits well with how BioTexCom has recently marketed its services, and it might be precisely such a disturbing image as the baby factory that speaks to the hopes of those who are desperate to finally have a child of their own. There is a new quality to this kind of marketing that explicitly foregrounds how reproduction has been turned into production.

By early June 2020, the English version of the video had received over one million views on YouTube and had been discussed widely in the Western and Ukrainian media, where the incident was often placed among the succession of scandalous stories around commercial surrogacy. Already in July 2018 the Ukrainian attorney general Yuri Luzenko had made serious allegations against BioTexCom. The owner as well as the medical director were accused of child trafficking, tax offenses, and document forgery and could face up to fifteen years of imprisonment. These accusations were based on the case of an Italian couple who became parents through BioTexCom in 2011. A DNA test proved that neither of them was genetically related to the child, even though Ukrainian law requires that the genetic material of at least one of the parents must be used in the context of IVF treatments (Klimchuk and Cheretski 2018). Only weeks later, BioTexCom again made headlines, when the media reported about a little girl, Bridget, who was left behind by her U.S.-American parents because she was born prematurely and with a number of disabilities (Hawley 2018)—a story reminiscent of the Baby Gammy case in Thailand a few years previously. A further case of supposed trafficking was reported in 2020, when the Ukrainian authorities announced that they had arrested a group of individuals that had organized surrogacy arrangements for single men. Since (heterosexual) marriage is a legal requirement, the group had set up illicit marriages with Ukrainian women, who were then inseminated with the men's sperm and, upon birth, resigned their motherhood rights. Many such arrangements included Chinese men, who were struggling to find partners due to China's long-term one-child policy and preference for male offspring, which have resulted in a massive gender imbalance (Neal 2020).

These incidents—primarily the events surrounding BioTexCom and the pandemic—sparked a renewed discussion on the ethics and regulation of surrogacy within and beyond Ukraine. Sociologist Alya Guseva, who closely follows the developments in Ukraine's fertility market, has argued that the current debates reflect different stakeholders' competition over control of the reproductive market. The many surrogacy agencies that have mushroomed in the past ten years pose a serious threat to the clinics' long-standing hegemony. Among these new actors, BioTexCom—agency and clinic in one—has for long had a bad reputation within the surrogacy sphere, as Guseva (2020, 7) writes. Directed by an entrepreneur with pronounced commercial interests, BioTexCom differs considerably from other actors in the field, particularly from medical professionals, represented by the Ukrainian Association for Reproductive Medicine (UARM). Being aware that the commercial character of reproductive services causes moral unease within society, the association has instead adopted a low-key approach to promoting and upholding the legitimacy of surrogacy (9): On the one hand, the UARM publicly de-emphasizes the scale and rapid development of surrogacy, and explicitly distances itself from wanting to turn Ukraine into the new India or Thailand, as it puts it. On the other hand, and building on this stance, the UARM has repeatedly argued that there is no need for more comprehensive legislation (Guseva 2020). As such, the association tries hard to preserve its position as "truth bearer" within ongoing debates and offers a counternarrative to the image of the reproductive assembly line presented by BioTexCom.

Despite the UARM's efforts, several draft bills have been submitted to the Ukrainian Parliament, and if legal changes are decided upon, it is likely that these will include banning surrogacy for foreign citizens. Some draft laws also envision licensing for the many surrogacy agencies, with the aim of improving accountability (Vlasenko 2020). To date, however, not much has advanced in this regard, and insiders doubt that a new law will be adopted (Grytsenko 2020). Bearing in mind past propositions, Guseva concludes that "moral panics eventually died down, fertility clinics that were accused of violations, including, most recently, BioTexCom, never ceased their activities, and everything eventually went back to normal" (2020, 9).

In the unlikely event that a comprehensive surrogacy ban is implemented, BioTexCom owner and director Albert Tochilovsky has already announced that he would shift his center's focus to providing embryo donations instead (Grytsenko 2020). While he does not go into further detail concerning these plans, they point to an interesting parallel to recent developments in India. In light of the approved, but yet to be passed, Surrogacy (Regulation) Bill, which limits surrogacy to its altruistic form, provided exclusively for citizens, Amrita Pande observes that the country has evolved into a "grey zone of pre-conception assemblage" (2021, 396). In this assemblage, egg cells extracted from Indian and global providers are fertilized with the sperm cells of intended fathers, and then exported to countries with more liberal regulations, where the embryos are implanted into the wombs of surrogate workers. "The world's future is in biotechnology, and most of the money will come into biotechnologies," Tochilovsky comments on his plans (Grytsenko 2020)—implying that he does not think much of the UARM's call for "self-restraint" (Guseva 2020) but is set to support the ways in which the reproductive market might, once again, prove that it constitutes a "shifting global form that disperses and realigns in response to new situations and conditions" (Whittaker 2019, 9–10). Besides prompting Ukraine—or at least BioTexCom—to transform into a center for embryo fertilization and export, the proposed legal changes, if implemented, could also lead Russian and Ukrainian women to become surrogates in other countries, where surrogacy is legal, such as neighboring Kazakhstan or Georgia (Vertommen and Barbagallo 2021)—a dynamic similar to those observed in other global areas of the surrogacy market (Pande 2021; Rudrappa 2018; Whittaker 2019).[3]

Protecting "Our" Children: The Legal Crackdown on Russian Surrogacy

In Russia, too, there have been several attempts to curtail the existing surrogacy legislation (see chapter 2). Although none of these were successful, fresh legal efforts are underway. In June 2021, a group of Duma deputies led by deputy chairman and United Russia member Pyotr Tolstoy submitted a new bill to regulate surrogacy to the State Duma. At the time of making final updates to this conclusion in autumn 2022, the bill had been—almost unanimously—passed in its first reading (Reuters 2022). If accepted, it would restrict surrogacy to couples who have either Russian citizenship or a residence permit in Russia, who have been in a heterosexual marriage for at least a year, who have a medical indication for infertility, and who are between the ages of twenty-five and fifty-five. The new law would also prescribe that surrogacy contracts need to be notarized, and it would prohibit advertising surrogacy as well as the involvement of intermediary agencies (Kuznetsova and Gubernatorov 2021).[4]

Tolstoy's bill was developed in response to the death of a surrogate baby in January 2020, in an apartment in the Odintsovo district, close to Moscow. Different explanations for the infant's death circulated in the media: some sources spoke of sudden infant death, others of a cephalohematoma (a hemorrhage between a newborn's skull and scalp) that was inadequately treated (Petrov 2020; TASS 2020). The boy was one of four children born a few months previously who were being looked after by a Ukrainian couple. The Thai and Filipino parents, some of whom were single men, had worked with the firm Rosjurconsulting, directed by lawyer Konstantin Svitnev, who—as previously discussed—is one of the central figures in Russia's surrogacy market. Svitnev defended the parents' absence, arguing that the clients in question were busy and successful politicians and businessmen who did not have time to wait around in Moscow until all the paperwork was done and their children were strong enough for the long flight "home." Following the infant's death and further investigations, Svitnev and several other professionals involved were charged under the Criminal Code with a total of eleven cases of child trafficking as an organized group, resulting, in one case, in death by negligence (Reiter and Rothrock 2020).

In June 2020, amid the COVID-19 pandemic, a further story attracted the attention of the Russian authorities and media, when five surrogate babies, some without documents, were found in an apartment in Moscow's Ostankino district. The children had been born for Chinese parents, who could not enter the country due to the travel restrictions, and were thus being looked after by two Chinese women. This must have been the case for several other children as well: a month later, *The Guardian* reported that up to one thousand surrogate babies were "stranded" in Russia, waiting for their foreign parents, most of whom were Chinese citizens (Roth 2020).[5]

A new trafficking case was opened, which was later merged with the earlier one, and in July 2020, eight people were arrested, including the director of the European Surrogacy Center in Moscow, several doctors, as well as a lawyer, a translator, and a courier. In addition, two of the surrogates involved have been accused of child trafficking, as they had carried babies for single men and put their own names on the birth certificates in order to facilitate the bureaucratic steps (Zatari 2020). Svitnev—who is seen as "leader" of the criminal group by the authorities—could only be arrested in absentia: In January 2020, he left for Prague, apparently on a vacation that he had not returned from at the time of writing up this conclusion (Kolesnikova 2021a).

According to the accused individuals, they had acted in accordance with the law and—even though this was not a legal requirement at the time (though it has been since January 2021)—the parents in question were all genetically related to the surrogate children, making it unclear why they were charged with child trafficking. Svitnev has suggested that the case was simply good ammunition for the authorities, because it could be cast as a scandal involving a "gang of foreigners, gays, and pedophiles" (Torocheshnikova 2021). While there certainly are aspects that cause moral unease—such as the fact that seven of the supposedly "trafficked" children were commissioned by just one couple, a famous Filipino politician and his wife (Reiter and Rothrock 2020)—it is likely that the two cases did present a welcome opportunity for a politically motivated state crackdown. As previously mentioned, Konstantin Svitnev was the first lawyer to push for a single father's "right" to parenthood through a court decision in 2010 and has, ever since, assisted many single and gay men in fulfilling their wish for a child (Svitnev 2012). Moreover, he himself is a single father to four children born through surrogacy (Zatari 2020)—a fact he has, however, not broadcast loudly. The criminal charges against Svitnev are thus certainly an attempt to spread fear and bring down certain sectors of Russia's reproductive market. Along these lines, in September 2020, it was reported that authorities were planning to arrest ten single and gay men on grounds of child trafficking and threatened to put their surrogacy-born children into foster care (Korelina 2020). Several men have since fled Russia with their children (Zatari 2020), but no recent reports could be found as to whether or not the authorities have translated their plans into action.

Debates around the new draft bill—as well as about the preceding alleged trafficking cases—once again reflect how different stakeholders negotiate and circulate truths about surrogacy and how these tie into larger bio- and geopolitical issues. More generally, ongoing debates about revising the surrogacy law reflect broader discourses that have come to characterize Russian politics. "Foreigners, gays, and pedophiles"—the three categories mentioned by Svitnev—are often lumped together within these discourses and have become popular targets. While gay men are generally cast as pedophiles, homosexuality is framed as imported and as a "Western neo-imperial project" (Persson 2015, 267). Conservatives in Russia have even warned against a "gay revolution" leading to the nation's moral collapse, and have characterized gay men and lesbian women as "a small but very influential minority," backed by a global network and pursuing distinct economic interests (264). These discourses facilitated implementing laws such as the so-called Gay Propaganda Law (Federal Law No. 135, 2013) in the name of protecting children (see chapter 2).[6] Against the background of apocalyptic scenarios, such laws thus become a matter of national urgency and interest—be it in the case of the Gay Propaganda Law or the new draft bill to restrict surrogacy. In regard to the latter, the need for stricter regulation was legitimized by the need to protect children born in Russia. According to the draft bill's authors, for instance, there were "a lot of reports coming from overseas about unenviable fates of children born by surrogate mothers who end up in sexual slavery or subjected to humiliations" (TASS 2021) or who become victims of organ traffickers (Kuznetsova and Gubernatorov 2021). Moreover, Pyotr Tolstoy problematized single men's wish for a child, comparing it to "getting a puppy," thus echoing a widespread skepticism about the true motives behind single or gay men's wish for a child of their own (see chapter 2).

The geopolitical component of the current debates is even more evident when considering the similarities between the ongoing discussions and those preceding the so-called Dima Yakovlev Law. Passed in 2012, the law bans U.S.-American citizens from adopting Russian children. The law was named after a Russian toddler who died of heatstroke in Virginia after his adoptive parents forgot him in the car. This incident provoked a heated debate about the dangers Russian children face when "bought" by U.S.-American families and was explicitly backed by over half of Russia's population (Fischer 2012).[7] Despite the fact that many children live in dire conditions in Russian orphanages (Disney 2015, 2017; Fujimura 2005; Human Rights Watch 2014), the Dima Yakovlev Law was presented as an act of child protection. In 2013, Putin signed a further law that bans the adoption of Russian children by same-sex couples or unmarried citizens in countries where same-sex marriage is legally recognized, in order to protect children "from possible unwanted influence such as artificial forcing of non-traditional sexual behavior" (Brennan 2014). The lawmakers also warned that the existing surrogacy legislation offers the opportunity to circumvent the new adoption restrictions and access "Russian" children through assisted reproduction (Kolesnikova 2021b). Several politicians have previously commented that it was "humiliating" for the country that foreigners "ordered" their children in Russia (Grigoryan and Zainitdinova 2019), and the draft bill's explanatory note states that providing surrogacy for foreigners damages the country's reputation (Kuznetsova and Gubernatorov 2021). These debates frame surrogacy as necessary and justified for Russian heterosexual couples but as dangerous and irresponsible for foreigners and single men.

The lawmakers had feared that the draft bill would not be easy to pass, as there is lively and strong opposition to the proposal from the "huge lobby" of those who profit from "exporting" surrogacy (Yasakova 2021). In fact, the Russian Association of Human Reproduction has clearly opposed the bill, arguing that it is unacceptable to exclude foreign patients from necessary medical treatments and a violation of Russia's international obligations. It did, however, endorse limiting surrogacy to married couples with a medical indication, banning advertisement, and introducing stricter control of surrogacy programs for foreigners (Kolesnikova 2021a, 2021b). Thus, while having long claimed that there was no need to develop any further regulation, it seems that in light of comprehensive restrictions on the practice of surrogacy—similar to the developments in Ukraine (Guseva 2020)—the medical community is prepared to make concessions.

Opposition to the draft bill was also voiced from within the Duma: Oksana Pushkina—deputy and vice-chair of the State Duma Committee for Family, Women, and Children—stated that no one should be deprived of the opportunity to become a parent, and surrogacy should therefore remain accessible for everyone, especially if Russia wanted to tackle the dire demographic situation (Kuznetsova and Gubernatorov 2021), reflecting a popular argument *for* surrogacy, which is often brought forward by market actors (see chapter 1). Pushkina is a member of the ruling party, United Russia, but she is known for her liberal stances and has repeatedly criticized the overinvolvement of the Russian Orthodox Church when it comes to questions around assisted conception (Korelina 2020). The "side" politicians take in relation to surrogacy is thus not always as clear as one might expect.[8]

While the outcomes of the legal debates around surrogacy are foreseeable but not yet finally decided upon, it is evident that the truths of surrogacy remain highly contested. Susan Markens has argued that reproductive politics offer "an unusually clear view of the ideological and structural foundation of societies as well as insight into the basis of specific social conflicts" (2007, 5). The discussions and developments detailed in this book thus reflect the contemporary tenor of a state that has become paranoid about its position in global politics, possessive about its territories and citizens, and strategically obsessed with moralized apocalyptic scenarios.

From Legal Void to Workers' Rights

A revision of the surrogacy laws in Russia and Ukraine is long overdue, but restricting commercial surrogacy to a country's citizens does nothing to improve the safety of those involved in the numerous "national" programs (see also Vlasenko 2020; Weis 2021a). Though some of the draft bills do envision more regulation and control, the comprehensive revision needed would probably not make it past the influential lobby of doctors and agency owners, who are clearly the biggest winners in the reproductive marketplace. As I have shown in this book, the legal void is often filled by precisely these actors, who set their own rules and frequently play intended parents and surrogates off against each other. Mainly promoting anonymous or at least heavily restricted surrogacy programs gives them considerable power, particularly in the context of transnational surrogacy, when intended parents and surrogates do not share a common language. Agencies and clinics profit from the lack of regulation. Thus it is no surprise that most professionals I spoke with—prior to the eruption of debates about changing surrogacy laws—said they were happy with the current laws and did not see any reason for amendments: the state should provide possibilities for their citizens rather than hinder them with "stupid laws" (see chapter 6).

From this perspective, surrogacy should merely be subject to the laws of the free market that individuals enter at their own risk. Based on the acceptance of economic inequalities and bodily commercialization in the post-Soviet space, surrogacy emerges as just another intimate economy. Here, "unfortunate" (*nyeudachniye*) women make a living by selling their reproductive capital to infertile couples who enter the market as medical consumers. This economy rests on a biopolitical discourse that grounds the right to a child in a supposedly universal and biological desire of humankind—particularly of women—and a crucial element in securing the future of the nation. At the same time, reproduction is cast as a space that is and should be free of politics. In this context, questions of power and economic inequalities are either accepted as entirely unproblematic, as unfortunate but part and parcel of capitalist life, or they are covered up altogether. In this sense, the moral economy of surrogacy rests on moving questions around (assisted) reproduction from the sphere of politics and ethics into an individual and private sphere of a "choice" that should not be interfered with.

In this bioeconomy, fully acknowledging the surrogates as feeling persons with their own rights threatens to destabilize the carefully choreographed programs. They are rather cast as uniform, unskilled workers, who offer their bodies as vases, fridges, or incubators for the embryos they receive. Professionals such as agency and clinic staff render the surrogates anonymous. They need to remain "intimate strangers," and their labor is dismissed as marginal and their bodies as in need of tight regulation and control. The surrogates and their subjectivities are continuously erased, and it comes as no surprise that the BioTexCom video shows the clinic's representative, lawyer, pediatrician, and the nannies, while the surrogates themselves are not even mentioned. This invisibility is facilitated by the stigmatization of surrogacy in Russia and Ukraine, which means that surrogacy is practiced in secrecy, that surrogates often live in isolation (from the intended parents but also from other surrogates), and that they need to stay invisible in the lives of the new families. Under these circumstances, "doing it business-style" and parting ways after the completion of the surrogacy program emerges as an ethical way of practicing surrogacy.

Surrogates and their concerns are also fairly invisible within the current debates about the legislation restricting surrogacy in Russia and Ukraine. It thus might well be that they need to stand up for their own rights; however, under the above-mentioned conditions it is, of course, much more challenging to develop an "identity" as a surrogate that is strong and proud enough, as in the United States (Berend 2016; Jacobson 2016) or Israel (Teman 2010), to do so. But incentives in this direction have been provided by the Ukrainian nongovernmental organization The Power of Mothers (Sila Materey) (Vlasenko 2020). Founded by former surrogate Svetlana Sokolova in 2018, the organization has called for adequately regulating the practice, so as to legally protect surrogates (Grytsenko 2020). Moreover, the organization offers legal counseling and regularly shares information and advice on issues of reproductive labor and health via social media. Thus, while the NGO might not have the power to affect legal outcomes right away, its work toward raising consciousness among surrogates about their own rights and obligations could enable them to undermine the system from within. The widespread understanding of surrogacy as work in the post-Soviet context might offer an effective starting point for surrogates to demand recognition and workers' rights for their reproductive labor.

Truth claims are often seductive: they appear as shiny "offerings," as easy answers that distract us from complex questions. In contexts in which interlocutors have a great personal and political interest in making researchers adopt their truths, they come to see us as "harbingers," who provide their stories "with the halo of objectivity" (Robben 2012, 186). But if we question their truths, if we do not retell their stories in the way we were supposed to, we are quickly accused of being biased and corrupted.

In the course of writing this book, my thoughts repeatedly returned to my interview with Larissa Osipovna, at the *inviTRA* International Fertility Fair in Barcelona, in May 2015. I kept wondering what she would make of my book: Would she dismiss all critical parts as "stupid mistakes"? Would she claim that I simply did not understand what surrogacy was about, because I myself had not experienced infertility? Or because I identify as a feminist researcher and, therefore, as some of the intended parents suggested, I must already be an ideologically tainted surrogacy opponent? "Who in the world can judge?" she had asked me without expecting an answer. "Who can blame a woman for wanting to be a mother?"

My book is not about judging or blaming. Instead, it offers an empathic account of commercial surrogacy, in which I take the anxieties, hopes, and desires of my research participants seriously. This, however, does not mean that I take them as absolute and universal truths. I am also devoted to offering a critical account, to contextualizing my findings in broader structural settings, attentive to the intersecting and shifting power relations at stake. Moreover, as a feminist anthropologist, I regard the personal and the intimate as inherently political and economic spheres. Entering the surrogacy market as an intended parent or reproductive worker is not a private decision made in a social vacuum—the "personal troubles" that move individuals to do so are connected to broader "public issues" (Markens 2007, 5). Consequently, the meanings attached to surrogacy and the experiences made by its participants are contingent on this broader context, accounting for stark differences between surrogacy arrangements in different parts of the world. Acknowledging the broader context also means that debates about surrogacy are always about more than simply a reproductive technique. They touch upon fundamental aspects of identity and human existence, raising controversial questions at the intersection of free choice and coercion, inclusion and exclusion, individual and structure, nature and technology, of the doable and its limits. These debates are, ultimately, about the kind of future we want to live in. As such, a public discussion on the subject is crucial and cannot be silenced by dismissing those with undesirable opinions.

I hope that this book will contribute to such a discussion and that readers will not evaluate it through the prism of true and false or right and wrong, but rather acknowledge it as offering new insights that bring us one step closer to understanding how intimate economies are negotiated, explained, challenged, and controlled. The case of surrogacy offers a lens through which to explore how contested practices become normalized and are made economically profitable. I have proposed that practices of ethical labor and "regimes of truth" (Foucault 1987) play a crucial role in this process, because commercial access to the intimate requires new intellectual, emotional, and corporeal understandings. Truths thus form an integral and indispensable part of the surrogacy market, lubricating its expansion into morally contentious arenas. Despite their fragility, these truths hold great power, since they are of existential necessity and are therefore diligently defended by those who desperately want a child, those who rent their wombs in order to cover their living expenses or secure stable housing conditions, and those who have found a profitable niche in nurturing and facilitating other people's existential hopes.

There is also another party involved in surrogacy arrangements—at least in "successful" ones: the children born through such arrangements. Considering that surrogacy only became more widely available in the 2000s, most of them are still young and little is known about their experiences, thoughts, and feelings. However, as the cases of (international) adoption and gamete provision have shown, the voices of the children at stake can have profound impacts on laws, discourses, and practices. As the surrogacy-born children grow older, some of them will surely enter the discussion, potentially unsettling the moral economy of surrogacy by contributing a perspective that up to now remains speculative.

Afterword

SURROGACY IN TIMES OF WAR

In early 2022, as the end of the COVID-19 pandemic seemed to be moving closer, another critical event unsettled the global order: On February 24, Russian troops invaded Ukraine. According to the Russian state news agency TASS (2022), the so-called "special military operation" was launched in response to a plea for help by leaders of the Donbass republics. Its aim, according to Putin, was to "protect the people that are subjected to abuse, genocide from the Kyiv regime." This protection was to be achieved by "demilitarizing and denazifying" Ukraine and—as Putin later added—by obliging Ukraine to remain neutral (Berger 2022). In other words: Ukraine was leaning too far westward, and Russia was afraid of losing its scope of influence, while feeling threatened by NATO's expansion toward the East.

The invasion came as a big shock to many, even though several incidents foreshadowed the increasing tensions between the two countries and between Russia and "the West" in more general terms: Putin's repeated lamentations regarding the collapse of the Soviet Union and the demise of Russian power; the insurgency war in eastern Ukraine and the annexation of Crimea in 2014; Putin's controversial 2021 essay "On the Historical Unity of Russians and Ukrainians" and his later denial of Ukrainian statehood; or his demands in late 2021 that Ukraine would not join NATO and that the latter would reverse its eastward expansion—demands that were rejected by the West (Bilefsky, Pérez-Peña, and Nagourney 2022; Rachman 2022; Schwirtz, Varenikova, and Gladstone 2022).

At the time of writing, in late April 2022, the war has been raging for two months. Russian warfare has been characterized by ruthless attacks on civilians and brutal destruction of vital infrastructure, causing a major humanitarian crisis. According to the United Nations High Commissioner for Refugees, almost eight million people have been internally displaced and more than five million have fled Ukraine.[1] The invasion constitutes the largest military offense and refugee movement within Europe since the end of World War II (Al Jazeera 2022).

The Russian invasion has also significantly impacted the Ukrainian surrogacy industry and the lives of the surrogates. Since I completed my book several months before the outbreak of war, it seems crucial to add this afterword and to briefly reflect on the status quo and the future prospects for surrogacy in Ukraine and beyond.

Bunker Babies

Unsurprisingly, it was the fertility center BioTexCom that again drew attention to the issue of surrogacy, when it posted a YouTube video three days prior to the Russian invasion.[2] Titled "Newborns in a Bombshelter," the video aims to show intended parents that BioTexCom has made emergency provisions. It gives viewers a tour through the center's bomb shelter on the outskirts of Kyiv, accompanied by siren sounds and dramatic music. While set in an entirely different scene, the images and rhetoric are strikingly similar to those in BioTexCom's COVID-19 video (discussed in this book's conclusion). And like the earlier video, the more recent one also unleashed a controversial debate about global surrogacy. However, early concerns that around one hundred newborns would accumulate in bunkers by the end of March 2022 (Heut and Davlashyan 2022) were not confirmed: In an interview dated March 19, 2022, a BioTexCom employee stated that there were only thirty-five surrogate babies in the (by now) two bomb shelters, as most intended parents were finding ways to pick up their newborns, either by themselves or with the help of others, such as the private, nonprofit rescue organization Project Dynamo, run by a group of "humanitarians," as they state on their website, many of whom have served in the U.S. military (Moore 2022). Only the children of Shanghai parents have to endure a longer waiting period, as the latter are not allowed to leave their city due to the renewed COVID-related lockdown there (Abé 2022). However, the number of these children is unlikely to be small: the end of the one-child policy and the economic rise of the middle class in China have made Chinese intended parents important players in the surrogacy market in recent years (Weis 2021b).

To date, the media has mainly focused on the situation of these intended parents. Many reports are written like "hero stories," depicting in great detail the parents' dangerous pick-up missions, the manifold legal obstacles they face, and their subsequent flight over the Polish or Moldovan borders (e.g., Baker 2022; CNN 2022). The courage of these couples is admirable and their desperation more than understandable. Many intended parents who opt for surrogacy have already spent years, if not decades, trying to have a child. To them, surrogacy is their last chance. What is striking and problematic, however, is that the surrogates are often invisible in these narratives or mentioned only in passing. We do not learn the current circumstances of their and their families' lives or their whereabouts after the birth; in some reports it seems as if there had never been a surrogacy. As this book has shown, the invisibility of the surrogate workers is no coincidence: It is inscribed in the Ukrainian surrogacy market and upheld by agencies, clinics, and intended parents. In this sense the current situation is reminiscent of the discussions surrounding the earthquake in Nepal in 2015. Following the earthquake, which claimed the lives of some nine thousand people, the Israeli state evacuated over twenty-six newborns born to Israeli male couples, while the surrogates themselves were left behind—a move that led to much international criticism (Duttagupta 2015).

Between Reproductive Autonomy and Contractual Obligation

So where are the women who carry foreign couples' children, and how are they doing? What does it mean that they can't just leave their work in Ukraine, but have to take it with them wherever they go? Can they decide for themselves whether to stay in Ukraine—at home with family and friends or (alone) in a hospital bunker? Or whether they want to flee the country and, if so, where they want to go? Do their contractual obligations force them to prioritize the welfare of the child in their womb? And would they be obligated to look after those children after birth if the legal parents cannot enter Ukraine? As Canadian journalist Alison Motluk (2022) states in an excellent article for *The Atlantic*, the war situation turns the spotlight onto potential conflicts of interest between different stakeholders.

Trying to find answers to these questions in the media, I read of intended parents pressuring surrogates to leave the country (Heut and Davlashyan 2022); agencies "offering" surrogates to relocate to L'viv or Moldova (Callaghan 2022; Garner-Purkis 2022); and centers demanding that women return to Kyiv, at least for the birth (Kato 2022). In a Facebook post, BioTexCom even explicitly warns intended parents against giving birth abroad, because "the surrogate mother will be considered a mother and the attempt to hand over the child will be called child trafficking, you will never be recognized as the child's parents. Such acts are punishable by imprisonment or fines."³ Such drastic language deters intended parents who would like to support the surrogates by facilitating their flight abroad or even taking them into their homes. The legal ambiguity could also force surrogates who would like to flee to stay in the country. More recently, a new alternative has emerged, as several agencies seem to have been offering childbirth in Georgia—a country where surrogacy is legal and where contracts therefore remain in place. A good solution, as two surrogates report in *Le Monde*: Viktoria, who fled to a Spanish city near the intended parents, and Marina, who is carrying twins for an Italian couple and who has found refuge in Poland—both are relieved that they will be able to give birth in Georgia (Pascual 2022). It nevertheless remains unclear how many weeks prior to their due date surrogates must fly to Georgia, how they will be accommodated, and whether they will be allowed to take their own children with them. Regardless of the place of delivery, there is the additional question of how well the surrogates are protected afterward: The German news outlet *Deutsche Welle*, for example, reported that a surrogate was put out on the street by BioTexCom just one day after giving birth (Carthaus 2022). Little is also known about the situation of women who are only "in preparation" for an embryo transfer (i.e., already taking hormones) or who are still in the early weeks of pregnancy. According to media reports, some of these women are also being transferred westward; one woman even reported that the agency was trying to pressure her into an abortion.

Surrogacy on Hold?

While everyday life is at a standstill for many people in Ukraine, the intended parents' clocks continue to tick. Even in the run-up to the war, many cancelled their planned fertility treatments in Ukraine and looked around for alternatives. Georgia would be an option, says Sam Everingham of the international organization Growing Families, but he fears the small country won't be able to meet the high demand. This could lead to a rise in the popularity of countries like Cyprus and Albania, where surrogacy is even more poorly regulated, if at all (Heut and Davlashyan 2022). For most Western intended parents, Russia is not likely to be an alternative they would feel comfortable with, and it is probable that those who had been considering Russia as a destination will also change their plans. The extensive economic sanctions with which many countries reacted to the Russian invasion (BBC 2022) also unsettle the foundations of local demand, while the fact that Ukrainian surrogates will no longer cross the border to work in Russia is likely to impact the "supply side" (Weis and Kirpichenko 2022).

The war will not only lead to a geopolitical reshuffling but could once again reveal the reproductive market's capacity to "realign" itself in new geographic areas under changing circumstances (Whittaker 2019). However, the Ukrainian reproductive industry is not entirely on hold. Private intermediaries continue to advertise arrangements in Ukraine on social media, and BioTexCom has announced on its website (in April 2022) that the war "has not stopped" them and that they have already returned to recruiting potential surrogates and egg providers. With few good alternatives, it is possible that the Ukrainian market will revive after the war and that intended parents will choose this destination "out of solidarity," casting their payments as a contribution to restoring the country and "helping" Ukrainian women in need.

Appendix
RESEARCH PARTICIPANTS

Interviews with representatives of European consulates only indirectly informed my research, so their names are not included in the following tables.

TABLE 1 Surrogates (39)

NO.[a]	NAME OF RESEARCH PARTICIPANT	AGE	FAMILY CONSTELLATION	NO. OF OWN CHILDREN	EDUCATION OR JOB	HOMETOWN	PLACE OF RESIDENCE DURING PREGNANCY	FORMS OF REPRODUCTIVE LABOR	TYPE OF PROGRAM (MA/DA)[c]	TYPE OF RESEARCH PARTICIPATION
1	Katya Yefimovna	31	married	1	Translator	Donetsk, UKR	Moscow	Egg provider (1) and surrogate (1)	MA	Continuous
2	Lena Mironovna	29	married	1	Educated as lawyer; works as wedding photographer	Nizhnij Novgorod, RU	Moscow	Surrogate (1)	MA	Continuous
3	Zhenya Pavlovna	29	married	2	—	Smolensk, RU	At home	Surrogate (1)	MA	Continuous
4	Sonya Vitalyevna	—	married	2	Higher technical education; works in a canteen	Lipetsk, RU	At home	Surrogate (1)	MA	Continuous
5	Lyuba Dmitriyevna	25	single	1	—	Greater Minsk, BLR	At home	Surrogate (1)	MA	Continuous
6	Anya Kirillovna	27	single	1	Educated as cook and baker; works as cashier (supermarket)	Moscow, RU	At home	Surrogate (1)	MA	Continuous
7	Diliara Eduardovna[b]	—	married	2	Surrogacy agent	Krasnodar, RU	Moscow	Egg provider (1), surrogate (2)	DA	Interview (1)
8	Olga Georgyevna	27	married	2	—	Belgorod, RU	At home	Surrogate (1)	MA	Continuous
9	Ekaterina Antipovna	24	—	1	Hairdresser	—	Moscow	Surrogate (1)	MA	Interview (1)
10	Raya Antonovna	30	married	2	Educated as cook and pastry chef; additional education in advertisement design	Saratov Oblast, RU	At home	Surrogate (1)	DA	Interview (1)
11	Ksenia Demyanovna	21	single	1	—	Ulyanovsk, RU	At home	Surrogate (1)	MA	Continuous

#	Name	Age	Marital status	Children	Occupation	Location	Where interviewed	Role	DA/MA	Interview type
12	Sveta Valentinovna	27	married	2	Cashier (supermarket)	Volgodonsk, RU	At home	Surrogate (1)	DA	Interview (1), text messages
13	Masha Arkadyevna[b]	37	married	2	Surrogacy agent	Ukraine	At home	Surrogate (2)	DA	Interview (1)
14	Polina Davidovna	–	married	1	–	Penza, RU	At home	Surrogate (1)	MA	Continuous
15	Alla Filippovna	25	married	2	Manicurist	Chelyabinsk, RU	At home	Egg provider (2), surrogate (1)	MA	Interview (1)
16	Venera Igorevna	31	single	1	Cook	Orenburg, RU	At home	Surrogate (1)	MA	Interview (1)
17	Anya Gennadyevna	32	married	3	Secretary	Tolyatti, RU	At home	Surrogate (1)	MA	Interview (1)
18	Anastasia Leonidovna	–	single	1	Saleswoman (clothing store)	Moscow, RU (but from Ulyanovsk)	Moscow	Surrogate (1)	MA	Continuous
19	Sasha Stepanovna	22	married	1	–	Volgograd, RU	Moscow	Surrogate (1)	DA/MA	Interview (1)
20	Oksana Yevgenyevna	35	married	2	Educated as seamstress; works in various jobs	Mariupol, UKR	At home	Surrogate (1)	MA	Continuous
21	Antonina Semyonovna	21	married	1	Saleswoman (supermarket)	Greater Moscow (but from Siberia)	Moscow	Surrogate (1)	MA	Interview (1)
22	Marina Nikitichna	–	married	1	–	Moldavia (but lives in Moscow)	At home	Egg provider (7), Surrogate (1)	MA	Interview (1)
23	Alyona Timofeyevna	28	single	1	–	Kharkiv, UKR	At home	Egg provider (1), surrogate (1)	MA	Continuous
24	Lidiya Radionovna	20	married	1	–	Kazan, RU	Moscow	Surrogate (1)	MA	Continuous
25	Vika Yeremeyevna	–	married	2	Cashier (supermarket)	Voronesh, RU	At home	Surrogate (1)	MA	Continuous
26	Elena Glebovna	–	married	2	–	Ryazan, RU	At home	Surrogate (1)	DA/MA	Interview (1)
27	Inessa Borislavnovna	28	married	4	Cook	Ufa, RU	Moscow	Surrogate (1)	MA	Interview (1)
28	Diana Tarasovna	25	married	2	–	Buryatia, RU	Moscow	Egg provider (1), Surrogate (1)	MA	Interview (1)
29	Yana Timurovna	–	single	1	–	Volgograd, RU	Moscow	Surrogate (1)	DA	Interview (1)

(*Continued*)

TABLE 1 (Continued)

NO.[a]	NAME OF RESEARCH PARTICIPANT	AGE	FAMILY CONSTELLATION	NO. OF OWN CHILDREN	EDUCATION OR JOB	HOMETOWN	PLACE OF RESIDENCE DURING PREGNANCY	FORMS OF REPRODUCTIVE LABOR	TYPE OF PROGRAM (MA/DA)[c]	TYPE OF RESEARCH PARTICIPATION
30	Carine Lvovna	–	–	2	Factory worker	Kostroma, RU (but from Armenia)	At home	Surrogate (1)	MA	Interview (1)
31	Alevtina Leontyevna	–	single	1	–	Moscow, RU (but from Cheboksary)	Moscow	Egg provider (1), Surrogate (1)	MA	Continuous
32	Yuliya Grigoryevna	22	married	1	Saleswoman	Volgograd, RU	At home	Surrogate (1)	MA	Interview (1)
33	Ulyana Iosifovna	–	–	–	Midwife	Kemerovo, RU	At home	Surrogate (1)	MA	Interview (1)
34	Nina Feodorovna	–	–	–	–	Belorussia	Moscow	Egg provider (1), Surrogate (1)	DA/MA	Interview (1)
35	Kira Konstantinovna	–	single	3	–	Greater Moscow, RU (but from Ulyanovsk)	Moscow	Surrogate (1)	DA/MA	Interview (1)
36	Lyuda Arkadyevna	34	married	2	Educated as chemist, works as saleswoman	Kharkov, UKR	–	Egg provider (1), Surrogate (1)	MA	Interview (1)
37	Sofiya Stanislavovna	21	married	2	–	Yaroslavl, RU	Moscow	Surrogate (1)	MA	Interview (1)
38	Valeriya Ilyinichna	30	single	1	Student of medicine	Moscow, RU (but from Ukraine)	Moscow	Surrogate (1)	MA	Interview (1)
39	Mariya Yegorovna	–	single	1	Saleswoman (flower shop)	Moscow, RU (but from Cheboksary)	Moscow	Surrogate (1)	MA	Interview (1)

[a] This list of surrogates comprises women who were "surrogacy candidates" (thus, women who had not yet entered a program), who were in a program at the time of my research, or who have already completed one or two programs.

[b] Interviewed as both a surrogate and an agent, so listed in both table 1 and table 3.

[c] MA = mediated arrangement, DA = direct arrangements. "DA/MA" does not indicate that the respective surrogate has completed two programs but rather that she first tried finding a DA or already was in a DA (but without successfully getting pregnant) and then opted for an MA.

TABLE 2 Intended parents (18)

NAME OF RESEARCH PARTICIPANT/S	AGE	FAMILY CONSTELLATION	COUNTRY OF RESIDENCE	COUNTRY OF (PLANNED) FERTILITY PROGRAM	FERTILITY PROGRAM PLANNED/CHOSEN	TYPE AND STAGE OF FERTILITY PROGRAM (UPON FIRST CONTACT)	TYPE OF RESEARCH PARTICIPATION
Olessia Valeryevna	52	Heterosexual couple	Russia	Russia	Surrogacy with egg donation	DA, completed, 1 child (9y.)	Interview (1)
Galya Yanovna	40	Heterosexual couple	Russia	Russia	Surrogacy	DA, completed, 1 child (5y.)	Interview (2)
Alisa Serafimovna	36	Heterosexual couple	Russia	Russia	Surrogacy	DA, completed, 3 children (3y. and—twins—1y.)	Interview (1)
Vera Romanovna	44	Heterosexual couple	Russia	Russia	Surrogacy	DA, in planning stage	Interview (1)
Rita Tikhonovna	—	Heterosexual couple	Russia	Russia	Surrogacy	DA, ongoing (4th month of pregnancy)	Interview (1)
Dina Antonovna	45	Heterosexual couple	Russia	Russia	Egg donation	MA, completed, 1 child (5y.)	Interview (1)
Juan Romero	36	Homosexual couple	Spain	Ukraine or Poland	Surrogacy with egg donation	DA, in planning stage	Interview (1), e-mails
Anna Martín	—	Heterosexual couple	Spain	Ukraine	Surrogacy	MA, in planning stage	Interview (1)
Marta Pérez	—	Heterosexual couple	Spain	Ukraine	Surrogacy	MA, in planning stage (later: completed, 1 child)	Interview (2), e-mails
Diego Torres	—	Heterosexual couple	Spain	USA	Surrogacy with egg donation	MA, completed	Interview (1)
Hannes & Simon Braschke	—	Homosexual couple	Germany	Yet unclear	Surrogacy with egg donation	In planning stage	Interview (1)
Alejandro Morales	—	Homosexual couple	Spain	USA	Surrogacy with egg donation	MA, completed, 2 children	Interview (1)
Sara Blanco	—	Heterosexual couple	Spain	Ukraine	Surrogacy with egg donation	MA, in planning stage	Interview (1), e-mails
Teresa & Stefan Wagner	39 (T.), 45 (S.)	Heterosexual couple	Germany	Ukraine	Surrogacy with egg donation	MA, in planning stage (later: completed, 2 children)	Continuous
David & Christoph Hauser	—	Homosexual couple	Austria	Russia	Surrogacy with egg donation	MA, completed, 1 child (another program in planning stage)	Interview (1)

TABLE 3 Professionals

NAME	OCCUPATION/JOB	LOCATION OF AGENCY/ CLINIC/OFFICE	TYPE OF RESEARCH PARTICIPATION
Doctors (14) and psychologists (2)			
Sergej Yakovenko (real name)	Doctor and clinic director	Moscow	Continuous
Pavel Viktorovich	Doctor	Moscow	Interview (1)
Valentina Maximovna	Doctor	Moscow	Interview (2)
Anton Feodorovich	Doctor	Moscow	Interview (1)
Mariya Alexeyevna	Doctor	Moscow	Interview (1)
Alexej Ivanovich	Doctor	Moscow	Interview (1)
Natalya Nikolayevna	Doctor	Moscow	Interview (1)
Valeriy Ivanovich	Doctor	Moscow	Interview (1)
Elena Yuryevna	Doctor and clinic director	Moscow	Interview (1), written
Anton Vladimirovich	Doctor	Moscow	Interview (2)
Galya Olegovna	Doctor	Moscow	Interview (1)
Alina Danilovna	Doctor	Moscow	Interview (1)
Aleksandra Denisovna	Infertility psychologist	Moscow	Interview (2)
Evgeniya Yanovna	Infertility psychologist	Moscow	Interview (1)
Kira Aleksandrovna	Doctor and clinic director	Kyiv	Interview (1)
Ludmila Petrovna	Doctor	L'viv	Interview (1)
Agents, managers, lawyers (22)			
Natasha Sergeyevna	Surrogate manager	Moscow	Continuous
Anna Semyonovna	Surrogate manager	Moscow	Continuous
Yelena Mikhailovna	Agency employee	Moscow	Interview (1)
Maksim Antonov	Lawyer	Moscow	Interview (1)
Konstantin Pavlovich	PR-representative of agency	Moscow	Interview (1)
Alina Ruslanovna	Agency employee	Moscow	Interview (1)
Ljuda Feodorovna	Agency employee	St. Petersburg	Interview (1)
Diliara Eduardovna[a]	Agency director (and former surrogate)	Krasnodar	Interview (1)
Masha Arkadyevna[a]	Agency director (and former surrogate)	Ukraine	Interview (1)
Nikolai Kirillovich	Agency director	Kharkov	Interview (1)
Larissa Osipovna	Agency director	Kyiv	Interview (1)
Anastasia Anatolyevna	Agency director	Kyiv	Interview (1)
Oksana Ivanovna	Agency employee	Kyiv	Interview (1)
Sergej Petrovich	Agency director	Kyiv	Interview (1)
Oleksandra Vadimovna	Agency employee	Kyiv	Interview (1)
Lara Gavrilovna	Agency employee	Kyiv	Interview (1)
Álvaro Fuentes	Agency director (and doctor)	Las Palmas de Gran Canaria	Interview (1)
Pedro Monte	Lawyer	Barcelona	Interview (1)
Ricardo Delmonte	Agency director	Barcelona	Interview (1)
Alejandro Garcia	Agency employee	Barcelona	Continuous
Nina Popov	Agency employee	Barcelona	Interview (1)
Lorenzo Rivera	Agency director	Barcelona	Interview (1)

[a] Interviewed as both a surrogate *and* an agent, so listed in both table 1 and table 3.

TABLE 4 Surrogacy opponents and advocates (4)

NAME	OCCUPATION/JOB	PLACE OF RESIDENCE	TYPE OF RESEARCH PARTICIPATION
Tatyana Vasilyevna	Former embryologist and surrogacy opponent	Moscow	Interview (1)
Dimitri Anatolyevich	Priest and surrogacy opponent	Moscow	Interview (1)
Anahi Molina	Surrogacy advocate	Barcelona	Interview (1)
Alberto Cabello	Surrogacy advocate	Barcelona	Interview (1)

Notes

INTRODUCTION

1. I use the terms "intended parents," "commissioning parents," and "client parents" interchangeably and, for reasons of convenience, also for those actors who have already become parents through surrogacy. I mostly write of "intended parents" in order to stress that their wish to become parents predates their involvement in surrogacy.

2. According to *Al Jazeera*, the share held by Ukrainian fertility centers could equal over a quarter of the global surrogacy market (Roache 2018).

3. I use the term "agent"—interchangeably with the term "intermediary"—for all sorts of actors who facilitate surrogacy arrangements from an organizational and bureaucratic point of view.

4. According to Spanish law, surrogacy as well as its facilitation are not explicitly banned, but domestic surrogacy contracts are void. As a consequence, many intended parents travel abroad for such arrangements. Spanish authorities have assumed a fairly tolerant approach when it comes to registering the intended parents as legal parents of the child (Orejudo Prieto de los Mozos 2013).

5. I use the terms "research participants" and "interview partners" almost interchangeably.

6. Today, this is by far the most widespread form of surrogacy, especially in the context of commercial surrogacy.

7. Committee on Foreign Affairs, "Report on the Annual Report on Human Rights and Democracy in the World 2014 and the European Union's Policy on the Matter," European Parliament, November 30, 2015, https://www.europarl.europa.eu/doceo/document/A-8-2015-0344_EN.html.

8. According to several doctors and surrogacy agents, the number of Ukrainian women crossing the border to Russia slightly decreased after the start of the conflict between the two countries in February 2014. This was partly because some sections of the common border were closed and partly because ethnically Ukrainian women no longer wanted to work for the "enemy."

9. There are no more recent statistics to be found. The Center of Medical Statistics of the Ministry of Health in Ukraine states that this is the most recent data on surrogacy cycles (I thank Polina Vlasenko for this information!), while my request concerning the number of surrogate births remained unanswered.

10. Extrapolating the numbers mentioned in an article in *The Guardian* (Roth 2020), could mean that up to two thousand children were born for foreign parents alone in 2020. According to another *Guardian* article (Merz 2020), experts estimate that about 3,500 surrogate births took place each year. Likewise, relying on the numbers provided by the Ukrainian fertility center BioTexCom ("Surrogacy: Babies Are Waiting for Their Parents," YouTube, April 30, 2020, https://www.youtube.com/watch?v=xPdRx_L96C0) could mean that in 2020 roughly 370 surrogate babies were born for foreign intended parents alone who had worked with this center.

11. There have been reports of intended parents refusing to take the child, for instance because of genetic deficiencies or because they had two programs running at the same time and only wanted to keep one child (Sudakov 2011a); as well as reports of surrogates

who did not want to relinquish the child, for reasons of attachment or because they demanded more money (Bondar 2017; Chemodanova 2019). For more information see chapter 4, note 1.

12. This would equal €320–400 for the monthly payment and between €13,000 and 16,000 for the final payment.

13. Marital status is irrelevant; however, if the surrogate is married, she needs to provide written consent from her husband.

14. The State Duma is the lower house of the Russian Federal Assembly.

15. Following anthropologists such as Michael Lambek (2010) as well as my research participants, I use "ethics" and "morality" synonymously in this book.

16. The first aspect concerns the determination of *ethical substance*, by which Foucault means "the . . . part of ourselves, or of our behaviour, which is relevant for ethical judgment" (1997, 263), the "prime material of [our] moral conduct" (1990, 26). He gives the example of how fidelity can mean very different things to different people, depending on what part of themselves they relate fidelity to—for instance fidelity as control of acts or as control of desires (Foucault 1990). The second aspect is the *mode of subjection*, referring to the question of what rules and laws actors follow and what logic lies behind them. Again taking fidelity as an example, one would ask whether someone practices fidelity because she or he is part of a certain group or institution. The fourth aspect concerns the *telos*, the purpose or goal, of the ethical subject. An action cannot be moral in itself but always has to be seen as part of the overall conduct of a person (Foucault 1990, 1997).

17. Which is not to be reduced to wage labor.

18. In all of Russia, there were 219 registered IVF clinics in 2019, 114 of which conducted surrogacy programs (RAHR 2021).

19. I put the word "participant" in brackets, since my position in the clinic was often only that of an observer, with no or very limited participation.

20. Following the director's wish, I anonymized neither him nor his clinic.

21. I included interviews with intended parents who were not involved in a surrogacy program or at least not in a program in Russia or Ukraine, as these interviews provided important additional dimensions to the discussion of the biopolitics of motherhood as well as the discussion of Russia and Ukraine as surrogacy destinations—as opposed to other potential destinations.

1. THE BIOPOLITICS OF MOTHERHOOD

1. The state's appropriation of women's bodies was nowhere more extreme than in Romania during the 1970s and 1980s, where abortion remained illegal until 1990, childless people had to pay "celibacy tax," and Nicolae Ceausescu openly claimed the fetus to be the "socialist property of the whole society" and giving birth to be a "patriotic duty" (Verdery 2013, 21). In Russia as well, abortion—which was relegalized in 1955 after Stalin's ban—came under attack, while the state failed to sufficiently provide other forms of birth control (Rivkin-Fish 2003, 2004).

2. This statement resonated with one of my interviews, in which a psychologist mentioned that infertility often occurred among couples who had "swapped roles"—the woman being a "controlling and well-paid boss" and the man thus being "weak."

3. "Birth Rate, Crude (per 1,000 People) – Russian Federation, Ukraine, Austria, Spain, Germany," World Bank, https://data.worldbank.org/indicator/SP.DYN.CBRT.IN?end=2014&locations=RU-UA-AT-ES-DE&start=1960&view=chart, and "Mortality Rate, Adult, Male (per 1,000 Male Adults) – Russian Federation, Ukraine, Austria, Spain, Germany," World Bank, https://data.worldbank.org/indicator/SP.DYN.AMRT.

MA?end=2014&locations=RU-UA-AT-ES-DE&start=1960&view=chart (both accessed December 15, 2017).

4. The support was financial but given in the form of vouchers equivalent to ₽250,000 (around US$12,000 at the time). These vouchers could be used when the child turned three, to acquire or renovate an apartment, to be added to a mother's pension savings, or for the child's education (Rivkin-Fish 2005). In addition to these Soviet-inspired welfare measures, the Russian state presented another Soviet-inspired move: in 2008, the "Order of Parental Glory" was introduced and awarded to families with seven or more children.

5. Feminist scholars (e.g., Rivkin-Fish 2005; Avdeyeva 2011) have furthermore criticized these policies for ultimately enforcing gender inequalities. Firstly, they remain concentrated on women, while men are not given responsibility and duties within the family. Secondly, extended leave policies and cash payments do little to tackle the problems mothers face in the labor market and are not directed at increasing women's reproductive decision-making.

6. "Natsional'nye Proyekty: Tselevye Pokazateli I Osnovnye Rezul'taty," February 17, 2019, http://static.government.ru/media/files/p7nn2CS0pVhvQ98OOwAt2dzCIAietQih.pdf, accessed October 7, 2022.

7. The COVID-19 pandemic has had a significant impact on the demographic situation, as Russia was (and still is) confronted with a high COVID-related mortality rate, an exceptionally low birth rate, as well as a slowdown of migration due to travel restrictions (Rogoża 2021).

8. See the sites for BioTexCom (biotexcom.com), VittoriaVita (vittoriavita.com), and Scandinavia AVA-PETER (avapeter.com).

9. In her media analysis of Russian newspaper articles on ARTs between 1996 and 2006, Tkach (2009, 152) argues that that these articles reassert notions of "real" parenthood and the nuclear family.

2. SECRET CONCEPTIONS

1. This is also the case concerning the discussion around LGBTQI+ rights in Russia (Persson 2015).

2. LGBTQI+ = lesbian, gay, bisexual, transgender, queer/questioning, intersex, plus.

3. Counterintuitively, Mizulina's statement was part of a debate about how to *counter* Russia's demographic problem.

4. I could find no proof to back up this statement through online research.

5. She was referring in particular to a procedure called ICSI (intracytoplasmic sperm injection), in which a sperm cell is injected directly into the cytoplasm of an egg cell—a treatment that has "revolutionized" treating male infertility (Inhorn and Birenbaum-Carmeli 2018, 1).

6. "Propaganda," *Oxford English Dictionary*, https://en.oxforddictionaries.com/definition/propaganda, accessed May 12, 2019.

7. In post-Soviet times, *kul'turnost'* is also employed as a marker of distinction in regard to the "new rich" and their supposed lack of culture, taste, and morality (Patico 2005).

8. Lack of mutual respect is also a concern in many other studies that look at morals and values in the Russian context (e.g., Patico 2005; Zigon 2009).

9. At the same time, the private was also a crucial site of political contestation and activity (Ritter 2001).

10. See Korolczuk (2014) for a discussion of infertility forums in Poland, as well as Gunnarsson Payne and Korolczuk (2016) for a comparison of Swedish and Polish online forums concerning ARTs.

11. While the American Society of Reproductive Medicine (Ethics Committee of the American Society for Reproductive Medicine 2018) and the European Society of Human Reproduction and Embryology ("Good Practice Recommendations for Information Provision for Those Involved in Reproductive Donation," https://www.eshre.eu/Guidelines-and-Legal/Guidelines/Information-provision-in-donation) have issued best practice guidelines or are in the process of doing so, to my knowledge, no such document has been issued by the Russian Association of Human Reproduction.

12. None of the women I interviewed had had abortions.

13. In her book *Lies that Bind*, Susan Blum (2007) deconstructs "truth" as a value in itself as rooted in a specific Western context and shows how her interlocutors in China evaluated questions of telling the truth or not in relation to the possible consequences and with regard to notions of responsibility and relationships.

3. CHOREOGRAPHING SURROGACY

1. There is no strict rule on this, but most clinics mentioned a waiting period of five days.

2. This would equal roughly €800.

3. According to the surrogates, a one-room apartment in one of the smaller cities in Russia cost at least ₽1.5 million, meaning that the salary they received for the surrogacy covered a maximum of two-thirds of the total costs.

4. Oblast refers to an administrative region in the Russian Federation.

5. I assume that "Blood +" refers to the wish for a surrogate who is rhesus (Rh) positive. The rhesus factor is a protein on the surface of red blood cells. This protein can be inherited, in which case a person is Rh positive (which most people are). Having a negative Rh factor and being pregnant with a child that is Rh positive can lead to complications during the pregnancy (which can, however, be medically prevented).

6. She actually said "*shtuk syem'desyat*," which can be translated as "around seventy pieces."

7. One of the doctors stated that Ukrainian surrogates were usually from central, southern, and eastern Ukraine, not from the western parts that were more religious.

8. After the second embryo transfer, Ksenia Demyanovna did get pregnant. She gave birth in 2016 and started working as a private broker for several agencies and clinics in 2017.

9. We did not want to enter Katya Yefimovna's flat without her being there, as this would have felt like an intrusion into her private space. Ultimately, the flat manager—while still not understanding our position—offered for us to go to Lena Mironovna's flat, who had consented to Sarah taking pictures in her flat and who was also at home when we visited her.

4. DOING IT BUSINESS-STYLE

1. There have been several such cases. In 2010, for instance, a surrogate from the Ulyanovsk region secretly registered the baby in her name, claiming that she had developed attachment. In the subsequent court case, she was given custody over the child. According to the director of a large surrogacy center in Moscow, however, court practices have been changing since then (Chemodanova 2019). One more recent case that made headlines was that of *Frolov v. Suzdaleva* in St. Petersburg, when surrogate Tatyana Suzdaleva refused to relinquish the twins she had given birth to, because the intended parents were not willing (and able) to meet her demands. She argued that since she had carried twins, she should also be entitled to double the salary. The court ultimately ruled in favor of the Frolovs, and many intended parents and professionals hope that this case will set a precedent (Bondar

2017). Moreover, in 2017, the Plenum of the Supreme Court of the Russian Federation issued a resolution, stating that in cases of disputes over legal parenthood a court should carefully evaluate the surrogacy contract and explore why the surrogate refuses to relinquish the child. The lack of written consent by the surrogate is thus no longer viewed as an absolute obstacle to acknowledging the intended parents' parental status (Mouliarova 2019, 413).

2. "Case of Paradiso and Campanelli v. Italy," HUDOC, European Court of Human Rights, January 24, 2017, https://hudoc.echr.coe.int/eng?i=001-170359.

5. TECHNOLOGIES OF ALIGNMENT

1. In an article entitled "Back Stage of the Global Free Market: Nannies and Surrogates," Hochschild (2012) explicitly addresses emotional labor in the context of surrogacy.

2. I draw on translations from the *Oxford Concise Russian Dictionary* in addition to the online dictionaries Linguee (linguee.com), bab.la (en.bab.la), PONS (pons.com), and Multitran (multitran.ru).

6. LABORING WITH HAPPINESS

1. English quotes taken from agency/clinic websites, online forums, etc. often contain spelling and grammatical mistakes. I nevertheless use the exact citations throughout this chapter.

2. Modern Family Surrogacy Center, http://www.modernfamilysurrogacy.com/, accessed November 25, 2017.

3. My point of departure is the conviction that there is no "outside" of affect, particularly not in the intimate sphere of surrogacy. As such, affective labor permeates all spheres of life; even the production and circulation of the understanding of surrogacy as "business-style" (as a sphere supposedly without affect) happens through affective labor.

4. In those states in which surrogacy is legalized and regulated.

5. Numerous interview partners assumed this association to have been founded and funded by one of Spain's largest surrogacy agencies, meaning that the association had commercial rather than altruistic interests, as suggested by Alberto Cabello.

6. According to an article in *Al Jazeera*, around half of all children born in Ukraine through surrogacy are conceived through arrangements mediated by BioTexCom (Roache 2018).

7. "BioTexCom in International Mass Media: What Does European Press Say about Kyiv Reproductive Center," BioTexCom, http://biotexcom.com/biotexcom-international-mass-media/, accessed November 20, 2017.

8. Sarah12, "Other side of Biotexcom," Egg donation and surrogacy forum at BioTexCom, September 11, 2014, http://forum.mother-surrogate.info/viewtopic.php?f=135&t=3860.

9. Among German intended parents, Ukraine was one of the two most important destinations for surrogacy, besides the United States (König, Majumdar, and Jacobson 2020).

10. One and a half years after our interview, Sara Blanco wrote me that they finally had an arrangement and a great surrogate in Ukraine.

11. In Russian, there is an equivalent for "compensation" but mostly the term "salary" (*gonorar*) is used.

12. VittoriaVita (https://vittoriavita.com), testimonies accessed on November 23, 2017 (the testimonials are rotating, so those cited cannot be found anymore on VittoriaVita's website).

13. For reasons of convenience, I nevertheless use "agency" as an umbrella term for all agencies that facilitated surrogacy arrangements from an organizational point of view.

14. "Gestational Carrier. Surrogate Mother Meaning," VittoriaVita, http://vittoriavita.it/surrogate-mother-gc/, accessed November 20, 2017.

15. Anna Lisnichenko, "Is Surrogacy Ethical?," Perfect Surrogacy Coordination Center, March 16, 2017, https://www.perfect-surrogacy.com/post/2017/03/16/is-surrogacy-ethical.

7. AMBIVALENCES OF FREEDOM

1. I do not have the data to thoroughly comment on this question in regard to my own research. However, it is safe to say that under the economic conditions women encountered in 2014 and 2015 (the financial crisis and the fall of the Russian ruble), surrogacy was certainly not life-changing for many of them.

2. Nevertheless, they made clear that they would not want their daughters to become surrogates.

3. Nirmala George, "Surrogates Feel Hurt by India's Ban," February 29, 2016, http://news.com.au/finance/business/surrogates-feel-hurt-by-indias-ban/news-story/800583bb0d9a16b29c38404ae4e51671.

4. The veracity of these claims could be neither proven nor refuted. However, a search on Google and on the website of the Ukrainian parliament (http://zakon.rada.gov.ua/laws) revealed no information about the legal changes mentioned by the agent.

5. See the preceding note.

CONCLUSION

1. BioTexCom, "Surrogacy: Babies Are Waiting for Their Parents," YouTube, April 30, 2020, https://www.youtube.com/watch?v=xPdRx_L96C0.

2. In the following months, the Ukrainian state allowed many parents to pick up their children—which was also visually documented by BioTexCom: BioTexCom, "Babies Born at Biotexcom, Ukraine, Are Reunited with Their Parents from Argentina and Spain," YouTube, June 15, 2020, https://www.youtube.com/watch?v=czNGl918tbw.

3. For instance, after India announced banning surrogacy for gay men in 2012, parts of the industry "shifted" to other countries in Southeast Asia, e.g., to Nepal, where Indian surrogates were then moved for the course of their pregnancies (Pande 2021; Rudrappa 2018; Whittaker 2019).

4. The draft bill has been published on the Duma's website (where the status quo can also be checked): "Bill No. 1191971-7," Legislative Support System, https://sozd.duma.gov.ru/bill/1191971-7, accessed September 14, 2021.

5. Lately, these have comprised the majority of all foreign parents traveling to Russia for surrogacy (Weis 2021b).

6. The latest step regarding homophobic legal measures is a controversial bill, entailing several constitutional changes, signed by Putin in April 2021. Besides allowing Putin to run for president for another two legislative periods (meaning that he might stay in power until 2036), the bill also constitutionally precludes same-sex marriage by stating that only a man and a woman can enter into a marriage (Luxmoore 2020).

7. Unarguably, the bill was also a response to the Sergei Magnitsky Rule of Law Accountability Act passed in the United States in late 2012, named after a Russian tax lawyer who had investigated fraud by the Russian state, was subsequently arrested, and died in police custody. The Magnitsky Act prohibits certain individuals that are known to have committed gross human rights violations to enter the country (Lally and Englund 2012).

8. Update: In mid-December 2022, President Putin signed legislation that will ban surrogacy for foreigners and allow the service for only heterosexual, married couples (of which at least one partner must have Russian citizenship) and single Russian women. In addition, children born through surrogacy will automatically obtain Russian citizenship. According to the Chairman of the State Duma, the new law shall "prevent the trafficking of our children [and] protect babies from falling into same-sex couples or becoming victims of crimes, including organ sales." (*Moscow Times*, "Putin Bans Surrogacy for Foreigners," December 19, 2022, https://www.themoscowtimes.com/2022/12/19/putin-bans-surrogacy-for-foreigners-a79738)

AFTERWORD

1. "Ukraine Situation Flash Update #10," United Nations High Commissioner for Refugees, April 28, 2022, https://data2.unhcr.org/en/documents/download/92353.

2. BioTexCom, "Newborns in a Bombshelter," YouTube, February 21, 2022, https://www.youtube.com/watch?v=fAPsvA9zzrw.

3. https://www.facebook.com/klinik.biotexcom/posts/pfbid0SPcLjh4nQDysuesA76PB2tGztyc85CMv5S844b4TGXStpaNAxExHem2f9YtjwT39l, accessed on March 5, 2022 (my translation).

References

Abé, Nicola. 2022. "Bleiben Sie ruhig: Das Lebens Ihres Kindes hängt davon ab." *Der Spiegel*, March 19. https://www.spiegel.de/ausland/leihmutterschaft-in-der-ukraine-ein-bunker-voller-babys-a-4a514c55-097a-4818-b379-98e5a82c7a67.

Adrian, Stine Willum, and Charlotte Kroløkke. 2018. "Passport to Parenthood: Reproductive Pathways in and out of Denmark." *NORA—Nordic Journal of Feminist and Gender Research* 26 (2): 112–28.

Agustín, Laura María. 2008. *Sex at the Margins: Migration, Labour Markets and the Rescue Industry*. London: Zed Books.

Ahmed, Sara. 2004a. "Affective Economies." *Social Text* 22 (2): 117–39.

———. 2004b. *The Cultural Politics of Emotion*. Edinburgh: Edinburgh University Press.

———. 2010. *The Promise of Happiness*. Durham, NC: Duke University Press.

Al Jazeera. 2022. "UN: Over 5 Million People Have Fled Ukraine since Russia Invasion." April 20. https://www.aljazeera.com/news/2022/4/20/more-than-5-million-ukrainians-have-fled-since-russian-invasion.

Almeling, Rene. 2007. "Selling Genes, Selling Gender: Egg Agencies, Sperm Banks, and the Medical Market in Genetic Material." *American Sociological Review* 72 (3): 319–40.

Anderson, John. 2016. "Religion, State and 'Sovereign Democracy' in Putin's Russia." *Journal of Religious and Political Practice* 2 (2): 249–66.

Appadurai, Arjun. 1986. "Introduction: Commodities and the Politics of Value." In *The Social Life of Things: Commodities in Cultural Perspective*, edited by Arjun Appadurai, 3–63. Cambridge: Cambridge University Press.

Arendt, Hannah. 1958. *The Human Condition*. Chicago: University of Chicago Press.

Arvidsson, Anna, Sara Johnsdotter, and Birgitta Essén. 2015. "Views of Swedish Commissioning Parents Relating to the Exploitation Discourse in Using Transnational Surrogacy." *PLoS ONE* 10 (5): e0126518.

Ashwin, Sarah. 2000. "Introduction: Gender, State and Society in Soviet and Post-Soviet Russia." In *Gender, State and Society in Soviet and Post-Soviet Russia*, edited by Sarah Ashwin, 1–29. London: Routledge.

———. 2002. "The Influence of the Soviet Gender Order on Employment Behavior in Contemporary Russia." *Sociological Research* 41 (1): 21–37.

Attwood, Lynne, Elisabeth Schimpfössl, and Marina Yusupova. 2018. "Introduction." In *Gender and Choice after Socialism*, edited by Lynne Attwood, Elisabeth Schimpfössl, and Marina Yusupova, xiii–xxiii. Cham: Springer International.

Avdeyeva, Olga A. 2011. "Policy Experiment in Russia: Cash-for-Babies and Fertility Change." *Social Politics: International Studies in Gender, State & Society* 18 (3): 361–86.

Baker, Jordan. 2022. "The Desperate Mission to Get an Australian Baby out of Ukraine." *Sydney Morning Herald*, March 4. https://www.smh.com.au/world/europe/the-desperate-mission-to-get-an-australian-baby-out-of-ukraine-20220303-p5a1hj.html.

Bandak, Andreas, and Manpreet K. Janeja. 2018. "Introduction: Worth the Wait." In *Ethnographies of Waiting: Doubt, Hope and Uncertainty*, edited by Manpreet K. Janeja and Andreas Bandak, 1–39. Oxford: Bloomsbury.

Banerjee, Amrita. 2010. "Reorienting the Ethics of Transnational Surrogacy as a Feminist Pragmatist." *The Pluralist* 5 (3): 107–27.

Bärnreuther, Sandra. 2019. "When Time Stretches: Waiting and in Vitro Fertilization in India." *Collection Puruṣārtha* 36: 269–85.

———. 2021. *Substantial Relations: Making Global Reproductive Medicine in Postcolonial India*. Ithaca, NY: Cornell University Press.

BBC. 2022. "What Are the Sanctions on Russia and Are They Hurting Its Economy?" June 27. https://www.bbc.com/news/world-europe-60125659.

Becker, Gay. 2000. *The Elusive Embryo: How Women and Men Approach New Reproductive Technologies*. Berkeley: University of California Press.

———. 2002. "Deciding Whether to Tell Children about Donor Insemination: An Unresolved Question in the United States." In *Infertility around the Globe: New Thinking on Childlessness, Gender, and Reproductive Technologies*, edited by Marcia C. Inhorn and Frank van Balen, 119–33. Berkeley: University of California Press.

Becker, Gay, Anneliese Butler, and Robert D. Nachtigall. 2005. "Resemblance Talk: A Challenge for Parents Whose Children Were Conceived with Donor Gametes in the US." *Social Science & Medicine* 61 (6): 1300–1309.

Berend, Zsuzsa. 2016. *The Online World of Surrogacy*. New York: Berghahn Books.

Berger, Miriam. 2022. "Putin Says He Will 'Denazify' Ukraine: Here's the History behind That Claim." *Washington Post*, February 25. https://www.washingtonpost.com/world/2022/02/24/putin-denazify-ukraine/.

Bergmann, Sven. 2012. "Resemblance that Matters: On Transnational Anonymized Egg Donation in Two European IVF Clinics." In *Reproductive Technologies as Global Form: Ethnographies of Knowledge, Practices, and Transnational Encounters*, edited by Michi Knecht, Maren Klotz, and Stefan Beck, 331–55. Frankfurt a.M.: Campus Verlag.

———. 2014. *Ausweichrouten der Reproduktion: Biomedizinische Mobilität und die Praxis der Eizellspende*. Wiesbaden: VS Verlag für Sozialwissenschaften.

Bernstein, Anya. 2013. "An Inadvertent Sacrifice: Body Politics and Sovereign Power in the Pussy Riot Affair." *Critical Inquiry* 40 (1): 220–41.

Berntsen, Sine, Viveca Söderström-Anttila, Ulla-Britt Wennerholm, Hannele Laivuori, Anne Loft, Nan B. Oldereid, Liv Bente Romundstad, Christina Bergh, and Anja Pinborg. 2019. "The Health of Children Conceived by ART: 'The Chicken or the Egg?'" *Human Reproduction Update* 25 (2): 137–58.

Beskaravajnaya, Tatyana. 2020. "EKO den'gi." *Medvestik*, April 20. https://medvestnik.ru/content/articles/EKO-dengi.html.

Bharadwaj, Aditya. 2006. "Sacred Modernity: Religion, Infertility, and Technoscientific Conception around the Globe." *Culture, Medicine and Psychiatry* 30 (4): 451–65.

Bilefsky, Dan, Richard Pérez-Peña, and Eric Nagourney. 2022. "The Roots of the Ukraine War: How the Crisis Developed." *New York Times*, April 21. https://www.nytimes.com/article/russia-ukraine-nato-europe.html.

Blum, Susan D. 2007. *Lies that Bind: Chinese Truth, Other Truths*. Lanham: Rowman & Littlefield.

Bondar, Yuliya. 2017. "Sud obyazal surrogatnuyu mat' otdat' detej zakazchikam." *Medportal*, August 10. https://medportal.ru/mednovosti/sud-obyazal-surrogatnuyu-mat-otdat-detey-zakazchikam/.

Boris, Eileen, and Rhacel Salazar Parreñas. 2010. "Introduction." In *Intimate Labors: Cultures, Technologies and the Politics of Care*, 1–17. Stanford: Stanford University Press.

Borozdina, Ekaterina, Anna Rotkirch, Anna Temkina, and Elena Zdravomyslova. 2016. "Using Maternity Capital: Citizen Distrust of Russian Family Policy." *European Journal of Women's Studies* 23 (1): 60–75.

Bourdieu, Pierre. 2007. *Distinction: A Social Critique of the Judgement of Taste*. Cambridge, MA: Harvard University Press.

Bowdler, Neil. 2020. "Russia Hopes 'Test-Tube Babies' Will Boost Birthrates." *Radio Free Europe*, February 15. https://www.rferl.org/a/russia-hopes-test-tube-babies-will-boost-birthrates/30434656.html.

Brednikova, Olga, Nadya Nartova, and Olga Tkach. 2009. "Assisted Reproduction in Russia: Legal Regulations and Public Debates." In *Making Bodies, Persons and Families: Normalising Reproductive Technologies in Russia, Switzerland and Germany*, edited by Willemijn de Jong and Olga Tkach, 43–56. Berlin: LIT Verlag.

Brennan, Christopher. 2014. "Russia Bans Adoptions to Countries Where Gay Marriage Is Legal." *Moscow Times*, February 13. https://www.themoscowtimes.com/2014/02/13/russia-bans-adoptions-to-countries-where-gay-marriage-is-legal-a32064.

Butler, Judith. 2015. *Bodies that Matter: On the Discursive Limits of "Sex."* New York: Routledge.

Callaghan, Louise. 2022. "Surrogate Mothers Fear Pressure to Flee Ukraine." *The Times*, February 20. https://www.thetimes.co.uk/article/surrogate-mothers-fear-pressure-to-flee-ukraine-gsntx9z7f.

Carthaus, Anna. 2022. "Ukrainische Leihmütter zwischen den Fronten." *Deutsche Welle*, March 23. https://www.dw.com/de/ukrainische-leihm%C3%BCtter-zwischen-den-fronten/a-61263581.

Chak, Kerry. 2013. "Ukraine Has the Worst Roads and the Best Reproductive Medicine in the World." *News Europe*, February 6. http://newseurope.info/ukraine-has-the-worst-roads-and-the-best-reproductive-medicine-in-theworld/.

Chemodanova, Ksenia. 2019. "Dorogo i opasno: Kak surrogatnye materi obmanyvayut zakazchikov." *Gazeta*, October 31. https://www.gazeta.ru/business/2019/08/28/12608059.shtml.

CNN. 2022. "'We Walked 8 Miles with a Newborn': US Couple Describes Their Dangerous Escape from Ukraine." March 3. https://www.youtube.com/watch?v=APhWmeRHgxc.

Cohen, Lawrence. 1999. "Where It Hurts: Indian Material for an Ethics of Organ Transplantation." *Daedalus* 128 (4): 135–65.

———. 2005. "Operability, Bioavailability, and Exception." In *Global Assemblages: Technology, Politics, and Ethics as Anthropological Problems*, edited by Aihwa Ong and Stephen J. Collier, 79–90. Malden, MA: Blackwell.

Constable, Nicole. 2006. "Brides, Maids, and Prostitutes: Reflections on the Study of 'Trafficked' Women." *PORTAL: Journal of Multidisciplinary International Studies* 3 (2): 1–25.

———. 2009. "The Commodification of Intimacy: Marriage, Sex, and Reproductive Labor." *Annual Review of Anthropology* 38 (1): 49–64.

Cooper, Melinda, and Catherine Waldby. 2014. *Clinical Labor: Tissue Donors and Research Subjects in the Global Bioeconomy*. Durham, NC: Duke University Press.

Corea, Gena. 1985. *The Mother Machine: Reproductive Technologies from Artificial Insemination to Artificial Wombs*. New York: Harper and Row.

Corrigan, Oonagh. 2003. "Empty Ethics: The Problem with Informed Consent." *Sociology of Health & Illness* 25 (7): 768–92.

Council for International Organizations of Medical Sciences and World Health Organization, eds. 2002. "International Ethical Guidelines for Biomedical Research Involving Human Subjects." CIOMS. https://cioms.ch/wp-content/uploads/2016/08/International_Ethical_Guidelines_for_Biomedical_Research_Involving_Human_Subjects.pdf.

Davis-Floyd, Robbie E. 1994. "The Technocratic Body: American Childbirth as Cultural Expression." *Social Science & Medicine* 38 (8): 1125–40.

De Lacey, Sheryl. 2002. "IVF as Lottery or Investment: Contesting Metaphors in Discourses of Infertility." *Nursing Inquiry* 9 (1): 43–51.

Dempsey, Deborah. 2015. "Relating across International Borders: Gay Men Forming Families through Overseas Surrogacy." In *Globalized Fatherhood*, edited by Marcia C. Inhorn, Wendy Chavkin, and José-Alberto Navarro, 267–90. New York: Berghahn Books.

Deomampo, Daisy. 2013a. "Transnational Surrogacy in India: Interrogating Power and Women's Agency." *Frontiers: A Journal of Women Studies* 34 (3): 167–88.

———. 2013b. "Gendered Geographies of Reproductive Tourism." *Gender & Society* 27 (4): 514–37.

———. 2016. *Transnational Reproduction: Race, Kinship, and Commercial Surrogacy in India*. New York: New York University Press.

Dionisius, Sarah. 2015. "Queer Matters: Family-Building Processes of Lesbian Couples Using Donor Insemination." *Distinktion: Journal of Social Theory* 16 (3): 283–301.

Disney, Tom. 2015. "Complex Spaces of Orphan Care—a Russian Therapeutic Children's Community." *Children's Geographies* 13 (1): 30–43.

———. 2017. "The Orphanage as an Institution of Coercive Mobility." *Environment and Planning A: Economy and Space* 49 (8): 1905–21.

Dow, Katharine. 2015. "'A Nine-Month Head-Start': The Maternal Bond and Surrogacy." *Ethnos* 82 (1): 1–19.

———. 2016. *Making a Good Life: An Ethnography of Nature, Ethics, and Reproduction*. Princeton, NJ: Princeton University Press.

Druzenko, Gennadiy. 2013. "Ukraine." In *International Surrogacy Arrangements: Legal Regulation at the International Level*, edited by Katarina Trimmings and Paul Beaumont, 357–65. Studies in Private International Law. Oxford: Hart Publishing.

Dumit, Joseph, and Robbie Davis-Floyd. 1998. "Cyborg Babies: Children from the Third Millennium." In *Cyborg Babies: From Techno-Sex to Techno-Tots*, edited by Joseph Dumit, 1–20. New York: Routledge.

Dushina, Anastasia, Yuliya Kersha, Tatyana Larkina, and Daria Provorova. 2016. "Legitimatsiya Kommercheskogo Surrogatnogo Materinstva v Rossii." *Ekonomicheskaya Sotsiologiya* 17 (1): 62–79.

Duttagupta, Ishani. 2015. "Why Surrogacy Issue Emerges after Nepal Earthquake." *Economic Times*, May 5. https://economictimes.indiatimes.com/blogs/globalindian/why-surrogacy-issue-emerges-after-nepal-earthquake/.

Ertman, Martha M. 2010. "The Upside of Baby Markets." In *Baby Markets: Money and the New Politics of Creating Families*, edited by Michele Goodwin, 23–40. Cambridge: Cambridge University Press.

Essig, Laurie. 1999. *Queer in Russia: A Story of Sex, Self, and the Other*. Durham, NC: Duke University Press.

Ethics Committee of the American Society for Reproductive Medicine. 2018. "Informing Offspring of Their Conception by Gamete or Embryo Donation: An Ethics Committee Opinion." *Fertility and Sterility* 109 (4): 601–5.

European Social Survey. 2017. *ESS Round 8 (2016/2017) Technical Report*. London: ESS ERIC.

Fassin, Didier. 2009. "Moral Economies Revisited." *Annales: Histoire, Sciences Sociales* 64 (6): 1237–66.

Fausto-Sterling, Anne. 2000. *Sexing the Body: Gender Politics and the Construction of Sexuality*. New York: Basic Books.

Feldman, Ilana. 2007. "The Quaker Way: Ethical Labor and Humanitarian Relief." *American Ethnologist* 34 (4): 689–705.

Ferguson, James. 1994. *The Anti-Politics Machine: Development, Depoliticization, and Bureaucratic Power in Lesotho*. Minneapolis: University of Minnesota Press.

Finch, Janet. 2007. "Displaying Families." *Sociology* 41 (1): 65–81.

Fine, Cordelia. 2017. *Testosterone Rex: Unmaking the Myths of Sex of Our Gendered Minds*. London: Icon Books.

Firestone, Shulamith. 1970. *The Dialectic of Sex: The Case for Feminist Revolution*. New York: William Morrow.

Fisher, Max. "The Real Reason Russia Wants to Ban Adoptions by 'Dangerous' American Families." *Washington Post*, December 28. https://www.washingtonpost.com/news/worldviews/wp/2012/12/28/the-real-reason-russia-wants-to-ban-adoptions-by-dangerous-american-families/.

Fixmer-Oraiz, Natalie. 2013. "Speaking of Solidarity: Transnational Gestational Surrogacy and the Rhetorics of Reproductive (In)Justice." *Frontiers: A Journal of Women Studies* 34 (3): 126–63.

Flatley, Jonathan. 2008. *Affective Mapping: Melancholia and the Politics of Modernism*. Cambridge, MA: Harvard University Press.

Førde, Kristin Engh. 2016. *Intimate Distance: Transnational Commercial Surrogacy in India*. Oslo: University of Oslo.

———. 2017. "Fair Play in a Dirty Field: The Ethical Work of Commissioning Surrogacy in India." In *Assisted Reproduction across Borders: Feminist Perspectives on Normalizations, Disruptions and Transmissions*, edited by Merete Lie and Nina Lykke, 37–48. New York: Routledge.

Foucault, Michel. 1980. *The History of Sexuality*. Vol. 1, *An Introduction*. New York: Vintage Books.

———. 1987. *The Foucault Reader*. Edited by Paul Rabinow. New York: Pantheon Books.

———. 1990. *The History of Sexuality*. Vol. 2, *The Use of Pleasure*. New York: Vintage Books.

———. 1997. *Ethics: Subjectivity and Truth*. Vol. 1 of *The Essential Works of Foucault, 1954–1984*. Edited by Paul Rabinow. London: Penguin Books.

Fourcade, Marion, and Kieran Healy. 2007. "Moral Views of Market Society." *Annual Review of Sociology* 33: 285–311.

France 24. 2020. "Russia Funds IVF Baby Boom to Battle Population Slump." January 20. https://www.france24.com/en/20200130-russia-funds-ivf-baby-boom-to-battle-population-slump.

Franklin, Sarah. 1997. *Embodied Progress: Cultural Account of Assisted Conception*. London: Routledge.

———. 1998. "Making Miracles: Scientific Progress and the Facts of Life." In *Reproducing Reproduction: Kinship, Power, and Technological Innovation*, edited by Sarah Franklin and Helena Ragoné, 102–17. Philadelphia: University of Pennsylvania Press.

———. 2012. "Five Million Miracle Babies Later: Biocultural Legacies of IVF." In *Reproductive Technologies as Global Form: Ethnographies of Knowledge, Practices, and Transnational Encounters*, edited by Michi Knecht, Maren Klotz, and Stefan Beck, 27–58. Frankfurt a.M.: Campus Verlag.

———. 2013. *Biological Relatives: IVF, Stem Cells, and the Future of Kinship*. Durham, NC: Duke University Press.

Franklin, Sarah, and Helena Ragoné. 1998. "Introduction." In *Reproducing Reproduction: Kinship, Power, and Technological Innovation*, edited by Sarah Franklin and Helena Ragoné, 1–14. Philadelphia: University of Pennsylvania Press.

Fujimura, Clementine K. 2005. *Russia's Abandoned Children: An Intimate Understanding*. Westport, CT: Praeger Publishers.

Funk, Nanette. 2004. "Feminist Critiques of Liberalism: Can They Travel East? Their Relevance in Eastern and Central Europe and the Former Soviet Union." *Signs: Journal of Women in Culture and Society* 29 (3): 695–726.

Gabowitsch, Mischa. 2013. *Putin kaputt!? Russlands neue Protestkultur*. Berlin: Suhrkamp.

Gal, Susan. 2002. "A Semiotics of the Public/Private Distinction." *Differences: A Journal of Feminist Cultural Studies* 13 (1): 77–95.

Gal, Susan, and Gail Kligman. 2000. *The Politics of Gender after Socialism: A Comparative-Historical Essay*. Princeton, NJ: Princeton University Press.

Garner-Purkis, Zak. 2022. "'We Hope No Missiles Hit Hospitals': The Ukrainian Woman Caught between Scared Surrogate Mums and Panicking Parents." *My London*, March 7. https://www.mylondon.news/news/uk-world-news/we-hope-no-missiles-hit-23317102.

Gershon, Ilana. 2011. "Neoliberal Agency." *Current Anthropology* 52 (4): 537–55.

Gilligan, Carol. 2003. *In a Different Voice: Psychological Theory and Women's Development*. Cambridge, MA: Harvard University Press.

Goffman, Erving. 1959. *The Presentation of Self in Everyday Life*. Edinburgh: University of Edinburgh Press.

———. 1989. "On Fieldwork." *Journal of Contemporary Ethnography* 18: 123–32.

Golombok, S., A. Brewaeys, M. T. Giavazzi, D. Guerra, F. MacCallum, and J. Rust. 2002. "The European Study of Assisted Reproduction Families: The Transition to Adolescence." *Human Reproduction* 17 (3): 830–40.

Grigoryan, Anzhelina, and Yana Zainitdinova. 2019. "Inostrantsy massovo zakazyvayut surrogatnoe materinstvo u rossiyanok za million rublej." *Riafan*, July 23. https://riafan.ru/1189990-inostrancy-massovo-zakazyvayut-surrogatnoe-materinstvo-u-rossiyanok-za-million-rublei.

Gryshchenko, Mykola, and Alexey Pravdyuk. 2016. "Gestational Surrogacy in Ukraine." In *Handbook of Gestational Surrogacy: International Clinical Practice and Policy Issues*, edited by E. Scott Sills, 250–65. Cambridge: Cambridge University Press.

Grytsenko, Oksana. 2020. "The Stranded Babies of Kyiv and the Women Who Give Birth for Money." *The Guardian*, June 15. https://www.theguardian.com/world/2020/jun/15/the-stranded-babies-of-kyiv-and-the-women-who-give-birth-for-money.

Gunnarsson Payne, Jenny. 2015. "Reproduction in Transition: Cross-Border Egg Donation, Biodesirability and New Reproductive Subjectivities on the European Fertility Market." *Gender, Place & Culture* 22 (1): 107–22.

———. 2016. "Grammars of Kinship: Biological Motherhood and Assisted Reproduction in the Age of Epigenetics." *Signs: Journal of Women in Culture and Society* 41 (3): 483–506.

Gunnarsson Payne, Jenny, and Elżbieta Korolczuk. 2016. "Reproducing Politics: The Politicisation of Patients' Identities and Assisted Reproduction in Poland and Sweden." *Sociology of Health & Illness* 38 (7): 1074–91.

Gunnarsson Payne, Jenny, Elżbieta Korolczuk, and Signe Mezinska. 2020. "Surrogacy Relationships: A Critical Interpretative Review." *Upsala Journal of Medical Sciences* 125 (0): 183–91.

Gupta, Jyotsna Agnihotri, and Annemiek Richters. 2008. "Embodied Subjects and Fragmented Objects: Women's Bodies, Assisted Reproduction Technologies and the Right to Self-Determination." *Journal of Bioethical Inquiry* 5 (4): 239–49.

Guseva, Alya. 2020. "Scandals, Morality Wars, and the Field of Reproductive Surrogacy in Ukraine." *Economic Sociology: The European Electronic Newsletter* 21 (3): 4–10.

Guseva, Alya, and Vyacheslav Lokshin. 2019. "Medical Conceptions of Control in the Field of Commercial Surrogacy in Kazakhstan." *Salute e Società* 1: 26–43.

Hage, Ghassan. 2009a. "Introduction." In *Waiting*, edited by Ghassan Hage, 1–12. Victoria: Melbourne University Press.

———. 2009b. "Waiting Out the Crisis: On Stuckedness and Governmentality." In *Waiting*, edited by Ghassan Hage, 97–106. Victoria: Melbourne University Press.

Halliday, Jane, Sharon Lewis, Joanne Kennedy, David P. Burgner, Markus Juonala, Karin Hammarberg, David J. Amor, Lex W. Doyle, Richard Saffery, Sarath Ranganathan, Liam Welsh, Michael Cheung, John McBain, Stephen J.C. Hearps, and Robert McLachlan. 2019. "Health of Adults Aged 22 to 35 Years Conceived by Assisted Reproductive Technology." *Fertility and Sterility* 112 (1): 130–39.

Hardt, Michael. 1999. "Affective Labor." *Boundary 2* 26 (2): 89–100.

Harrison, Laura. 2016. *Brown Bodies, White Babies: The Politics of Cross-Racial Surrogacy*. New York: New York University Press.

Hawley, Samantha. 2018. "Surrogacy in Ukraine in Spotlight after Disabled Child Abandoned." *ABC News*, August 20. https://www.abc.net.au/radio/programs/am/surrogacy-in-ukraine-in-spotlight/11430452.

Held, Virginia. 2006. *The Ethics of Care: Personal, Political, and Global*. Oxford: Oxford University Press.

Hellman, Andrew, and Glenn Cohen. 2017. "Prohibiting Sperm Donor Anonymity in the US and Possible Effects on Recruitment and Compensation." *BioNews* (blog), April 4. https://www.bionews.org.uk/page_95954.

Hemmings, Clare, and Amal Treacher Kabesh. 2013. "The Feminist Subject of Agency: Recognition and Affect in Encounters with 'the Other.'" In *Gender, Agency, and Coercion*, edited by Sumi Madhok, Anne Phillips, and Kalpana Wilson, 29–46. Basingstoke: Palgrave Macmillan.

Heut, Nathalia, and Naira Davlashyan. 2022. "Surrogate Mothers, Babies and Frozen Embryos Trapped by Ukraine War as IVF Parents Watch in Horror." *Euronews*, March 18. https://www.euronews.com/next/2022/03/11/surrogacy-in-crisis-as-ukraine-war-leaves-newborns-stranded-in-bomb-shelters-and-families-.

Hibino, Yuri, and Yosuke Shimazono. 2013. "Becoming a Surrogate Online: 'Message Board' Surrogacy in Thailand." *Asian Bioethics Review* 5 (1): 56–72.

Hildebrand, Sarah, Gerhild Perl, Julia Rehsmann, and Veronika Siegl, eds. 2018. *hope*. Basel: Christoph Merian Verlag. https://www.merianverlag.ch/produkt/fotografie/hope/b79ed4db-c980-4e41-b450-e13b75244e8e.html.

Hochschild, Arlie. 2012. "Back Stage of the Global Free Market: Nannies and Surrogates." In *Transnationale Vergesellschaftungen*, edited by Hans-Georg Soeffner, 1125–38. Wiesbaden: Springer Fachmedien Wiesbaden.

Hochschild, Arlie Russell. 2000. "Global Care Chains and Emotional Surplus Value." In *On the Edge: Living with Global Capitalism*, edited by Anthony Giddens and Will Hutton, 130–46. London: Jonathan Cape.

———. 2003. *The Managed Heart: Commercialization of Human Feeling.* Berkeley: University of California Press.

Hoeyer, Klaus, and Linda F. Hogle. 2014. "Informed Consent: The Politics of Intent and Practice in Medical Research Ethics." *Annual Review of Anthropology* 43 (1): 347–62.

Hofmann, Susanne, and Adi Moreno. 2016. "Introduction. Global Intimate Economies: Discontents and Debates." In *Intimate Economies: Bodies, Emotions, and Sexualities on the Global Market*, edited by Susanne Hofmann and Adi Moreno, 1–29. New York: Palgrave Macmillan.

Holmgren, Beth. 2013. "Toward an Understanding of Gendered Agency in Contemporary Russia." *Signs: Journal of Women in Culture and Society* 38 (3): 535–42.

Hovav, April. 2020. "Cutting out the Surrogate: Caesarean Sections in the Mexican Surrogacy Industry." *Social Science & Medicine* 256: 113–63.

Human Rights Watch. 2014. "Abandoned by the State: Violence, Neglect, and Isolation for Children with Disabilities in Russian Orphanages." https://www.hrw.org/sites/default/files/reports/russia0914_ForUploadweb.pdf.

Iarskaia-Smirnova, Elena, and Pavel Romanov. 2012. "Doing Class in Social Welfare Discourses: 'Unfortunate Families' in Russia." In *Rethinking Class in Russia*, edited by Suvi Salmenniemi, 85–106. Farnham: Ashgate.

Inhorn, Marcia C. 1994. *Quest for Conception: Gender, Infertility and Egyptian Medical Traditions.* Philadelphia: University of Pennsylvania Press.

———. 2003. *Local Babies, Global Science: Gender, Religion, and in Vitro Fertilization in Egypt.* London: Routledge.

———. 2004. "Privacy, Privatization, and the Politics of Patronage: Ethnographic Challenges to Penetrating the Secret World of Middle Eastern, Hospital-Based in Vitro Fertilization." *Social Science & Medicine* 59 (10): 2095–2108.

———. 2007. *Reproductive Disruptions: Gender, Technology, and Biopolitics in the New Millennium.* London: Berghahn Books.

———. 2011. "Globalization and Gametes: Reproductive 'Tourism,' Islamic Bioethics, and Middle Eastern Modernity." *Anthropology & Medicine* 18 (1): 87–103.

Inhorn, Marcia C., and Frank van Balen. 2002. "Introduction. Interpreting Infertility: A View from the Social Sciences." In *Infertility around the Globe: New Thinking on Childlessness, Gender, and Reproductive Technologies*, edited by Marcia C. Inhorn and Frank van Balen, 3–32. Berkeley: University of California Press.

Inhorn, Marcia C., and Daphna Birenbaum-Carmeli. 2018. "Assisted Reproductive Technologies." In *The International Encyclopedia of Anthropology*, edited by Hilary Callan, 1–6. New York: John Wiley & Sons.

Inhorn, Marcia C., and Pasquale Patrizio. 2012. "The Global Landscape of Cross-Border Reproductive Care: Twenty Key Findings for the New Millennium." *Current Opinion in Obstetrics and Gynecology* 24 (3): 158–63.

Interfax. 2009. "Glavnyj pediatr Rossii vystupayet protiv podderzhaniya na gosudarstvennom urovnye tekhnologii iskusstvyennogo oplodotvoreniya." September 28. https://www.interfax-russia.ru/siberia/report/

glavnyy-pediatr-rossii-vystupaet-protiv-podderzhaniya-na-gosudarstvennom-urovne-tehnologii-iskusstvennogo-oplodotvoreniya.

Issoupova, Olga. 2000. "From Duty to Pleasure? Motherhood in Soviet and Post-Soviet Russia." In *Gender, State and Society in Soviet and Post-Soviet Russia*, edited by Sarah Ashwin, 30–54. London: Routledge.

Isupova, Olga G. 2011. "Support through Patient Internet-Communities: Lived Experience of Russian in Vitro Fertilization Patients." *International Journal of Qualitative Studies on Health and Well-Being* 6 (3): no. 5907 (n.p.).

Jacobson, Heather. 2016. *Labor of Love: Gestational Surrogacy and the Work of Making Babies*. New Brunswick, NJ: Rutgers University Press.

Jadva, V., L. Blake, P. Casey, and S. Golombok. 2012. "Surrogacy Families 10 Years On: Relationship with the Surrogate, Decisions over Disclosure and Children's Understanding of Their Surrogacy Origins." *Human Reproduction* 27 (10): 3008–14.

Kahn, Susan Martha. 2000. *Reproducing Jews: A Cultural Account of Assisted Conception in Israel*. Durham, NC: Duke University Press.

Kato, Brooke. 2022. "Ukrainian Surrogates Must Return to War Zone to Give Birth to Westerners' Babies." *New York Post*, March 9. https://nypost.com/2022/03/09/ukrainian-surrogates-must-return-to-war-zone-to-give-birth/.

Kay, Rebecca. 2002. "A Liberation from Emancipation? Changing Discourses on Women's Employment in Soviet and Post-Soviet Russia." *Journal of Communist Studies and Transition Politics* 18 (1): 51–72.

Kempadoo, Kamala, and Jo Doezema, eds. 1998. *Global Sex Workers: Rights, Resistance, and Redefinition*. London: Routledge.

Khodyakov, Dmitry. 2007. "Trust as a Process: A Three-Dimensional Approach." *Sociology* 41 (1): 115–32.

Khvorostyanov, Natalia, and Daphna Yeshua-Katz. 2020. "Bad, Pathetic and Greedy Women: Expressions of Surrogate Motherhood Stigma in a Russian Online Forum." *Sex Roles* 83 (7): 474–84.

Kierans, Ciara, and Kirsten Bell. 2017. "Cultivating Ambivalence: Some Methodological Considerations for Anthropology." *HAU: Journal of Ethnographic Theory* 7 (2): 23–44.

Kirpichenko, Maria. 2017. "Russian Legislative Practices and Debates on the Restriction of Wide Access to ARTs." In *Assisted Reproduction across Borders: Feminist Perspectives on Normalizations, Disruptions and Transmissions*, edited by Merete Lie and Nina Lykke, 232–48. New York: Routledge.

——. 2020. "Ideology of Simulation: The Material-Semiotic Production of the Surrogate in the Web Worldings of Russian Surrogacy." *European Journal of Women's Studies* (online), June 9. https://doi.org/10.1177/1350506820922603.

Klimchuk, Oleg, and Viktor Cheretski. 2018. "Ukraine's Surrogacy Industry Leaves Parents in Limbo." *Deutsche Welle*, September 7. https://www.dw.com/en/ukraines-surrogacy-industry-leaves-parents-in-limbo/a-45371478.

Klomegah, Kester Kenn. 2021. "Moment of Truth: Russia Faces Demography Crisis." *Modern Diplomacy* (blog), February 3. https://moderndiplomacy.eu/2021/02/03/moment-of-truth-russia-faces-demography-crisis/.

Knecht, Michi, Maren Klotz, and Stefan Beck. 2012. "Reproductive Technologies as Global Form: Introduction." In *Reproductive Technologies as Global Form: Ethnographies of Knowledge, Practices, and Transnational Encounters*, edited by Michi Knecht, Maren Klotz, and Stefan Beck, 11–26. Frankfurt a.M.: Campus Verlag.

Knight, Frank H. 1921. *Risk, Uncertainty and Profit*. Boston: Riverside.
Kolesnikova, Varvara. 2021a. "RAHR nazvala zakonproyekt o surrogatnom materinstvye nekonstitutsionnym." *Vademecum*, February 2. https://vademec.ru/news/2021/02/02/rarch-nazvala-zakonoproekt-o-surrogatnom-materinstve-nekonstitutsionnym/.
———. 2021b. "V kakom regulirovanii nuzhdayetsya rynok surrogatnogo materinstva v Rossii." *Vademecum*, June 7. https://vademec.ru/article/v_kakom_regulirovanii_nuzhdaetsya_rynok_surrogatnogo_materinstva_v_rossii/.
König, Anika. 2018. "Parents on the Move: German Intended Parents' Experiences with Transnational Surrogacy." In *Cross-Cultural Comparisons on Surrogacy and Egg Donation: Interdisciplinary Perspectives from India, Germany and Israel*, edited by Sayani Mitra, Silke Schicktanz, and Tulsi Patel, 277–99. Cham: Springer International.
König, Anika, Anindita Majumdar, and Heather Jacobson. 2020. "'Pandemic Disruptions' in Surrogacy Arrangements in Germany, U.S.A., and India during COVID-19." *Medical Anthropology Quarterly* Rapid Response Blog Series, August 11. https://medanthroquarterly.org/rapid-response/2020/08/pandemic-disruptions-in-surrogacy-arrangements-in-germany-u-s-a/.
Konrad, Monica. 2005. *Nameless Relations: Anonymity, Melanesia and Reproductive Gift Exchange between British Ova Donors and Recipients*. London: Berghahn Books.
Korelina, Olga. 2020. "'A Flagrant Rights Violation': State Investigators in Russia Reportedly Plan to Arrest Single Gay Fathers on Child Trafficking Charges." *Meduza*, October 1. https://meduza.io/en/feature/2020/10/01/a-flagrant-rights-violation.
Korolczuk, Elżbieta. 2014. "Terms of Engagement: Re-defining Identity and Infertility On-line." *Culture Unbound: Journal of Current Cultural Research* 6 (2): 431–49.
———. 2016. "'The Purest Citizens' and 'IVF Children': Reproductive Citizenship in Contemporary Poland." *Reproductive Biomedicine & Society Online* 3: 126–33.
Krainova, Natalya. 2013. "Mizulina's Surrogacy Ban Idea Ridiculed." *Moscow Times*, November 11. http://www.themoscowtimes.com/2013/11/11/mizulinas-surrogacy-ban-idea-ridiculed-a29455.
Kroløkke, Charlotte Halmø. 2014. "West Is Best: Affective Assemblages and Spanish Oöcytes." *European Journal of Women's Studies* 21 (1): 57–71.
———. 2015. "Have Eggs, Will Travel: The Experiences and Ethics of Global Egg Donation." *Somatechnics* 5 (1): 12–31.
Kroløkke, Charlotte Halmø, and Saumya Pant. 2012. "'I Only Need Her Uterus': Neo-Liberal Discourses on Transnational Surrogacy." *NORA—Nordic Journal of Feminist and Gender Research* 20 (4): 233–48.
Kruglova, Anna. 2016. "Anything Can Happen: Everyday Morality and Social Theory in Russia." PhD thesis, University of Toronto.
Kurlenkova, Alexandra. 2018. "Ova Exchange Practices at a Moscow Fertility Clinic: Gift or Commodity?" In *Health, Technologies, and Politics in Post-Soviet Settings*, edited by Olga Zvonareva, Evgeniya Popova, and Klasien Horstman, 173–97. Cham: Springer International.
Kuznetsova, Yevgeniya, and Yegor Gubernatorov. 2021. "Deputaty podgotovili zapryet na surrogatnoe materinstvo dlya odinokikh lyudej." *RBC*, January 19. https://www.rbc.ru/politics/19/01/2021/6006e6759a79472e23983481.
Laidlaw, James. 2014. *The Subject of Virtue: An Anthropology of Ethics and Freedom*. Cambridge: Cambridge University Press.

Lally, Kathy, and Will Englund. 2012. "Russia Fumes as U.S. Senate Passes Measure Aimed at Human Rights." *Washington Post*, December 6. https://www.washingtonpost.com/world/europe/us-passes-magnitsky-bill-aimed-atrussia/2012/12/06/262a5bba-3fd5-11e2-bca3-aadc9b7e29c5_story.html.

Lambek, Michael. 2010. *Ordinary Ethics: Anthropology, Language, and Action*. New York: Fordham University Press.

Leibetseder, Doris. 2020. "Precarious Bodily Performances in Queer and Transgender Reproduction with ART." In *Bodily Interventions and Intimate Labour: Understanding Bioprecarity*, edited by Gabriele Griffin and Doris Leibetseder, 79–94. Manchester: Manchester University Press.

Lemke, Thomas. 2011. *Biopolitics: An Advanced Introduction*. New York: New York University Press.

Lettow, Susanne. 2015. "Population, Race and Gender: On the Genealogy of the Modern Politics of Reproduction." *Distinktion: Journal of Social Theory* 16 (3): 267–82.

Lewis, Sophie. 2019. "Surrogacy as Feminism: The Philanthrocapitalist Framing of Contract Pregnancy." *Frontiers: A Journal of Women Studies* 40 (1): 1–38.

Leykin, Inna. 2019. "The History and Afterlife of Soviet Demography: The Socialist Roots of Post-Soviet Neoliberalism." *Slavic Review* 78 (1): 149–72.

Lock, Margaret. 2001. "The Tempering of Medical Anthropology: Troubling Natural Categories." *Medical Anthropology Quarterly* 15 (4): 478–92.

Lock, Margaret, and Patricia Kauffert. 1998. "Introduction." In *Pragmatic Women and Body Politics*, edited by Margaret Lock and Patricia A Kauffert, 1–27. Cambridge: Cambridge University Press.

Loktionova, Maria. 2020. "Minzdrav RF nameren izmenit' zakon o surrogatnom materinstve s yanvarya." *Gazeta*, October 21. https://www.gazeta.ru/social/2020/10/20/13326049.shtml.

Lustenberger, Sibylle. 2016. "From Mumbai to Tel Aviv: Distance and Intimacy in Transnational Surrogacy Arrangements." *Journal of Middle East Women's Studies* 12 (2): 203–24.

Luxmoore, Matthew. 2020. "The Putin Constitution: How Will It Change Russia?" *Radio Free Europe*, July 1. https://www.rferl.org/a/the-putin-constitution-how-will-it-change-russia/30699899.html.

Maciejewska-Mroczek, Ewa. 2019. "Tactile Crease: The Embodiment of Anti-IVF Discourses in Poland." *Ethnologia Europaea* 49 (1): 91–102.

Maciejewska-Mroczek, Ewa, and Magdalena Radkowska-Walkowicz. 2017. "Between Monster Child and Innocent Baby: Managing Fear and Hope in Polish Debates on in Vitro Fertilization." In *Childhood, Literature and Science: Fragile Subjects*, edited by Jutta Ahlbeck, Päivi Lappalainen, Kati Launis, and Kirsi Tuohela, 184–95. London: Routledge.

Magnus, Maria C., Allen J. Wilcox, Elin A. Fadum, Håkon K. Gjessing, Signe Opdahl, Petur B. Juliusson, Liv Bente Romundstad, and Siri E. Håberg. 2021. "Growth in Children Conceived by ART." *Human Reproduction* 36 (4): 1074–82.

Mair, Jonathan, Ann Kelly, and Casey High. 2016. "Introduction: Making Ignorance an Ethnographic Object." In *Anthropology of Ignorance: An Ethnographic Approach*, edited by Casey High, Ann Kelly, and Jonathan Mair, 1–32. New York: Palgrave Macmillan.

Majumdar, Anindita. 2017. *Transnational Commercial Surrogacy and the (Un)Making of Kin in India*. Oxford: Oxford University Press.

Makarychev, Andrey, and Sergei Medvedev. 2015. "Biopolitics and Power in Putin's Russia." *Problems of Post-Communism* 62 (1): 45–54.

Malich, Lisa. 2017. *Die Gefühle der Schwangeren: Eine Geschichte somatischer Emotionalität (1780–2010)*. Bielefeld: Transcript.
Mamo, Laura. 2007. *Queering Reproduction: Achieving Pregnancy in the Age of Technoscience*. Durham, NC: Duke University Press.
Markens, Susan. 2007. *Surrogate Motherhood and the Politics of Reproduction*. Berkeley: University of California Press.
———. 2012. "The Global Reproductive Health Market: U.S. Media Framings and Public Discourses about Transnational Surrogacy." *Social Science & Medicine* 74 (11): 1745–53.
Martin, Emily. 2001. *The Woman in the Body: A Cultural Analysis of Reproduction*. Boston: Beacon Press.
Mattingly, Cheryl. 2019. "Waiting." *Cambridge Journal of Anthropology* 37 (1): 17–31.
Matza, Tomas. 2009. "Moscow's Echo: Technologies of the Self, Publics, and Politics on the Russian Talk Show." *Cultural Anthropology* 24 (3): 489–522.
———. 2012. "'Good Individualism'? Psychology, Ethics, and Neoliberalism in Postsocialist Russia." *American Ethnologist* 39 (4): 804–18.
Mauss, Marcel. 1966. *The Gift: Forms and Functions of Exchange in Archaic Societies*. London: Cohen & West.
Mayes, Christopher, Jane Williams, and Wendy Lipworth. 2018. "Conflicted Hope: Social Egg Freezing and Clinical Conflicts of Interest." *Health Sociology Review* 27 (1): 45–59.
Merz, Theo. 2020. "Single Fathers with Children via Surrogates Flee Russia amid Crackdown." *The Guardian*, October 15. https://www.theguardian.com/world/2020/oct/15/single-fathers-in-russia-with-surrogate-babies-become-official-target.
Mies, Maria. 1986. "Reproduktionstechnik als sexistische und rassistische Bevölkerungspolitik." In *Frauen gegen Gentechnik und Reproduktionstechnologien*, edited by A. K. Frauenpolitik, 44–47. Cologne: Kölner Volksblatt.
Mishtal, Joanna. 2012. "Irrational Non-Reproduction? The 'Dying Nation' and the Postsocialist Logics of Declining Motherhood in Poland." *Anthropology & Medicine* 19 (2): 153–69.
———. 2015. *The Politics of Morality: The Church, the State, and Reproductive Rights in Postsocialist Poland*. Athens: Ohio University Press.
Mitra, Sayani. 2017. "Disruptive Embodiments: A Study of Risks and Disruptions during Commercial Surrogacy in India." PhD thesis, Georg-August University of Göttingen.
Mitra, Sayani, and Silke Schicktanz. 2016. "Failed Surrogate Conceptions: Social and Ethical Aspects of Preconception Disruptions during Commercial Surrogacy in India." *Philosophy, Ethics, and Humanities in Medicine* 11 (1): 1–16.
Mitter, Vera R. 2020. *Obstetric and Perinatal Outcomes of Women Treated for Subfertility and Children Born after in Vitro Fertilisation*. Bern: University of Bern.
Mohanty, Chandra Talpade. 1984. "Under Western Eyes: Feminist Scholarship and Colonial Discourses." *Boundary 2* 12 (3) / 13 (1): 333–58.
Mol, Annemarie. 2008. *The Logic of Care: Health and the Problem of Patient Choice*. London: Routledge.
Moore, Cortney. 2022. "Surrogate Mothers Rescued from Ukraine War." *New York Post*, April 18. https://nypost.com/2022/04/18/project-dynamo-rescues-surrogate-mothers-from-ukraine-war/.

Moreno, Adi. 2016. "Families on the Market Front." In *Intimate Economies: Bodies, Emotions, and Sexualities on the Global Market*, edited by Susanne Hofmann and Adi Moreno, 233–59. New York: Palgrave Macmillan.

Morgan, Lynn, and Elizabeth Roberts. 2012. "Reproductive Governance in Latin America." *Anthropology & Medicine* 19 (2): 241–254.

Motluk, Alison. 2022. "Ukraine's Surrogacy Industry Has Put Women in Impossible Positions." *The Atlantic*, March 1. https://www.theatlantic.com/health/archive/2022/03/russia-invasion-ukraine-surrogate-family/623327/.

Mouliarova, Ekaterina. 2019. "The Legal Regulation of Surrogacy in Russia." *Italian Journal of Public Law* 11 (1): 393–433.

Murray, Clare, and Susan Golombok. 2003. "To Tell or Not to Tell: The Decision-Making Process of Egg-Donation Parents." *Human Fertility* 6 (2): 89–95.

Nahman, Michal. 2008. "Nodes of Desire: Romanian Egg Sellers, 'Dignity' and Feminist Alliances in Transnational Ova Exchanges." *European Journal of Women's Studies* 15 (2): 65–82.

———. 2010. "'Embryos Are Our Baby': Abridging Hope, Body and Nation in Transnational Ova Donation." In *Technologized Images, Technologized Bodies*, edited by Jeanette Edwards, Penelope Harvey, and Peter Wade, 185–210. New York: Berghahn Books.

———. 2011. "Reverse Traffic: Intersecting Inequalities in Human Egg Donation." *Reproductive BioMedicine Online* 23 (5): 626–33.

Narotzky, Susana. 2018. "Rethinking the Concept of Labour." *Journal of the Royal Anthropological Institute* 24 (S1): 29–43.

Narotzky, Susana, and Niko Besnier. 2014. "Crisis, Value, and Hope: Rethinking the Economy. An Introduction to Supplement 9." *Current Anthropology* 55 (S9): S4–16.

Nartova, Nadya. 2009. "Surrogate Motherhood and Sperm Donorship in the Russian Media: Normalising the Body." In *Making Bodies, Persons and Families: Normalising Reproductive Technologies in Russia, Switzerland and Germany*, edited by Willemijn de Jong and Olga Tkach, 75–94. Berlin: LIT Verlag.

Neal, Will. 2020. "Ukrainian Police in Baby-Mill Bust." Organized Crime and Corruption Reporting Project, April 29. https://www.occrp.org/en/daily/12226-ukrainian-police-in-baby-mill-bust.

Nebeling Petersen, Michael, Charlotte Kroløkke, and Lene Myong. 2017. "Dad and Daddy Assemblage: Resuturing the Nation through Transnational Surrogacy, Homosexuality, and Norwegian Exceptionalism." *GLQ: A Journal of Lesbian and Gay Studies* 23 (1): 83–112.

Nechepurenko, Ivan. 2013. "Rainbow Lamp Post Is Not Gay Propaganda, Prosecutors Say." *Moscow Times*, September 24. https://www.themoscowtimes.com/2013/09/24/rainbow-lamppost-is-not-gay-propagandaprosecutors-say-a27983.

Nordqvist, Petra. 2010. "Out of Sight, Out of Mind: Family Resemblances in Lesbian Donor Conception." *Sociology* 44 (6): 1128–44.

———. 2014. "The Drive for Openness in Donor Conception: Disclosure and the Trouble with Real Life." *International Journal of Law, Policy and the Family* 28 (3): 321–38.

———. 2021. "Telling Reproductive Stories: Social Scripts, Relationality and Donor Conception." *Sociology* 55 (4): 677–95.

Nordqvist, Petra, and Carol Smart. 2014. "Relational Lives, Relational Selves: Assisted Reproduction and the Impact on Grandparents." In *Relatedness in Assisted Production: Families, Origins and Identities*, edited by Tabitha Freeman,

Susanna Graham, Fatemeh Ebtehaj, and Martin Richards, 548–77. Cambridge: Cambridge University Press.

North, Douglass C. 2010. *Understanding the Process of Economic Change*. Princeton, NJ: Princeton University Press.

Onisenko, Kostas. 2020. "Russian Orthodox Church Expressed Opposition to in Vitro Fertilization." *Orthodox Times*, September 21. https://orthodoxtimes.com/russian-orthodox-church-expressed-opposition-to-in-vitro-fertilization.

Orejudo Prieto de los Mozos, Patricia. 2013. "Spain." In *International Surrogacy Arrangements: Legal Regulation at the International Level*, edited by Katarina Trimmings and Paul Beaumont, 347–55. Studies in Private International Law. Oxford: Hart Publishing.

Palomera, Jaime, and Theodora Vetta. 2016. "Moral Economy: Rethinking a Radical Concept." *Anthropological Theory* 16 (4): 413–32.

Panchenko, Alexander. 2012. "'Popular Orthodoxy' and Identity in Soviet and Post-Soviet Russia: Ideology, Consumption and Competition." In *Soviet and Post-Soviet Identities*, edited by Mark Bassin and Catriona Kelly, 321–40. Cambridge: Cambridge University Press.

Pande, Amrita. 2009. "'It May Be Her Eggs But It's My Blood': Surrogates and Everyday Forms of Kinship in India." *Qualitative Sociology* 32 (4): 379–97.

———. 2010. "Commercial Surrogacy in India: Manufacturing a Perfect Mother-Worker." *Signs: Journal of Women in Culture and Society* 35 (4): 969–92.

———. 2011. "Transnational Commercial Surrogacy in India: Gifts for Global Sisters?" *Reproductive BioMedicine Online* 23 (5): 618–25.

———. 2014. *Wombs in Labor: Transnational Commercial Surrogacy in India*. New York: Columbia University Press.

———. 2015. "Blood, Sweat and Dummy Tummies: Kin Labour and Transnational Surrogacy in India." *Anthropologica* 57 (1): 53–62.

———. 2016. "Surrogates Are Workers, Not Wombs." *The Hindu*, August 29. https://www.thehindu.com/opinion/op-ed/Surrogates-are-workers-not-wombs/article14594820.ece.

———. 2021. "Revisiting Surrogacy in India: Domino Effects of the Ban." *Journal of Gender Studies* 30 (4): 395–405.

Pande, Amrita, and Tessa Moll. 2018. "Gendered Bio-Responsibilities and Travelling Egg Providers from South Africa." *Reproductive Biomedicine & Society Online* 6: 23–33.

Parry, Bronwyn. 2015. "Narratives of Neoliberalism: 'Clinical Labour' in Context." *Medical Humanities* 41 (1): 32–37.

Pascual, Julia. 2022. "Des mères porteuses ukrainiennes prises au piège de la guerre." *Le Monde*, April 24. https://www.lemonde.fr/m-le-mag/article/2022/04/24/des-meres-porteuses-ukrainiennes-prises-au-piege-de-la-guerre_6123417_4500055.html.

Patico, Jennifer. 2005. "To Be Happy in a Mercedes: Tropes of Value and Ambivalent Visions of Marketization." *American Ethnologist* 32 (3): 479–96.

———. 2009. "For Love, Money, or Normalcy: Meanings of Strategy and Sentiment in the Russian-American Matchmaking Industry." *Ethnos* 74 (3): 307–30.

Paxson, Heather. 2003. "With or against Nature? IVF, Gender and Reproductive Agency in Athens, Greece." In "Reproduction Gone Awry," special issue, *Social Science & Medicine* 56 (9): 1853–66.

Pennings, Guido. 2004. "Legal Harmonization and Reproductive Tourism in Europe." *Human Reproduction* 19 (12): 2689–94.

———. 2009. "The Green Grass on the Other Side: Crossing Borders to Obtain Infertility Treatment." *Facts, Views & Vision in ObGyn* 1 (1): 1–6.

———. 2010. "The Rough Guide to Insemination: Cross-Border Travelling for Donor Semen Due to Different Regulations." In *Artificial Insemination: An Update*, edited by Willem Ombelet and Herman Tournaye, *Facts, Views & Vision in ObGyn* Monograph (Wetteren: Universa Press), 55–60.

Perler, Laura. 2022. *Selektioniertes Leben: Eine feministische Perspektive auf die Eizellenspende*. Münster: Edition Assemblage.

Perler, Laura, and Carolin Schurr. 2021. "Intimate Lives in the Global Bioeconomy: Reproductive Biographies of Mexican Egg Donors." *Body & Society* 27 (3): 3–27.

Persson, Emil. 2015. "Banning 'Homosexual Propaganda': Belonging and Visibility in Contemporary Russian Media." *Sexuality & Culture* 19 (2): 256–74.

Petropanagos, Angel. 2017. "Pronatalism, Geneticism, and ART." *International Journal of Feminist Approaches to Bioethics* 10 (1): 119–47.

Petrov, Ivan. 2020. "Materinskaya plata: SKR rasslefuyet smert' rebyonka surrogatnoj materi. Kak ustroyen biznes po prodazhe rozhdyennykh v Rossii detey inostrantsam." *Izvestia*, January 16. https://iz.ru/964655/ivanpetrov/materinskaia-plata-skr-rassleduet-smert-rebenka-surrogatnoi-materi.

Pfeffer, Naomi. 2011. "Eggs-Ploiting Women: A Critical Feminist Analysis of the Different Principles in Transplant and Fertility Tourism." In "Symposium: Cross-Border Reproductive Care—Ethical, Legal, and Socio-Cultural Perspectives," special issue, *Reproductive BioMedicine Online* 23 (5): 634–41.

Phillips, Anne. 2013. "Does the Body Make a Difference?" In *Gender, Agency, and Coercion*, edited by Sumi Madhok, Anne Phillips, and Kalpana Wilson, 143–56. Basingstoke: Palgrave Macmillan.

Ploeg, Irma van der. 2001. *Prosthetic Bodies: The Construction of the Fetus and the Couple as Patients in Reproductive Technologies*. Dordrecht: Kluwer Academic.

Rabinow, Paul, and Nikolas Rose. 2006. "Biopower Today." *BioSocieties* 1 (2): 195–217.

Rachman, Gideon. 2022. "Understanding Vladimir Putin, the Man Who Fooled the World." The Guardian, April 9. https://www.theguardian.com/world/2022/apr/09/understanding-vladimir-putin-the-man-who-fooled-the-world.

Radaev, Vadim. 2004. "How Trust Is Established in Economic Relationships When Institutions and Individuals Are Not Trustworthy: The Case of Russia." In *Creating Social Trust in Post-Socialist Transition*, edited by János Kornai, Bo Rothstein, and Susan Rose-Ackerman, 91–110. New York: Palgrave Macmillan.

Radin, Margaret Jane. 1987. "Market-Inalienability." *Harvard Law Review* 100 (8): 1849–1937.

———. 2005. "Contested Commodities." In *Rethinking Commodification: Cases and Readings in Law and Culture*, edited by Martha M. Ertman and Joan C. Williams, 81–95. New York: New York University Press.

Radkowska-Walkowicz, Magdalena. 2012. "The Creation of 'Monsters': The Discourse of Opposition to in Vitro Fertilization in Poland." *Reproductive Health Matters* 20 (40): 30–37.

Ragoné, Helena. 1994. *Surrogate Motherhood: Conception in the Heart*. Boulder: Westview Press.

———. 1996. "Chasing the Blood Tie: Surrogate Mothers, Adoptive Mothers and Fathers." *American Ethnologist* 23 (2): 352–65.

RAHR (Russian Association of Human Reproduction). 2016. *Registr VRT: Yubileynyj 20j Ochyot za 2014 God*. https://www.rahr.ru/d_registr_otchet/registr_BRT_RARCH16.pdf.

———. 2017. *Registr VRT: Ochyot za 2015 God.* https://www.rahr.ru/d_registr_otchet/RegistrVRT_2015.pdf.
———. 2021. *Registr VRT: Ochyot za 2019 God.* http://www.rahr.ru/d_registr_otchet/RegistrART2019.pdf.
Rapp, Rayna. 1999. *Testing Women, Testing the Fetus: The Social Impact of Amniocentesis in America.* New York: Routledge.
Readings, Jennifer, Lucy Blake, Polly Casey, Vasanti Jadva, and Susan Golombok. 2011. "Secrecy, Disclosure and Everything in-between: Decisions of Parents of Children Conceived by Donor Insemination, Egg Donation and Surrogacy." *Reproductive BioMedicine Online* 22 (5): 485–95.
Rehsmann, Julia. 2018. "Exciting Waiting: Exploring Liver Transplantation in Germany." *Medicine Anthropology Theory* 5 (1). http://www.medanthrotheory.org/article/view/5373.
Reiter, Svetlana, and Kevin Rothrock. 2020. "The Invention of 'Gay Mutilators.'" *Meduza*, October 5. https://meduza.io/en/feature/2020/10/05/the-invention-of-gay-mutilators.
Remington, Thomas F. 2011. *The Politics of Inequality in Russia.* Cambridge: Cambridge University Press.
Reuters. 2022. "Russia Moves to Bar Foreigners from Using Its Surrogate Mothers." May 24. https://www.reuters.com/world/europe/russia-moves-bar-foreigners-using-its-surrogate-mothers-2022-05-24/.
RIA Novosti. 2013. "Surrogatnoe materinstvo." October 7. https://ria.ru/20131007/968214798.html.
Richard, Analiese, and Daromir Rudnyckyj. 2009. "Economies of Affect." *Journal of the Royal Anthropological Institute* 15 (1): 57–77.
Riggs, Damien W. 2016. "Narratives of Choice amongst White Australians Who Undertake Surrogacy Arrangements in India." *Journal of Medical Humanities* 37 (3): 313–25.
Riggs, Damien W., and Clare Bartholomaeus. 2016. "The Desire for a Child among a Sample of Heterosexual Australian Couples." *Journal of Reproductive and Infant Psychology* 34 (5): 442–50.
———. 2018. "'It's Just What You Do': Australian Middle-Class Heterosexual Couples Negotiating Compulsory Parenthood." *Feminism & Psychology* 28 (3): 373–89.
Riggs, Damien W., and Clemence Due. 2013. "Representations of Reproductive Citizenship and Vulnerability in Media Reports of Offshore Surrogacy." *Citizenship Studies* 17 (8): 956–69.
———. 2017. "Constructions of Gay Men's Reproductive Desires on Commercial Surrogacy Clinic Websites." In *Babies for Sale? Transnational Surrogacy, Human Rights and the Politics of Reproduction*, edited by Miranda Davis, 33–45. London: Zed Books.
Ritter, Martina. 2001. "Müttermacht im Patriarchat—Geschlechterverhältnisse in Rußland." In *Zivilgesellschaft und Gender-Politik in Rußland*, edited by Martina Ritter, 21–40. Frankfurt: Campus-Verlag.
Rivkin-Fish, Michele. 2003. "Anthropology, Demography, and the Search for a Critical Analysis of Fertility: Insights from Russia." *American Anthropologist* 105 (2): 289–301.
———. 2004. "'Change Yourself and the Whole World Will Become Kinder': Russian Activists for Reproductive Health and the Limits of Claims Making for Women." *Medical Anthropology Quarterly* 18 (3): 281–304.

———. 2005. *Women's Health in Post-Soviet Russia: The Politics of Intervention.* Bloomington: Indiana University Press.

———. 2009. "Tracing Landscapes of the Past in Class Subjectivity: Practices of Memory and Distinction in Marketizing Russia." *American Ethnologist* 36 (1): 79–95.

———. 2010. "Pronatalism, Gender Politics, and the Renewal of Family Support in Russia: Toward a Feminist Anthropology of 'Maternity Capital.'" *Slavic Review* 69 (3): 701–24.

———. 2011. "Learning the Moral Economy of Commodified Health Care: 'Community Education,' Failed Consumers, and the Shaping of Ethical Clinician-Citizens." *Culture, Medicine, and Psychiatry* 35 (2): 183–208.

———. 2013. "Conceptualizing Feminist Strategies for Russian Reproductive Politics: Abortion, Surrogate Motherhood, and Family Support after Socialism." *Signs: Journal of Women in Culture and Society* 38 (3): 569–93.

———. 2018. "'Fight Abortion, Not Women': The Moral Economy Underlying Russian Feminist Advocacy." *Anthropological Journal of European Cultures* 27 (2): 22–44.

Rivkin-Fish, Michele, and Cassandra Hartblay. 2014. "When Global LGBTQ Advocacy Became Entangled with New Cold War Sentiment: A Call for Examining Russian Queer Experience." *Brown Journal of World Affairs* 21 (1): 95–111.

Roache, Madeline. 2018. "Ukraine's 'Baby Factories': The Human Cost of Surrogacy." *Al Jazeera*, September 13. https://www.aljazeera.com/features/2018/9/13/ukraines-baby-factories-the-human-cost-of-surrogacy.

Robben, Antonius C. G. M. 2012. "The Politics of Truth and Emotion among Victims and Perpetrators of Violence." In *Ethnographic Fieldwork: An Anthropological Reader*, edited by Antonius C. G. M. Robben and Jeffrey A. Sluka, 175–90. Malden, MA: Blackwell.

Roberts, Celia. 2007. *Messengers of Sex: Hormones, Biomedicine, and Feminism.* Cambridge: Cambridge University Press.

Roberts, Elizabeth. 2006. "God's Laboratory: Religious Rationalities and Modernity in Ecuadorian in Vitro Fertilization." *Culture, Medicine and Psychiatry* 30 (4): 507–36.

ROC (Russian Orthodox Church). 2000. *The Basis of the Social Concept.* https://old.mospat.ru/en/documents/social-concepts/.

Rogoża, Jadwiga. 2021. "The Pandemic Takes Its Toll: Russia's Demographic Crisis." *OSW Centre for Eastern Studies*, February 16. https://www.osw.waw.pl/en/publikacje/analyses/2021-02-16/pandemic-takes-its-toll-russias-demographic-crisis.

Rose, Nikolas. 2004. *Powers of Freedom: Reframing Political Thought.* Cambridge: Cambridge University Press.

———. 2007. *The Politics of Life Itself: Biomedicine, Power, and Subjectivity in the Twenty-First Century.* Princeton, NJ: Princeton University Press.

Roth, Andrew. 2020. "Up to 1,000 Babies Born to Surrogate Mothers Stranded in Russia." *The Guardian*, July 29. http://www.theguardian.com/lifeandstyle/2020/jul/29/up-to-1000-babies-born-to-surrogate-mothers-stranded-in-russia.

Rotkirch, Anna, Anna Temkina, and Elena Zdravomyslova. 2007. "Who Helps the Degraded Housewife? Comments on Vladimir Putin's Demographic Speech." *European Journal of Women's Studies* 14 (4): 349–57.

Rudrappa, Sharmila. 2010. "Making India the 'Mother Destination': Outsourcing Labor to Indian Surrogates." In *Gender and Sexuality in the Workplace*, edited by Christine L. Williams and Kirsten Dellinger, 253–85. Bingley: Emerald Group Publishing.

———. 2014. "Conceiving Fatherhood: Gay Men and Indian Surrogate Mothers." In *Globalized Fatherhood*, edited by Marcia C. Inhorn, Wendy Chavkin, and José-Alberto Navarro, 291–311. New York: Berghahn Books.

———. 2016a. *Discounted Life: The Price of Global Surrogacy in India*. New York: New York University Press.

———. 2016b. "Why India's New Surrogacy Bill Is Bad for Women." *Huffington Post*, August 26. https://www.huffpost.com/entry/why-indias-new-surrogacy-bill-is-bad-for-women_b_57c075f9e4b0b01630de83ad.

———. 2018. "Reproducing Dystopia: The Politics of Transnational Surrogacy in India, 2002–2015." *Critical Sociology* 44 (7–8): 1087–1101.

Rudrappa, Sharmila, and Caitlyn Collins. 2015. "Altruistic Agencies and Compassionate Consumers: Moral Framing of Transnational Surrogacy." *Gender & Society* 29 (6): 937–59.

Salmenniemi, Suvi, and Maria Adamson. 2015. "New Heroines of Labour: Domesticating Post-Feminism and Neoliberal Capitalism in Russia." *Sociology* 49 (1): 88–105.

Sandel, Michael. 2009. *Justice: What's the Right Thing To Do?* New York: Farrar, Straus and Giroux.

———. 2013. *What Money Can't Buy: The Moral Limits of Markets*. London: Penguin Books.

Sandelowski, Margarete. 1991. "Compelled to Try: The Never-Enough Quality of Conceptive Technology." *Medical Anthropology Quarterly* 5 (1): 29–47.

Sandelowski, Margarete, and Sheryl De Lacey. 2002. "The Uses of a 'Disease': Infertility as Rhetorical Vehicle." In *Infertility around the Globe: New Thinking on Childlessness, Gender, and Reproductive Technologies*, edited by Marcia C. Inhorn and Frank van Balen, 33–51. Berkeley: University of California Press.

Sänger, Eva. 2020. *Elternwerden zwischen "Babyfernsehen" und medizinischer Überwachung: Eine Ethnografie pränataler Ultraschalluntersuchungen*. Bielefeld: Transcript Verlag.

Scheper-Hughes, Nancy. 1985. "Culture, Scarcity, and Maternal Thinking: Maternal Detachment and Infant Survival in a Brazilian Shantytown." *Ethos* 13 (4): 291–317.

Schultz, Susanne. 2015. "Reproducing the Nation: The New German Population Policy and the Concept of Demographization." *Distinktion: Journal of Social Theory* 16 (3): 337–61.

Schurr, Carolin. 2017. "From Biopolitics to Bioeconomies: The ART of (Re-)Producing White Futures in Mexico's Surrogacy Market." *Environment and Planning D: Society and Space* 35 (2): 241–62.

———. 2019. "Multiple Mobilities in Mexico's Fertility Industry." *Mobilities* 14 (1): 103–19.

Schurr, Carolin, and Elisabeth Militz. 2018. "The Affective Economy of Transnational Surrogacy." *Environment and Planning A: Economy and Space* 50 (8): 1626–45.

Schwirtz, Michael, Maria Varenikova, and Rick Gladstone. 2022. "Putin Calls Ukrainian Statehood a Fiction: History Suggests Otherwise." *New York Times*, February 22. https://www.nytimes.com/2022/02/21/world/europe/putin-ukraine.html.

Shalev, Carmel. 1989. *Birth Power: The Case for Surrogacy*. New Haven, CT: Yale University Press.

Sharp, Lesley A. 2000. "The Commodification of the Body and Its Parts." *Annual Review of Anthropology* 29 (1): 287–328.

Shchurko, Tatsiana. 2017. "Women's Health—Nation's Health: The Policies of Reproduction in Post-Soviet Belarus." In *Gender Panic, Gender Policy*, edited by Vasilikie Demos and Marcia Texler Segal, 24:45–66. Advances in Gender Research. Bingley: Emerald Publishing.

Shenfield, F., J. de Mouzon, Guido Pennings, A. P. Ferraretti, A. Nyboe Andersen, G. de Wert, V. Goossens, and ESHRE Taskforce on Cross Border Reproductive Care. 2010. "Cross Border Reproductive Care in Six European Countries." *Human Reproduction* 25 (6): 1361–68.

Siegl, Veronika. 2015. "Märkte der guten Hoffnung." *PROKLA: Zeitschrift für kritische Sozialwissenschaft* 45 (178): 99–115. https://www.prokla.de/index.php/PROKLA/article/view/231.

———. 2018a. "Aligning the Affective Body: Commercial Surrogacy in Moscow and the Emotional Labour of 'Nastraivatsya.'" *Tsantsa: Journal of the Swiss Anthropological Association* 23: 63–72.

———. 2018b. "The Ultimate Argument: Evoking the Affective Powers of 'Happiness' in Commercial Surrogacy." *Anthropological Journal of European Cultures* 27 (2): 1–21.

———. 2018c. "Zehn Monate / Ten Months." In *hope*, edited by Sarah Hildebrand, 41–63. Basel: Christoph Merian Verlag. https://www.merianverlag.ch/produkt/fotografie/hope/b79ed4db-c980-4e41-b450-e13b75244e8e.html.

———. 2019. "There's a Crack in Everything. Or: How Leonard Cohen Inspired My Research on Commercial Surrogacy." *Medicine Anthropology Theory* 6 (1). http://www.medanthrotheory.org/article/view/5371/7356.

———. 2022. "Die 'Leihmütter' der Ukraine: Wer bestimmt über den schwangeren Körper?" *GeN-ethisches Netzwerk*, March 22. https://gen-ethisches-netzwerk.de/maerz-2022/die-leihmuetter-der-ukraine.

Siegl, Veronika, Carolin Schurr, Laura Perler, Christine Bigler, and Tina Büchler. 2022. "Transnationale reproduktive Mobilität – empirische Befunde zu einer umstrittenen Praxis." URPP Human Reproduction Reloaded, Working Paper 3. Zürich: Seismo. https://doi.org/10.33058/wpuzh.2022.8865.

Simoni, Valerio. 2016. "Economization, Moralization, and the Changing Moral Economies of 'Capitalism' and 'Communism' among Cuban Migrants in Spain." *Anthropological Theory* 16 (4): 454–75.

Smietana, Marcin. 2017a. "'Families Like We'd Always Known'? Spanish Gay Fathers' Normalization Narratives in Transnational Surrogacy." In *Assisted Reproduction across Borders: Feminist Perspectives on Normalizations, Disruptions and Transmissions*, edited by Merete Lie and Nina Lykke, 49–60. New York: Routledge.

———. 2017b. "Affective De-Commodifying, Economic De-Kinning: Surrogates' and Gay Fathers' Narratives in U.S. Surrogacy." *Sociological Research Online* 22 (2): 163–75.

———. 2018. "Procreative Consciousness in a Global Market: Gay Men's Paths to Surrogacy in the USA." *Reproductive Biomedicine & Society Online* 7: 101–11.

Smietana, Marcin, Sharmila Rudrappa, and Christina Weis. 2021. "Moral Frameworks of Commercial Surrogacy within the US, India and Russia." *Sexual and Reproductive Health Matters* 29 (1): 1–17.

Smyth, Regina, and Irina Soboleva. 2014. "Looking beyond the Economy: Pussy Riot and the Kremlin's Voting Coalition." *Post-Soviet Affairs* 30 (4): 257–75.

Soboleva, Irina V., and Yaroslav A. Bakhmetjev. 2015. "Political Awareness and Self-Blame in the Explanatory Narratives of LGBT People amid the Anti-LGBT Campaign in Russia." *Sexuality & Culture* 19 (2): 275–96.

REFERENCES

Spar, Debora. 2006. *The Baby Business: How Money, Science, and Politics Drive the Commerce of Conception*. Boston: Harvard Business School Press.

———. 2010. "Free Markets, Free Choice? A Market Approach to Reproductive Rights." In *Baby Markets: Money and the New Politics of Creating Families*, edited by Michele Goodwin, 177–90. Cambridge: Cambridge University Press.

Speier, Amy. 2011. "Brokers, Consumers and the Internet: How North American Consumers Navigate Their Infertility Journeys." *Reproductive BioMedicine Online* 23 (5): 592–99.

———. 2016. *Fertility Holidays: IVF Tourism and the Reproduction of Whiteness*. New York: New York University Press.

Speier, Amy, Kristin Lozanski, and Susan Frohlick. 2020. "Reproductive Mobilities." *Mobilities* 15 (2): 107–19.

Sputnik. 2013. "Most Russians Say Surrogate Motherhood Acceptable – Survey." December 19. https://sputniknews.com/20131219/Most-Russians-Say-Surrogate-Motherhood-Acceptable--Survey-185736619.html.

Starza-Allen, Antony. 2016. "Council of Europe Rejects Surrogacy Guidelines." *BioNews* (blog), October 18. https://www.bionews.org.uk/page_95737.

Strasser, Sabine, and Luisa Piart. 2018. "Intimate Uncertainties." *Anthropological Journal of European Cultures* 27 (2): v–xv.

Strathern, Marilyn. 1992a. *After Nature: English Kinship in the Late Twentieth Century*. Cambridge: Cambridge University Press.

———. 1992b. *Reproducing the Future: Essays on Anthropology, Kinship and the New Reproductive Technologies*. Manchester: Manchester University Press.

Stuvøy, Ingvill. 2018. "Accounting for the Money-Made Parenthood of Transnational Surrogacy." *Anthropology & Medicine* 25 (3): 280–95.

Sudakov, Dmitry. 2011a. "Market of Surrogate Motherhood Grows Like a Weed." *Pravda*, January 20. https://english.pravda.ru/society/116585-surrogate_motherhood/.

———. 2011b. "Surrogacy: A Form of Female Slavery?" *Pravda*, December 1. https://english.pravda.ru/society/119805-surrogate_motherhood/.

Svitnev, Konstantin. 2006. "The Right to Life (ART, Surrogate Motherhood and Demographics)." *The Scientific Expert Magazine* 1: n.p.

———. 2007. *ART Regulations in Russia and Elsewhere*. http://www.jurconsult.ru/en/publications/art_regulations_in_russia_and_elsewhere/. Accessed July 3, 2014 (no longer available).

———. 2012. "New Russian Legislation on Assisted Reproduction." *Open Access Scientific Reports* 1 (3). https://doi.org/10.4172/scientificreports.207.

———. 2016. "Gestational Surrogacy in the Russian Federation." In *Handbook of Gestational Surrogacy: International Clinical Practice and Policy Issues*, edited by E. Scott Sills, 232–40. Cambridge: Cambridge University Press.

Swader, Christopher S. 2013. *The Capitalist Personality: Face-to-Face Sociality and Economic Change in the Post-Communist World*. New York: Routledge.

Swader, Christopher S., and Vaida Obelene. 2015. "Post-Soviet Intimacies: An Introduction." *Sexuality & Culture* 19 (2): 245–55.

Swader, Christopher S., Olga Strelkova, Alena Sutormina, Viktoria Syomina, Volha Vysotskaya, and Irene Fedorova. 2013. "Love as a Fictitious Commodity: Gift-for-Sex Barters as Contractual Carriers of Intimacy." *Sexuality & Culture* 17 (4): 598–616.

Swader, Christopher S., and Irina D. Vorobeva. 2015. "Receiving Gifts for Sex in Moscow, Kyiv, and Minsk: A Compensated Dating Survey." *Sexuality & Culture* 19 (2): 321–48.

Tarabrin, Roman. 2020. "Orthodox Perspectives on in Vitro Fertilization in Russia." *Christian Bioethics: Non-Ecumenical Studies in Medical Morality* 26 (2): 177–204.

TASS. 2020. "Key Suspect in Russian Baby Trafficking Case Put on Wanted List." July 19. https://tass.com/emergencies/1180171.

———. 2021. "Russia to Grant Citizenship to Children Born through Surrogacy for Foreigners—Bill." June 11. https://tass.com/society/1301807.

———. 2022. "Decision Taken on Denazification, Demilitarization of Ukraine—Putin." February 23. https://tass.com/politics/1409189.

Teman, Elly. 2003. "The Medicalization of 'Nature' in the 'Artificial Body': Surrogate Motherhood in Israel." *Medical Anthropology Quarterly* 17 (1): 78–98.

———. 2008. "The Social Construction of Surrogacy Research: An Anthropological Critique of the Psychosocial Scholarship on Surrogate Motherhood." *Social Science & Medicine* 67 (7): 1104–12.

———. 2009. "Embodying Surrogate Motherhood: Pregnancy as a Dyadic Body-Project." *Body & Society* 15 (3): 47–69.

———. 2010. *Birthing a Mother: The Surrogate Body and the Pregnant Self*. Berkeley: University of California Press.

———. 2019. "The Power of the Single Story: Surrogacy and Social Media in Israel." *Medical Anthropology* 38 (3): 282–94.

Teman, Elly, and Zsuzsa Berend. 2018. "Surrogate Non-Motherhood: Israeli and US Surrogates Speak about Kinship and Parenthood." *Anthropology & Medicine* 25 (3): 296–310.

———. 2021. "Surrogacy as a Family Project: How Surrogates Articulate Familial Identity and Belonging." *Journal of Family Issues* 42 (6): 1143–65.

Temkina, Anna. 2010. "Childbearing and Work-Family Balance among Contemporary Russian Women." *Finnish Yearbook of Population Research* 45: 83–101.

Temkina, Anna, and Elena Zdravomyslova. 2015. "The Sexual Scripts and Identity of Middle-Class Russian Women." *Sexuality & Culture* 19 (2): 297–320.

———. 2018. "Responsible Motherhood, Practices of Reproductive Choice and Class Construction in Contemporary Russia." In *Gender and Choice after Socialism*, edited by Lynne Attwood, Elisabeth Schimpfössl, and Marina Yusupova, 161–86. Cham: Springer International.

Teschlade, Julia. 2019. "'Wenn das liebe Geld nicht wär': Zur Konstruktion von Intimität zwischen Tragemüttern und gleichgeschlechtlichen Männerpaaren." *Feministische Studien* 37 (1): 65–81.

Teschlade, Julia, and Almut Peukert. 2019. "Creating a Family through Surrogacy: Negotiating Parental Positions, Familial Boundaries and Kinship Practices." *GENDER: Zeitschrift für Geschlecht, Kultur und Gesellschaft* 11 (2): 56–70.

Tétrault-Farber, Gabrielle. 2014. "Russian Lawmaker Proposes Ban on Commercial Surrogate Motherhood." *Moscow Times*, April 24. http://www.themoscowtimes.com/2014/04/24/russian-lawmaker-proposes-ban-on-commercial-surrogate-motherhood-a34637.

Thompson, Charis. 2005. *Making Parents: The Ontological Choreography of Reproductive Technologies*. Inside Technology. Cambridge, MA: MIT Press.

Thompson, Edward P. 1971. "The Moral Economy of the English Crowd in the Eighteenth Century." *Past & Present* 50: 76–136.

Tickle, Jonny. 2020a. "Reproduce or Pay Up! Controversial Russian Communist Politician Backs Childlessness Tax on Citizens Who Don't Want to Have Kids." *Russia Today*, October 14. https://www.rt.com/russia/503490-childnessness-payment-tax-russia/.

———. 2020b. "Russian MP Zhirinovsky Suggests Government Offer Money to Discourage Women from Abortion, to Help Alleviate Demographic Crisis." *Russia Today*, December 24. https://www.rt.com/russia/510618-zhirinovsky-money-discourage-abortion/.

Ticktin, Miriam. 2013. "The Waiting Room." *Somatosphere* (blog), October 28. http://somatosphere.net/2013/the-waiting-room.html/.

Tkach, Olga. 2009. "Making Family and Unmaking Kin in the Russian Media: Reproductive Technologies and Relatedness." In *Making Bodies, Persons and Families: Normalising Reproductive Technologies in Russia, Switzerland and Germany*, edited by Willemijn de Jong and Olga Tkach, 135–57. Berlin: LIT Verlag.

Tober, Diane. 2018. *Romancing the Sperm*. New Brunswick, NJ: Rutgers University Press.

Tober, Diane, and Charlotte Halmø Kroløkke. 2021. "Emotion, Embodiment, and Reproductive Colonialism in the Global Human Egg Trade." *Gender, Work & Organization* 28 (5): 1766–86.

Toledano, Sarah Jane, and Kristin Zeiler. 2017. "Hosting the Others' Child? Relational Work and Embodied Responsibility in Altruistic Surrogate Motherhood." *Feminist Theory* 18 (2): 159–75.

Torocheshnikova, Maryana. 2021. "'Torgovlya det'mi' и 'delo reproduktologov.'" *Radio Svoboda*, July 15. https://www.svoboda.org/a/31360422.html.

Tronto, Joan C. 1994. *Moral Boundaries: A Political Argument for an Ethics of Care*. London: Routledge.

Tronto, Joan, and Berenice Fischer. 1990. "Toward a Feminist Theory of Caring." In *Circles of Care: Work and Identity in Women's Lives*, edited by Emily K. Abel and Margaret K. Nelson, 36–54. Albany: State University of New York Press.

Trubina, Elena. 2012. "Class Differences and Social Mobility amongst College-Educated Young People in Russia." In *Rethinking Class in Russia*, edited by Suvi Salmenniemi, 203–20. Farnham: Ashgate.

Tsing, Anna. 2013. "Sorting out Commodities: How Capitalist Value Is Made through Gifts." *HAU: Journal of Ethnographic Theory* 3 (1): 21–43.

Tuller, David. 1996. *Cracks in the Iron Closet: Travels in Gay & Lesbian Russia*. Chicago: University of Chicago Press.

Turbine, Vikki, and Kathleen Riach. 2012. "The Right to Choose or Choosing What's Right? Women's Conceptualizations of Work and Life Choices in Contemporary Russia." *Gender, Work & Organization* 19 (2): 165–87.

Twine, France Winddance. 2011. *Outsourcing the Womb: Race, Class and Gestational Surrogacy in a Global Market*. New York: Routledge.

United Nations, OHCHR (Office of the High Commissioner of Human Rights). 1989. "Convention on the Rights of the Child." November 20. https://www.ohchr.org/en/professionalinterest/pages/crc.aspx.

Utrata, Jennifer. 2015. *Women without Men: Single Mothers and Family Change in the New Russia*. Ithaca, NY: Cornell University Press.

Vaughn, Richard. 2020. "Is Sperm Donor Anonymity a Thing of the Past?" *International Fertility Law Group* (blog), October 30. https://www.iflg.net/is-sperm-donor-anonymity-a-thing-of-the-past/.

Verdery, Katherine. 2013. "From Parent-State to Family Patriarchs: Gender and Nation in Contemporary Eastern Europe." In *Eastern Europe: Women in Transition*, edited by Irena Grudzinska-Gross and Andrzej W. Tymowski, 15–44. Frankfurt a.M.: Peter Lang Verlag.

Vertommen, Sigrid. 2016. "Babies from Behind Bars: Stratified Assisted Reproduction in Palestine/Israel." In *Assisted Reproduction across Borders: Feminist Perspectives on Normalizations, Disruptions and Transmissions*, edited by Merete Lie and Nina Lykke, 207–18. New York: Routledge.

Vertommen, Sigrid, and Camille Barbagallo. 2021. "The In/Visible Wombs of the Market: The Dialectics of Waged and Unwaged Reproductive Labour in the Global Surrogacy Industry." *Review of International Political Economy*, January, 1–41.

Vitebsky, Piers. 1993. "Is Death the Same Everywhere? Contexts of Knowing and Doubting." In *An Anthropological Critique of Development: The Growth of Ignorance*, edited by Mark Hobart, 100–115. London: Routledge.

Vlasenko, Polina. 2014. "Governing through Precarity: The Experience of Infertile Bodies in IVF Treatment in Ukraine." *Journal of Social Policy Studies* 12 (3): 441–54.

———. 2015. "Desirable Bodies/Precarious Laborers: Ukrainian Egg Donors in Context of Transnational Fertility." In *(In)Fertile Citizens: Anthropological and Legal Challenges of Assisted Reproduction Technologies*, edited by Venetia Kantsa, Giulia Zanini, and Lina Papadopoulou, 197–216. Athens: (In)FERCIT.

———. 2020. "Ukraine's Surrogate Mothers Struggle under Quarantine." *OpenDemocracy*, June 10. https://www.opendemocracy.net/en/odr/ukraines-surrogate-mothers-struggle-under-quarantine/.

———. 2021. "Global Circuits of Fertility: The Political Economy of the Ukrainian Ova Market." PhD thesis, Indiana University.

Vora, Kalindi. 2009. "Indian Transnational Surrogacy and the Commodification of Vital Energy." *Subjectivity* 28 (1): 266–78.

———. 2013. "Potential, Risk, and Return in Transnational Indian Gestational Surrogacy." *Current Anthropology* 54 (S7): S97–106.

Vora, Kalindi, and Malathi Michelle Iyengar. 2017. "Citizen, Subject, Property: Indian Surrogacy and the Global Fertility Market." In *Assisted Reproduction across Borders: Feminist Perspectives on Normalizations, Disruptions and Transmissions*, edited by Merete Lie and Nina Lykke, 25–35. New York: Routledge.

Walker, Charles. 2012. "Re-inventing Themselves? Gender, Employment and Subjective Well-being amongst Young Working-Class Russians." In *Rethinking Class in Russia*, edited by Suvi Salmenniemi, 221–40. Farnham: Ashgate.

Waldby, Catherine, and Melinda Cooper. 2008. "The Biopolitics of Reproduction: Post-Fordist Biotechnology and Women's Clinical Labour." *Australian Feminist Studies* 23 (55): 57–73.

Weis, Christina. 2015. "Workers or Mothers? The Business of Surrogacy in Russia." *Open Democracy*, December 15. https://www.opendemocracy.net/beyondslavery/christina-weis/workers-or-mothers-business-of-surrogacy-in-russia.

———. 2021a. *Surrogacy in Russia: An Ethnography of Reproductive Labour, Stratification and Migration*. Bingley: Emerald Publishing.

———. 2021b. "Changing Fertility Landscapes: Exploring the Reproductive Routes and Choices of Fertility Patients from China for Assisted Reproduction in Russia." *Asian Bioethics Review* 13 (1): 7–22.

Weis, Christina, and Maria Kirpichenko. 2022. "The Impact of the War in Ukraine on the Russian Fertility Industry." *BioNews* (blog), April 4. https://www.bionews.org.uk/page_163451.

Whittaker, Andrea. 2019. *International Surrogacy as Disruptive Industry in Southeast Asia*. New Brunswick, NJ: Rutgers University Press.

Wichterich, Christa. 2018. "Transnational Reconfigurations of Re/Production and the Female Body: Bioeconomics, Motherhoods and the Case of Surrogacy in India." In *Feminist Political Ecology and the Economics of Care*, edited by Chiristine Bauhardt and Wendy Harcourt, 211–29. New York: Routledge.

Widdows, Heather. 2013. "Rejecting the Choice Paradigm: Ethical Framework of Prostitution and Egg Sale." In *Gender, Agency, and Coercion*, edited by Sumi Madhok, Anne Phillips, and Kalpana Wilson, 157–80. Basingstoke: Palgrave Macmillan.

Williams, Joan C., and Viviana A. Zelizer. 2005. "To Commodify or Not to Commodify: That Is Not the Question." In *Rethinking Commodification: Cases and Readings in Law and Culture*, edited by Martha M. Ertman and Joan C. Williams, 362–82. New York: New York University Press.

Wilson, Kalpana. 2008. "Reclaiming Agency, Reasserting Resistance." *IDS Bulletin* 39 (6): 83–91.

———. 2013. "Agency as 'Smart Economics': Neoliberalism, Gender and Development." In *Gender, Agency, and Coercion*, edited by Sumi Madhok, Anne Phillips, and Kalpana Wilson, 84–101. Basingstoke: Palgrave Macmillian.

Yasakova, Ekaterina. 2021. "Nye primut u chastnykh: Surrogatnow materinstvo predlozhili perevesti v goskliniki." *Izvestia*, August 16. https://iz.ru/1207641/ekaterina-iasakova/ne-primut-u-chastnykh-surrogatnoe-materinstvo predlozhili-perevesti-v-goskliniki.

Yurchak, Alexei. 2003. "Russian Neoliberal: The Entrepreneurial Ethic and the Spirit of 'True Careerism.'" *Russian Review* 62 (1): 72–90.

Yuval-Davis, Nira. 1997. *Gender and Nation*. Thousand Oaks, CA: SAGE Publishing.

Zatari, Amalia. 2020. "'My dazhe nye znaem, zhiv li on': SKR zayel delo o torgovle dyet'mi, ikh roditeli prosyat pomoshch u Putina." *BBC*, October 9. https://www.bbc.com/russian/features-54468421.

Zelizer, Viviana A. 2013. *Economic Lives: How Culture Shapes the Economy*. Princeton, NJ: Princeton University Press.

Zhurzhenko, Tatiana. 2012. "Mothering the Nation: Demographic Politics, Gender and Parenting in Ukraine." In *Gendering Post-Socialist Transition: Studies of Changing Gender Perspectives*, edited by Krassimira Daskalova, Caroline Hornstein Tomić, Karl Kaser, and Filip Radunović, 285–302. Vienna: LIT Verlag.

Ziff, Elizabeth. 2017. "'The Mommy Deployment': Military Spouses and Surrogacy in the United States." *Sociological Forum* 32 (2): 406–25.

———. 2019. "'Honey, I Want to Be a Surrogate': How Military Spouses Negotiate and Navigate Surrogacy with Their Service Member Husbands." *Journal of Family Issues* 40 (18): 2774–2800.

———. 2020. "Surrogacy and Medicalization: Navigating Power, Control, and Autonomy in Embodied Labor." *Sociological Quarterly* 62 (3): 510–27.

Zigon, Jarrett. 2009. "Developing the Moral Person: The Concepts of Human, Godmanhood, and Feelings in Some Russian Articulations of Morality." *Anthropology of Consciousness* 20 (1): 1–26.

———. 2011. "A Moral and Ethical Assemblage in Russian Orthodox Drug Rehabilitation." *Ethos* 39 (1): 30–50.

Index

abortion
  as alleged reason for infertility, 35, 79
  bodily autonomy and, 193, 196
  compensation and, 106–107
  opposition to, 40, 189
  screening process and, 86
adoption, 40–42, 179, 202, 230
advertising, 95–97, 99, 171
affect aliens, 143
affect/emotions
  hormones and maternal instinct and, 143, 149–155
  individualization and, 160–161
affective de-commodification, 166, 191
affective labor, 168–169, 171, 174–175, 185–186, 191
affective understanding, 222
agencies
  as protection, 123–128
  see also individual agencies
agents, interviews with, 25
Ahmed, Sara, 143, 167–168, 187
Albania, 238
Aleksandra Denisovna, 76–77, 114–115, 183
alienation, 134
alignment, technologies of, 136–161
alimony, 92
Alisa Serafimovna, 34, 41, 44–47, 53, 56, 70–71, 74, 79, 128–130
Altra Vita IVF Clinic, 19–25, 83–85, 104, 106–109, 144
altruism, 113, 130, 166, 177, 180, 183–184
Alyona Timofeyevna, 66, 182–183, 201, 203–211, 213–215, 221
Amapola, 173–174, 188
American Society of Reproductive Medicine, 252n11
Anastasia Anatolyevna, 118, 126, 159
anonymity, 31, 69, 72, 85, 128, 133–134, 220, 231–232
"Anthem" (Cohen), 217
antipolitics machine, 160
Anton Feodorovich, 75–77, 117

anxiety about pregnancy outcomes, 105–106
Arendt, Hannah, 15–16
Ashwin, Sarah, 37
assisted reproductive technologies (ART)
  agencies and, 32
  development of, 5, 12
  disinformation regarding children born via, 60–62, 64
  overview of research on, 7–9
  public discourse on, 5
attachment
  emotional articulation and, 157–158
  lack of, 143

Baby Gammy, 6–7, 225
Baby M case, 194–195
Bakhmetjev, Yaroslav, 69
ban, call for, 198–199
Baranov, Alexander, 61
Basis of the Social Concept, The (ROC), 35, 60
Becker, Gay, 76
Bell, Kirsten, 218
bellies, strap-on, 56, 70–71
Belyakov, Anton, 60
Berend, Zsuzsa, 9
Bharadwaj, Aditya, 103
biopolitical turn, 17, 57, 59, 63–64
biopower, 32, 53
BioTexCom, 171–175, 224–227, 232, 236–239, 249n10
birth rates, 38–40
blackmail, 121, 125
Blanco, Sara, 170, 179–180, 182
body maps, 145
bonding, between surrogate and child, 136–137, 143–144
Bourdieu, Pierre, 201

Cabello, Alberto, 169–170, 190
Cambodia, 7
capitalism, 54, 180, 189–199
capriciousness, 122–124
care, ethics of, 57–58, 79–80

INDEX

caring communities, 187
Catholic Church, 57, 62
Center of Medical Statistics, Ministry of Health (Ukraine), 249n9
chance, element of, 101–102
child trafficking, allegations of, 14, 225, 228–229, 237–238
China/Chinese parents, 225, 227–228, 236
choreographing surrogacy, 83–111
class, 52–54, 170
coercion critique, 6, 191
Cohen, Lawrence, 197
Cohen, Leonard, 217
Collins, Caitlyn, 9, 198
commissions, 100
commodities, gifts versus, 134
compensated dating, 94–96
constructing phrases, 74
contact, restriction of, 125–128, 146
contracts, 13, 86, 106–107, 111, 132, 208–209
Cooper, Melinda, 117
Corea, Gena, 6
corruption critique, 6, 191
cosmopolitanism, 63
costs of surrogacy, 11–12, 52, 96, 100–101, 180–181
Council for International Organizations of Medical Sciences, 209
couvade-like practices, 78
COVID-19 pandemic, 224, 228, 236, 251n7
cravings, 122–123
"crystal vase" metaphor, 84, 101, 105, 107, 110
C-sections, 206–207
"culturedness," 65
cutting ties, 134–135
Cyprus, 238
Czech Republic, 203

deep acting, 168
delegitimization of critique, 222
deliveries, 149–150, 153–154, 160
Delmonte, Ricardo, 124, 185, 187
demographic crisis, discourse of, 32, 36–40, 51, 54
Deomampo, Daisy, 106
dependency, mutual, 219
detachment, 113–114, 143–144
Diliara Eduardovna, 120–121
Dima Yakovlev Law, 229–230
Dimitri Anatolyevich, 35–36, 43, 63, 71
Dina Antonovna, 34, 48, 52, 65, 68–70
direct arrangements, 24–25, 95, 127–129, 132, 147–148, 158
disclosure to children, 74–76, 80

discrimination, 73–74, 92, 189, 211–212
"dis-emotionalizing," 160
diversity among surrogates, 21–22
divorce due to infertility, 34
doctors, interviews with, 25. *see also individual doctors*
Donbass republics, 235
donor conception, 41
double bind, 198–201
dyadic body-project, 78

"echo chambers," 186
economic imbalance/inequality, 4–5, 54, 92
economies of affect, 168
egg providers, 90, 100, 104, 200
embodied labor, 119
embryo donations, 226
embryo transfers, 86–87, 101
emotional entanglements, prevention of, 133
emotional labor, 137–143, 145, 158–159, 168
emptiness, feelings of, 149–150, 152, 155–156, 160
Ertman, Martha, 192
Essig, Laurie, 69
ethical labor, 3, 10, 15–16, 57–58
ethics, 15
ethnography, definition of, 23
ethnonationalism, 39, 51, 54
European Council, 7, 223
European Court of Human Rights, 129
European Parliament, 223
experience, benefits and disadvantages of, 121
exploitation, 95–96, 165–166, 170, 191, 195, 212, 214

Facebook, 186
Family Code of the Russian Federation, 13, 120
Family Code of Ukraine, 14
Fassin, Didier, 10
Federal Laws and Orders (Russia), 13
feeling rules, 137–138, 159, 168, 218
feminist criticism, 6–7, 193–196
Ferguson, James, 160
fertilization process, 86–87
fieldwork
  access difficulties, 16–20
  clinic fieldwork, 84–88
  definition of ethnography, 23
  overview of research, 25
financial struggles, 52
FINRRAGE (Feminist Interventional Network of Resistance to Reproductive and Genetic Engineering), 6
Firestone, Shulamith, 6

INDEX

Fischer, Berenice, 79–80
Flatley, Jonathan, 144
Førde, Kristin Engh, 16
forgetting about surrogacy, 77–79
foster care, 202
Foucault, Michel, 15, 32, 53, 137
fragmentation of "motherhood," 5–6
fraud, 119–120
free choice, 166–167, 193–194, 215–216
freedom, ambivalences of, 193–216
fridge metaphor, 116
Frolov v. Suzdaleva, 252n1
Fuentes, Álvaro, 125, 185, 187, 199–201

Gal, Susan, 67
Galkin, Maksim, 58
Galya Yanovna, 33, 41, 47, 52, 64, 66–67, 70–71, 74, 77–78, 120, 122, 130
gay men/couples, 14, 49–50, 175–178, 211–212, 228–230. *see also* LGBTQI+ community
Gay Propaganda Law, 63–64, 175, 229
gender differences, 54
gender roles/norms, 36–38
gendered altruism, 166
gendered empowerment, 166, 194
genetic links
 absence of, 129, 139–140, 143
 importance of, 41–42, 44
 intent and, 139–140
 requirements involving, 13
genetics, fragmentation and, 5–6
Georgia, 227, 238
gestational surrogacy, 5
gifts/gift metaphor, 134, 197–198
Goffman, Erving, 168
Gorbachev, Mikhail, 38
grief, 157
group attitudes, 144
Guseva, Alya, 49, 225–226

habitus, 201
happiness
 finding, 191–192
 as human right, 187–191
 narratives of, 166–167
 promise of, 167–169, 171
"happy objects," 136
Hardt, Michael, 168
Hauser, David and Christoph, 175–179, 218–219
Heidegger, Martin, 144
Held, Virginia, 80
heroism, maternal, 44–48
Hildebrand, Sarah, 109

Hochschild, Arlie, 137, 168
Hoeyer, Klaus, 209–210
Hogle, Linda F., 209–210
homophobia, 60
hope, 46, 48
hormonal stimulation, 86–87, 104
hormones, risk and, 122, 124
housing, 107–110

ICSI (intracytoplasmic sperm injection), 251n5
income inequality, 92
incubator metaphor, 116
indebtedness, feelings of, 133–134
indexical recalibration, 67–68
India
 comparison with, 5, 140, 144, 161, 174, 220
 costs of surrogacy in, 12
 economic factors and, 197–199
 economic motives and, 89
 ethical work and, 16
 exploitation and, 170, 191
 gay men/couples and, 7–8, 175, 254n3
 housing in, 107
 invisibility of surrogate and, 127, 134–135
 "mother-worker" and, 118
 negative pregnancy outcomes and, 103, 106, 157
 neocolonialism and, 169
 private agents and, 100
 restrictions in, 226
infantilization, 123, 131
infertility
 as disability, 31, 53
 divorce due to, 34
 male, 43, 251n5
 as medical issue, 49–50, 53
 ROC on, 35–36
 as self-inflicted, 35, 79
 as women's problem, 43
infertility psychologists, interviews with, 25
informed consent, 209–210, 214–216
Inhorn, Marcia, 43
insurance, 208–209
intended parents
 deliveries and, 153–154
 direct arrangements and, 147–148
 interviews with, 25
 lack of contact with, 146–149, 159
 Russian invasion of Ukraine and, 236–238
 see also individual parents
intent, importance of, 139
Internet, role of, 24–25, 69–70
interviews, overview of, 25–26
intimate economies, 195

intimate labor, definition of, 4
inviTRA International Fertility Fair, 1, 24, 169, 233
Isupova, Olga, 64–65, 68
IVF, uncertainty and, 103

Katya Yefimovna, 21, 42, 72, 90–93, 100, 108–110, 123, 138, 146–147, 149–152, 155–156, 158–161
Kauffert, Patricia, 53
Kay, Rebecca, 38
Kazakhstan, 227
Khvorostyanov, Natalia, 96
Kierans, Ciara, 218
Kirill, Patriarch, 59
Kirkorov, Philipp, 50–51, 58
Kirpichenko, Maria, 184
Konstantin Pavlovich, 51, 115–118, 124–125, 128, 156–158
Korolczuk, Elżbieta, 251n10
Korsak, Vladislav, 49
KrolØkke, Charlotte, 200
Kruglova, Anna, 74
Ksenia Demyanovna, 73, 102–104

Laidlaw, James, 15
Lambek, Michael, 250n15
Larissa Osipovna, 1–3, 16, 122, 125–128, 133–134, 161, 222, 233
lawyers, interviews with, 25. *see also individual lawyers*
legislation
  adaptability and, 1–2
  on disclosure, 75
  gray areas in, 50
  medical indication requirement and, 141
  minimalistic, 188–189
  proposals for, 226–227, 230, 232
  in Russia and Ukraine, 11–15
  see also regulation; *individual laws*
legitimization, quests for, 47
Lena Mironovna, 21, 72, 79, 89–90, 93, 108–109, 111, 115, 132, 138, 146–147, 149, 153–161, 218–219
Levada Center, 58–59
Lewis, Sophie, 198
LGBTQI+ community, 69, 229–230, 254n6.
  see also gay men/couples
lie detectors, 115
Lock, Margaret, 53
Lokshin, Vyacheslav, 49
Lustenberger, Sibylle, 135

Luzenko, Yuri, 225
lying, not telling versus, 67–68
Lyuba Dmitriyevna, 91, 103, 140–141, 148–149

Makarychev, Andrey, 56–57
Maksim Antonov, 40–41, 127
male infertility, 43, 251n5
Malich, Lisa, 160
Marina Nikitichna, 139–140, 143, 145–146, 149, 152
Marina Romanovna, 182–183, 206
Mariya Alexeyevna, 44, 46, 65–66
Markens, Susan, 9, 231
Martin, Emily, 117
Masha Arkadyevna, 99–100, 105, 120, 124, 132, 143–144, 148, 150–151, 159
Masha Radionovna, 204–205, 207–208
Maslennikova, Galina, 61
maternal rights
  legislation on, 120
  payment tied to relinquishing, 13, 106
Maternity Capital, 39
Matza, Tomas, 160–161
Mauss, Marcel, 134
Meddesk, 24, 56, 95, 131
media coverage, 9
mediated arrangements
  agencies' role in, 123–124
  direct versus, 24–25, 95, 158
Medvedev, Sergei, 56–57
men
  genetic links and, 42–44
  lack of involvement of, 34, 43
  male infertility, 43, 251n5
  marital consent and, 141–142
  single, 14, 50–51, 98, 228–230
  see also gay men/couples; *individual men*
metaphorical thinking, 116–117, 140
Mexico, 169–170, 174, 191, 197
Mies, Maria, 6
Milonov, Vitaly, 60
"miracle stories," 46–47
Mishtal, Joanna, 57
Mitra, Sayani, 157
Mizulina, Yelena, 60
modes of subjection, 137
Mohanty, Chandra, 195
monetary sanctions, 106–107
Monte, Pedro, 171, 186
moods, 144
moral economy/economies, 10, 24, 26–27, 94, 217, 220

INDEX

moral framings, 8–9
moral governance, 57, 62, 79
moral middle ground, 169–171, 175, 193
mortality rates, 38
Mother-Heroines, 38
motherhood
   biopolitics of, 31–55
   deserving, 47
   importance of, 31–36
   norm of, 32, 40
   pressures regarding, 33–34
   state support for, 37–39
   timing of, 33
"mother-worker," 118–119
Motluk, Alison, 237

nanny metaphor, 140, 143
Narotzky, Susana, 16
nastraivat'sya, 138–143
Natalya Nikolayevna, 112–113, 117
Natasha Sergeyevna, 20, 22, 83–88, 114, 122–123
nationalism, 36
naturalization of ART, 53–54
neoliberal discourses, 193
neoliberal subjects, 142
Nepal, 7, 254n3
No Somos Vasijas ("We are not containers"), 7
Nordqvist, Petra, 75

Odnoklassniki, 95
Oksana Yevgenyevna, 71–72
Olessia Valeryevna, 31, 33–34, 41–42, 48, 52–53, 56, 62, 67–70, 73–74, 76, 78–79, 121–122, 129–130, 135
Olga Georgyevna, 72, 144
online forums/platforms, 9, 69–70, 96, 99
Oprah Winfrey Show, 198
Order of Maternal Glory (Russia), 38
Order of the Ministry of Health on Assisted Reproductive Technologies (Ukraine), 14
orphanages, 41–42
Ostrov Kenguru, 24, 95
othering, 59–64
othering of surrogate child, 140–141

Pande, Amrita, 107, 118–119, 197, 226
Paradiso and Campanelli v. Italy, 129
Patel, Nayna, 198
Patico, Jennifer, 95
Pavel Viktorovich, 50–51
Payne, Gunnarsson, 251n10

Pérez, Marta, 126, 195, 197
"philanthrocapitalism," 198
photographs, as evidence, 186–187
Poland, 57, 62, 251n10
Polina Davidovna, 122–123
population decline, 38–39
postbirth narratives, 149–159
posthumous surrogacy, 12, 58
poverty, exploitation and, 6, 199–201
Power of Mothers, The, 232
practical realism, 92–93, 104, 146, 215
pregnancies
   anxiety about outcomes of, 105–106
   element of chance in, 101–102
   hiding, 71–73
   simulated, 56, 70–73, 77–78
   visibility of, 70–73
"pregnant in the head," 77–78
privacy, 17–18
private agents, 100
Probirka, 24, 64, 68–69, 95
"propaganda," 63–64, 76–77
psychological counseling, lack of, 157
psychological screening, 86, 114–115
public opinion on surrogacy, 58–59
Pugacheva, Alla, 12, 58
Pushkina, Oksana, 230
Pussy Riot, 59
Putin, Vladimir, 36–37, 39, 59, 230, 235, 254n6

race, issues involving, 12
Radin, Margaret, 199
Ragoné, Helena, 139
Rapp, Rayna, 15
Raya Antonovna, 66, 74, 94–96, 131, 147–148, 160
reductions, 87, 107
regime of truth, 27
regrets, 155–159, 218
regulation
   lack of in Spain, 212–213
   minimalistic, 188–189
   see also legislation
religion
   Catholic Church, 57, 62
   uncertainty and, 103
   see also Russian Orthodox Church (ROC)
reproductive governance, 31–32, 57
resemblance, as validating, 41
resistance, small acts of, 110–111
Riach, Kathleen, 93
"right understanding," 3, 117, 143, 221–222

INDEX

Rita Tikhonovna, 33, 35, 42, 52, 66, 70, 98–99, 102, 130–132, 147–148
Rivkin-Fish, Michele, 14, 39, 54, 160–161
Robben, Antonius, 3
Roberts, Elizabeth, 32, 103
Romania, 250n1
Romero, Juan, 120, 169–170, 181–182, 184, 193, 196, 211–212, 216
Rose, Nikolas, 194
Rosjurconsulting, 227
Rudrappa, Sharmila, 9, 15, 127, 134–135, 187, 198
rules/guidelines during pregnancy, 84, 105, 107
Russian Association of Human Reproduction (RAHR), 12, 16, 49, 230
Russian invasion of Ukraine, 235–239
Russian Orthodox Church (ROC)
  condemnation of surrogacy by, 71, 73
  criticism of, 230
  growing influence of, 56
  on infertility, 34–35, 53
  on motherhood, 36
  political importance of, 17, 32
  push for surrogacy ban and, 60
  Putin and, 59
  role of, 79
Russian Public Opinion Research Center (VCIOM), 58–59

salaries
  commissions from, 100
  conversion rates for, xvi
  nationalities and, 100–101
  terminations and, 106–107
  timing of, 106–107
  see also costs of surrogacy
Sandel, Michael, 6
Schicktanz, Silke, 157
screening process, 86, 114–115, 199
secrecy, 5, 17, 25, 56–80, 113, 161
selection criteria, surrogate, 13–14
selective reduction, 107
self
  technologies of, 137, 168
  work on, 142–143
self-commodification, 94, 96
self-formation, 15
self-government, narratives of, 160
separate-spheres and hostile-worlds doctrine, 218
Sergei Magnitsky Rule of Law Accountability Act, 254n7
Sergej Petrovich, 49, 53, 118, 127, 157–158
sex selection, 189–190

Shalev, Carmel, 195
simulated pregnancies, 56, 70–73, 77–78
single motherhood, 92–93
Smyth, Regina, 59
Soboleva, Irina, 59, 69
Sokolova, Svetlana, 232
Sonya Vitalyevna, 88–89, 91, 93
Speier, Amy, 186
Stalin, Joseph, 38
Stop Surrogacy Now campaign, 7, 195, 223
structural inequalities, 160–161
superstitions, 103
surrogacy
  costs of, 11–13, 52, 96, 100–101, 180–181
  feminist positions toward, 6–7, 193–196
  forgetting about, 77–79
  market, global, 1–2, 8, 16–170, 224–227, 238–239
  as medical solution, 48–50
  number of children born through, 12, 249n9, 249n10
  public opinion on, 58–59
  as work, 89, 112–114, 119, 130, 133–135, 144, 220, 232
Surrogacy (Regulation) Bill (India), 226
surrogates
  control of, 84, 105, 107, 124–126
  decisions to become, 94–101
  description of perfect, 112
  with experience, 121
  first visits of, 85–86
  "happy," 182–187
  inner alignment and, 138–143
  interviews with, 87
  invisibility of, 232, 237
  limited exchange among, 161
  marital consent for, 141–142
  motives of, 89–92, 113, 129–130, 166, 188, 196–197, 199
  questions from, 87–88
  recruiting perfect, 114–119
  riskiness and, 119–123
  screening of, 86
  see also individual surrogates
surveillance, 108–109
Svitnev, Konstantin, 14, 51–52, 54, 189–190, 221, 227–228
Swader, Christopher, 94–96
switch metaphor, 139, 145, 156, 158–159

Tatyana Vasilyevna, 36, 43, 60–61, 63–64, 71, 136, 140
Teman, Elly, 5, 9, 41, 78, 137, 143, 145, 158
Temkina, Anna, 94

terminations, 106–107. *see also* abortion
Teschlade, Julia, 177
testimonials, 184
Thailand, 6–7, 170, 191, 220, 225
"Third World Women," 195
Thompson, Charis, 43, 53
Thompson, Edward P., 10
Ticktin, Miriam, 108
Tkach, Olga, 251n7
Tochilovsky, Albert, 226
Tolstoy, Pyotr, 60, 227, 229
Torres, Diego, 180–181, 195–197, 212–213, 216
transnational surrogacy arrangements, 6–8, 123–124, 165–167, 191
travelling donors, 104
Trisomy 21, 6–7
Tronto, Joan, 79–80
trust, lack of, 18–19, 64–66, 128, 130
truth
  fragile, 218–221
  regimes of, 221–224
  truth claims, 10–11
  truth discourses, 57
  truthfulness, 67–68
Tsing, Anna, 134
Tuller, David, 69
Turbine, Vikki, 93

Ukrainian Association for Reproductive Medicine (UARM), 226
uncertainty
  dealing with, 101–104
  managing, 110–111
unenforceability of contracts, 13
United Russia, 59, 227, 230

United States, 169–171, 177–179, 191, 197, 212, 220, 254n7
Utrata, Jennifer, 40, 92–93

Valeriy Ivanovich, 189, 192
Venera Igorevna, 175–179
Vera Romanovna, 43, 52, 66, 68, 103, 123
victim discourse, 127
visibility of pregnancies, 70–73
Vittoria Vita, 184
Vkontakte, 95, 155
Vlasenko, Polina, 33
Vora, Kalindi, 197
Vorobeva, Irina, 94–96

Wagner, Stefan and Teresa, 120, 170, 182–183, 201–211, 213–214, 216, 221
Waldby, Catherine, 117
Weis, Christina, 22
"what if" sensibility, 74
Whittaker, Andrea, 10
Williams, Joan, 7
win-win argument, 196–197, 201
World Health Organization, 209

Yakovenko, Sergej, 19–20, 22–23
Yana Timurovna, 141, 145
Yeshua-Katz, Daphna, 96
Yurchak, Alexei, 142
Yushchenko, Viktor, 37

Zdravomyslova, Elena, 94
Zelizer, Viviana, 7, 218
Zhenya Pavlovna, 88–91, 100–102, 138–141

Printed in the USA
CPSIA information can be obtained
at www.ICGtesting.com
CBHW031351290424
7729CB00002B/46